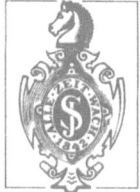

Jiro Suzuki (Ed.)

Treatment of Glioma

With 137 Figures

Springer-Verlag

Tokyo Berlin Heidelberg New York London Paris

Prof. Jiro Suzuki, MD
Division of Neurosurgery
Institute of Brain Diseases
Tohoku University
School of Medicine
Sendai, 980 Japan

ISBN-13: 978-4-431-68455-8   e-ISBN-13: 978-4-431-68453-4
DOI: 10.1007/978-4-431-68453-4

Typesetting: Asco Trade Typesetting, Hong Kong/Fujicom, Tokyo

Preface

The world's first successful diagnosis and treatment of a glioma was done on a 24-year-old man on 25 November 1884. This historic achievement was made possible by the collaboration of a diagnostician, Bennett, who diagnosed the disease on the basis of local neurological signs, and a London neurosurgeon, Godlee, who performed a craniotomy and excision of the glioma located in the right premotor cortex. Unfortunately, the patient died of meningitis 4 weeks postoperatively and Godlee's name is not to be found in the history of neurosurgery. Thereafter, White and others argued that gliomas were not suitable for surgical excision and treated glioma patients for syphilis, which was believed to be the source of the brain disorder. In 1892, Keen maintained that gliomas should be removed using the fingers, but Cushing in 1908 rejected this as being too invasive a procedure. Conversely, Dandy argued that there were many cases in which such treatment was effective and, moreover, that a portion of the surrounding normal tissue should also be excised. Dandy also reported a case of complete hemispherectomy.

Clearly, the early history of surgical treatment of gliomas is characterized by uncertainty, but by 1926 Bailey and Cushing had provided a histological classification of gliomas which has since been recognized as a major contribution to the initial research and treatment of these tumors. It is also noteworthy that Ewing first discussed the possibility of radiation treatment in 1921, and Olivecrona, Tönnis, and others maintained that even when the effectiveness of radiation therapy could not be completely assured, it should nonetheless be implemented.

Following the Second World War, the clinical application of anticancer drugs began and, more recently, immunopotentiators have been employed. Research into combined radiation and drug therapy has advanced considerably, particularly with respect to the timing, dosage, and administrative methods.

Since 1977, the Sendai Group of Neurosurgeons (originally under the leadership of Dr. Teruaki Mori) has used the so-called RAFP therapy for the treatment of glioma. This therapy involves the administration of radiation treatment and three chemical compounds:

ACNU (a nitrosourea agent), Futraful (a masked compound of 5-FU), and PSK (an immunopotentiator). Following Dr. Mori's academic promotion to Associate Professor at Oita University, the responsibility for basic research and clinical applications of RAFP therapy fell on the shoulders of Dr. Ryuichi Katakura and his team. They have produced remarkable results, both with regard to elucidation of the theoretical foundations of the timing of these drugs and to their clinical use.

With the cooperation of the neurosurgeons of northern Japan, extensive statistics on gliomas have been collected for this region's population of 10 million. The statistics include the incidence of gliomas, symptoms, diagnosis, effectiveness of RAFP therapy, and histological, CT, and angiographic findings in such cases. These statistics and data from follow-up studies have been collected and recorded in a computer database and constitute an important source of basic information on gliomas.

The effectiveness of RAFP therapy has been found to vary in the different histological subcategories of gliomas: It is particularly effective for medulloblastoma and anaplastic astrocytoma, but glioblastoma multiforme has thus far proven resistant to all forms of therapy. Even if dissolution of a glioblastoma has been confirmed in CT scans, recurrence is frequent and RAFP therapy can be expected to prolong life by only a few months. Therapy for this form of glioma has thus progressed little since the days of Cushing and Dandy. As a consequence, glioblastoma multiforme is a reminder to neurosurgeons of the limitations of current therapies. It is the duty, therefore, of researchers in this field, to meet the challenge of glioblastoma multiforme and to find a cure for this disease.

The present volume deals with many aspects of gliomas, including factors related to the incidence and epidemiology, and surveys the history of glioma therapies. Experimental studies carried out by the Sendai Group of Neurosurgeons are reported, together with the results of many clinical studies and clinical experience. A recent technique for evaluating the effectiveness of therapy based upon the MRI diagnostic method is introduced.

I hope that this book will make an important contribution to the continuing development of therapies for glioma. Through such efforts, I fully expect that glioblastoma multiforme will, before long, be included among the human cancers which are capable of being cured.

I wish to express my heartfelt thanks to Drs. Teruaki Mori, Ryuichi Katakura, and Masakazu Kitahara, whose efforts have been central both to the research described herein and the completion of the book itself. I also wish to thank the team of researchers whose dedicated efforts have made this book possible and Mr. Norman D. Cook, who has translated this work into such fine English.

Sendai, Japan, January 1988   JIRO SUZUKI

Table of Contents

Part I. Statistical Analysis

  1. Epidemiology and Statistical Analysis of Gliomas.
     R. KATAKURA, T. YOSHIMOTO. 3

  2. Statistical Considerations of Therapeutic Results in
     Glioblastoma. K. MINEURA.
     With 3 Figures 17

Part II. Basic Studies

  3. Combined Effects of Radiation, ACNU, and 5-FU on
     Gliomas: An Experimental Combination Therapy.
     S. MASHIYAMA, S. SUGIYAMA, K. KUWAHARA,
     M. KITAHARA, K. TAKAHASHI, T. SASAKI.
     With 71 Figures 37

  4. The Pharmacokinetics of ACNU in Patients with
     Malignant Brain Tumor. T. MORI.
     With 3 Figures 109

  5. The Effects of Induced Hypertension on the Uptake of
     ACNU in Experimental Brain Tumor. Y. TSURUMI.
     With 5 Figures 117

  6. A Study of Intratumoral Oxygen Pressure in Brain
     Tumors. T. KAYAMA.
     With 6 Figures 125

Part III. Clinical Studies

  7. An Outline of RAFP Therapy. T. MORI.
     With 5 Figures 137

  8. Results of RAFP Therapy on CT Scan.
     J. SHINGAI. 149

9. Clinical Analysis of Glioma: Anaplastic Astrocytoma and
    Glioblastoma. J. SHINGAI, M. KANNO.
    With 10 Figures 153

10. Clinical Analysis of Glioma: Low-Grade Astrocytoma.
    M. KITAHARA.
    With 9 Figures 173

11. Clinical Analysis of Glioma: Oligodendroglioma.
    M. KITAHARA.
    With 5 Figures 187

12. Clinical Analysis of Glioma: Ependymoma.
    M. KITAHARA.
    With 6 Figures 197

13. Clinical Analysis of Glioma: Medulloblastoma.
    Y. TAKAHASHI.
    With 3 Figures 209

14. Side Effects of RAFP Therapy. M. KITAHARA.
    With 2 Figures 221

15. Clinical Study Using MRI in Patients Treated with
    RAFP Therapy. S. FUJIWARA.
    With 9 Figures 231

Subject Index 241

List of Contributors

FUJIWARA, SATORU   Division of Neurosurgery, Institute of Brain Diseases, Tohoku University School of Medicine, Sendai, 980 Japan

KANNO, MITSUNOBU   Division of Neurosurgery, Institute of Brain Diseases, Tohoku University School of Medicine, Sendai, 980 Japan

KATAKURA, RYUICHI   Division of Neurosurgery, Institute of Brain Diseases, Tohoku University School of Medicine, Sendai, 980 Japan

KAYAMA, TAKAMASA   Department of Neurosurgery, National Hospital, Sendai, 980 Japan

KITAHARA, MASAKAZU   Division of Neurosurgery, Institute of Brain Diseases, Tohoku University School of Medicine, Sendai, 980 Japan

KUWAHARA, KENJI   Division of Neurosurgery, Institute of Brain Diseases, Tohoku University School of Medicine, Sendai, 980 Japan

MASHIYAMA, SHOJI   Division of Neurosurgery, Institute of Brain Diseases, Tohoku University School of Medicine, Sendai, 980 Japan

MINEURA, KATSUYOSHI   Neurosurgical Service, Akita University Hospital, Akita, 010 Japan

MORI, TERUAKI   Department of Neurosurgery, Medical College of Ohita, Ohita, 870 Japan

SASAKI, TAKEHITO   Department of Radiation Research, Tohoku University School of Medicine, Sendai, 980 Japan

SHINGAI, JUNJI   Division of Neurosurgery, Institute of Brain Diseases, Tohoku University School of Medicine, Sendai, 980 Japan

SUGIYAMA, SATORU   Department of Neurosurgery, Medical
                           College of Ohita, Ohita, 870 Japan

TAKAHASHI, KO   Division of Neurosurgery, Institute of Brain
                           Diseases, Tohoku University School of
                           Medicine, Sendai, 980 Japan

TAKAHASHI, YASUHIRO   Division of Neurosurgery, Institute of Brain
                           Diseases, Tohoku University School of
                           Medicine, Sendai, 980 Japan

TSURUMI, YUJI   Division of Neurosurgery, Institute of Brain
                           Diseases, Tohoku University School of
                           Medicine, Sendai, 980 Japan

YOSHIMOTO, TAKASHI   Division of Neurosurgery, Institute of Brain
                           Diseases, Tohoku University School of
                           Medicine, Sendai, 980 Japan

Part I
Statistical Analysis

Chapter 1

Epidemiology and Statistical Analysis of Gliomas

R. KATAKURA and T. YOSHIMOTO

Introduction

There have been a great many studies on the epidemiology and statistical analysis of brain tumors [1, 4–6, 9, 18, 22], but most of them have been concerned with tumors of the entire central nervous system. There have been few detailed studies on gliomas alone. One reason for the scarcity of such work is the fact that, starting with the classification of Bailey and Cushing [3], several classification schemes have been devised [11, 17, 25–27] based upon various criteria—often by the degree of malignancy, as seen in the Kernohan and Sayre classification [11]. No unified schema has yet been developed. Schoenberg has emphasized that when undertaking an epidemiological investigation the most important factor is the classification of distinct disease entities [18]. For both epidemiological study and analysis of operative results, if uniformity of the histological classification has not been achieved, it is impossible to make use of the survey results. International uniformity of the histological classification is all the more essential because the incidence of glioma is low and the number of cases treated at any given institute is small.

In the present chapter, we report the results of a statistical analysis of glioma cases experienced over the 5-year period between 1980 and 1984 in the Tohoku (northeastern) district of Japan. This statistical analysis was reported by the Tohoku Brain Tumor Registry in 1984 [20]. The Tohoku area is comprised of six prefectures containing a population of about ten million people. With the collaboration of the 66 neurosurgical clinics in this region, records of glioma cases have been kept and the therapeutic results analyzed. The histological classification used in these records is that advocated by the World Health Organization (WHO; Table 1.1) [27], primarily because it is the most widely used in the world today.

Incidence of Glioma

The incidence of primary central nervous system tumors has been reported to be between 1 and 8/100 000 of the population and is generally taken to be about 4 or 5/100 000. Between 40% and 60% of such tumors are gliomas, which means an incidence of glioma between 1 and 5/100 000.

In a study by Barker et al. [4] on the incidence of brain tumors in the Wessex

Table 1.1. Histological classification of neuroepithelial tumors by WHO

A. Astrocytic tumors
   1. Astrocytoma
      a. Fibrillary
      b. Protoplasmic
      c. Gemistocytic
   2. Pilocytic astrocytoma
   3. Subependymal giant cell astrocytoma
      (ventricular tumor of tuberous
      sclerosis)
   4. Astroblastoma
   5. Anaplastic (malignant) astrocytoma
B. Oligodendroglial tumors
   1. Oligodendroglioma
   2. Mixed oligoastrocytoma
   3. Anaplastic (malignant)
      oligodendroglioma
C. Ependymal and choroid plexus tumors
   1. Ependymoma
      a. Myxopapillary ependymoma
      b. Papillary ependymoma
      c. Subependymoma
   2. Anaplastic (malignant) ependymoma
   3. Choroid plexus papilloma
   4. Anaplastic (malignant) choroid
      plexus papilloma

D. Pineal cell tumors
   1. Pineocytoma (pinealocytoma)
   2. Pineoblastoma (pinealoblastoma)
E. Neuronal tumors
   1. Gangliocytoma
   2. Ganglioglioma
   3. Ganglioneuroblastoma
   4. Anaplastic (malignant) gangliocytoma
      and ganglioglioma
   5. Neuroblastoma
F. Poorly differentiated and embryonal
   tumors
   1. Glioblastoma
      a. Glioblastoma with sarcomatous
         component (mixed glioblastoma
         and sarcoma)
      b. Giant cell glioblastoma
   2. Medulloblastoma
      a. Desmoplastic medulloblastoma
      b. Medullomyoblastoma
   3. Medulloepithelioma
   4. Primitive polar spongioblastoma
   5. Gliomatosis cerebri

region of southern England, the age-adjusted incidence of glioma was 3.94/100 000. Heshmat et al. [9] reported that in the metropolitan area of Washington DC over a 10-year period between 1960 and 1969, the crude incidence rates were 6.5/100 000 among Caucasians and 3.3/100 000 among Negroes. The incidence found in the Tohoku district of Japan was 1.5/100 000, well below that reported in the West. These differences may be due to racial factors, as suggested by the incidences in whites and blacks in America, but sufficient data on the Mongoloid races are still not available.

Epidemiological Study of Glioma

Study was made of the relationship between the histological type and site of the glioma in relation to the age and sex of the patients among the 662 glioma cases in the Tohoku district between 1980 and 1984. In the WHO classification, glioblastomas and medulloblastomas are classified with poorly differentiated and embryonal tumors; they are also treated together in the present study.

Age and Sex

Table 1.2 shows the age and sex of the 662 glioma patients at the time of admission to hospital. There were 40 patients between 0 and 4 years of age (6.0%) and 50

Table 1.2. Distribution of 662 glioma cases by age and sex, Tohoku brain tumor registry (1980–1984)

Age (years)	Sex		Total	
	Male	Female	No.	Percent
0–4	20	20	40	6.0
5–9	27	23	50	7.6
10–14	20	18	38	5.7
15–19	13	10	23	3.5
20–29	28	28	56	8.4
30–39	55	39	94	14.3
40–49	55	40	95	14.4
50–59	55	54	109	16.5
60–69	65	41	106	16.0
70–79	28	22	50	7.6
80–	1	0	1	0.2
Total	367 (55.4%)	295 (44.6%)	662	100

between 5 and 9 years (7.6%), giving a total of 13.6% (90 cases) in the first decade of life. The incidence then decreased for the second and third decades (9.2% and 8.4%, respectively) but showed an increase thereafter: 14.3% between the ages of 30 and 39 and 14.4% between 40 and 49. The highest incidence was for patients between 50 and 59 years of age (16.5%), followed by those between 60 and 69 (16.0%). There was then a sharp decline for those between 70 and 79 (7.6%) and only one patient in his 80s.

The overall sex ratio was 1.24 : 1 (55.4% males and 44.6% females). The predominance of males was particularly strong in the 30- to 39-year-old group (1.41 : 1), the 40- to 49-year-old group (1.38 : 1), and the 60- to 69-year-old group (1.59 : 1), but the sex ratios for the other age-groups were near 1 : 1.

Age Distribution of Supra- and Infratentorial Cases

The distribution according to the supra- or infratentorial location of the tumor is shown in Table 1.3. The overall ratio of supra- to infratentorial lesions was approximately 4 : 1 (528 supratentorial and 123 infratentorial cases or 81.1% and 18.9%, respectively). The distribution according to age was as follows: Among the youngest patients (0–4 years), there were twice as many infratentorial as supratentorial gliomas, whereas among the 5–9 year olds there were about four times as many. Among the 10–14 year olds, however, there was a slight excess of supratentorial cases and thereafter the vast majority of cases were supratentorial: 92% in the 50- to 59-year-old group, 97% in the 60- to 69-year-old group and 98% among patients over 70.

Histological Distribution of the Glioma

Table 1.4 shows the number of cases with each of the WHO histological characteristics among the 451 cases for which histological diagnosis was possible. The highest

Table 1.3. Age and distribution of supra- and infratentorial glioma, Tohoku brain tumor registry (1980–1984)

Age (years)	Supratentorial	Infratentorial	Total
0–4	13	25	38
5–9	10	39	49
10–14	22	16	38
15–19	17	5	22
20–29	47	9	56
30–39	85	9	94
40–49	85	8	93
50–59	100	8	108
60–69	99	3	102
70–	50	1	51
Total	528 (81.1%)	123 (18.9%)	651

Table 1.4. Histological distribution of 451 glioma cases by sex, Tohoku brain tumor registry (1980–1984)

Finding	Sex		Total	
	Male	Female	No.	Percent
Astrocytoma	9	7	16	3.5
Pilocytic astrocytoma	14	10	24	5.3
Subependymal giant cell astrocytoma	0	1	1	0.2
Fibrillary astrocytoma	20	22	42	9.3
Gemistocytic astrocytoma	3	5	8	1.7
Protoplasmic astrocytoma	3	1	4	0.9
Mixed oligoastrocytoma	5	4	9	2.0
Anaplastic astrocytoma	82	71	153	33.9
Glioblastoma	80	57	137	30.4
Giant cell glioblastoma	2	3	5	1.1
Oligodendroglioma	12	8	20	4.4
Anaplastic oligodendroglioma	6	2	8	1.8
Ependymoma	2	6	8	1.8
Medulloblastoma	7	7	14	3.1
Desmoplastic medulloblastoma	2	0	2	0.4
Total	247	204	451	100

incidence was found for anaplastic astrocytoma (33.9%), followed by glioblastoma (30.4%) and fibrillary astrocytoma (9.3%). Following the WHO subclassification of astrocytoma, there were 25 grade I cases (5.5%; pilocytic astrocytoma and subependymal giant cell astrocytoma) and 79 grade II cases (17.5%; fibrillary astrocytoma, gemistocytic astrocytoma, protoplasmic astrocytoma). The majority of the gliomas were highly malignant, i.e., 33.9% were grade III anaplastic astrocytomas and 31.5% were grade IV glioblastomas. Oligodendrogliomas accounted for 6.2%, ependymomas for only 1.8%, and medulloblastomas for 3.5%.

With regard to previous reports on the incidence of astrocytoma and glioblastoma, Hirano found that among gliomas glioblastomas accounted for some 55% and astrocytomas (including anaplastic astrocytoma) for 20% in the USA. According to the Japan Brain Tumor Registry [22], glioblastomas have arisen less frequently in Japan than in the USA, accounting for 29% in Japan, whereas astrocytomas have accounted for 45%. In the Tohoku Brain Tumor Registry [20] as well, glioblastomas accounted for 31.5% of gliomas suggesting that the incidence in Japan is in the vicinity of 30%. In contrast, with regard to the rate of high-grade astrocytoma (anaplastic astrocytoma together with glioblastoma) among glioma cases, it was found in the Wessex study that grade III and IV astrocytomas accounted for 428 of the total 611 gliomas (64.7%). In the Tohoku Brain Tumor Registry, this value was 65.4%.

A problem which arises, however, in any study of the incidence of astrocytoma according to differences in malignancy concerns the time during therapy at which the histological diagnosis is made. That is, since one of the characteristics of astrocytomas is their tendency for malignant transformation, if histological diagnosis is made in an advanced stage of the lesion, a large number of glioblastoma cases will be found, whereas early diagnosis of the same disease will lead to a higher incidence of the more benign lesions.

With regard to the number of oligodendroglioma cases, most studies have found incidences in the vicinity of 4%–6%, specifically 6.2% in the Japan Brain Tumor Registry, 6.2% in the Tohoku Brain Tumor Registry, 5.0% in the USA study, and 4.5% in the Wessex study.

The incidence of medulloblastoma, however, shows a marked difference between the Japan Brain Tumor Registry value of 8.8% and the Tohoku Brain Tumor Registry value of 3.5%. One possible explanation for this difference is that there are regional differences in viral infection. Thus, medulloblastoma should be more prevalent in southern and warmer regions, where viral infections in general are more common. It must be emphasized that the responsible virus has not been identified, but the low incidence of medulloblastoma in the more northerly Tohoku district is certainly a suggestive finding.

Histological Findings and Patient Age

Table 1.5 presents the age distribution for each of the histological types. The incidence of low-grade astrocytoma (grades I and II) was highest (23.3%) for the 0- to 9-year-old group. One reason for this high incidence is that more than half of the low-grade astrocytoma cases (12/23) were pilocytic astrocytomas arising in the cerebellum. The incidence between the ages of 10 and 50 remained fairly constant (15%–18%), but decreased thereafter. In contrast, the incidence of anaplastic astrocytoma was low in the first and second decades of life (5.9% and 8.5%, respectively) but was relatively high between the ages of 30 and 70. Glioblastomas were quite rare among the young (2.9%, 2.2%, and 2.2% in the first three decades), but showed a rise at about 30 years of age and reached a peak of 34% at 50–59 years. In comparison with the other types of glioma, the incidence of the more malignant glioma was high for the elderly: For low-grade astrocytoma it was 5.0%, but for anaplastic astrocytoma it was 29.4% and for glioblastoma it was 35.5%. On the other hand, in the 0- to 9-year-old group, the incidence of malignant glioma was

Table 1.5. Correlation of glioma by age and histological findings, Tohoku brain tumor registry (1980–1984)

Age (years)	Low-grade astrocytoma	Anaplastic astrocytoma	Glioblas- toma	Oligodendro- glioma	Ependy- moma	Medullo- blastoma
0–4	7 (7.1)	7 (4.6)	3 (2.2)	—	5 (62.5)	6 (37.5)
5–9	16 (16.2)	2 (1.3)	1 (0.7)	—	1 (12.5)	6 (37.5)
10–14	8 (8.1)	10 (6.5)	3 (2.2)	—	—	1 (6.3)
15–19	7 (7.1)	3 (2.0)	—	3 (10.7)	—	—
20–29	15 (15.2)	15 (9.8)	3 (2.2)	—	1 (12.5)	2 (12.5)
30–39	18 (18.2)	25 (16.3)	14 (10.3)	6 (21.4)	—	1 (6.3)
40–49	15 (15.2)	28 (18.3)	18 (13.2)	8 (28.6)	—	—
50–59	8 (8.1)	18 (11.8)	47 (34.3)	7 (25.0)	1 (12.5)	—
60–69	4 (4.0)	33 (21.6)	30 (22.1)	3 (10.7)	—	—
70–	1 (1.0)	12 (7.8)	18 (13.2)	1 (3.6)	—	—
Total	99 (100)	153 (100)	137 (100)	28 (100)	8 (100)	16 (100)

Percentages in *Parentheses*

low, i.e., the incidence of low-grade astrocytoma was 23.3%, anaplastic astrocytoma 5.9%, and glioblastoma 2.9%. Clearly, the malignancy of astrocytic tumors increases with age.

Glioma in Children and Adults

The incidence of the various types of glioma in children (0–14 years of age) and adults (15 years and over) is shown in Table 1.6. In both groups, the highest incidence was for the anaplastic astrocytoma cases. The next most common gliomas among the juvenile cases were pilocytic astrocytoma (21%), so-called astrocytoma grade II (18.4%), and medulloblastoma (17.1%). In contrast, in the adult cases, anaplastic astrocytoma and glioblastoma accounted for similar percentages (36.2% and 35.1%, respectively) and together these accounted for some 71.3% of all adult cases. Next, there followed astrocytoma grade II (17.6%) and oligodendroglioma (7.6%).

A comparison with the results of Schoenberg's Connecticut study of 1935–1964 is informative. The most common glioma among the Connecticut children was medulloblastoma (35%), followed by low-grade astrocytoma (28.5%) and anaplastic astrocytoma and glioblastoma (28.0%). In the Tohoku data, the incidence of medulloblastoma was relatively high, whereas ependymoma (7.9%) showed an incidence similar to that in the Connecticut children (9.0%). Among the Connecticut adults, anaplastic astrocytoma and glioblastoma accounted for 79.2%, whereas low-grade astrocytoma accounted for 15.3%. In adults of the Tohoku district, similar rates were found (71.3% and 17.6%, respectively). As seen by these reports, there are differences apparently in the incidence of medulloblastoma according to geographical locality.

Histological Distribution of Supra- and Infratentorial Giloma

Table 1.7 shows the histological types of the glioma classified according to their

Table 1.6. Frequency of glioma in children and adults, Tohoku brain tumor registry (1980–1984)

Histological type	Adults		Children	
	No.	Percent	No.	Percent
Anaplastic astrocytoma	134	36.2	19	25.0
Glioblastoma	130	35.1	7	9.2
Astrocytoma (GII)	65	17.6	14	18.4
Fibrillary	34		8	
Astrocytoma	12		4	
Mixed oligoastrocytoma	9			
Gemistocytic	8			
Protoplasmic	2		2	
Oligodendroglioma	28	7.6		
Pilocytic astrocytoma	8	2.2	16	21.0
Medulloblastoma	3	0.8	13	17.1
Ependymoma	2	0.5	6	7.9
Subependymal giant cell astrocytoma			1	1.3
Total	370	100	76	100

Children were aged up to 14 years, adults 15 years and over

Table 1.7. Histological distribution of supra- and infratentorial glioma, Tohoku brain tumor registry (1980–1984)

Location	Low-grade astrocytoma	Anaplastic astrocytoma	Giloblas-toma	Oligodendro-glioma	Ependy-moma	Medullo-blastoma	Total
Supratentorial	63 (69.2)	134 (90.5)	135 (98.5)	28 (100)	3 (37.5)	——	363
Infratentorial	28 (30.8)	14 (9.5)	2 (1.5)	——	5 (62.5)	16 (100)	65
Total	91	148	137	28	8	16	428

Percentages in *Parentheses*

supra- or infratentorial location. Since 69.2% of the low-grade astrocytoma were supratentorial and 30.8% infratentorial, a ratio considerably higher than that seen in the high-grade astrocytoma cases was obtained. More than 90% of the anaplastic astrocytoma and glioblastoma cases were located supratentorially, and all 28 of the oligodendroglioma cases were supratentorial.

Incidence of Giloma at Various Sites

Tables 1.8–1.12 shows the histological types of glioma in relation to the incidence of the lesions at various cerebral sites, namely the frontal lobe, temporal lobe, parietal lobe, occipital lobe, and cerbellum and fourth ventricle. There were a large number of cases (133) located in the frontal lobe, followed by the temporal lobe (60 cases), the cerebellum and fourth ventricle (50 cases), the parietal lobe (30 cases), and the occipital lobe (13 cases).

With regard to the histological types of these cases, glioblastoma and anaplastic

Table 1.8. Incidence of glioma in frontal lobe, Tohoku brain tumor registry (1980–1984)

Finding	Cases	
	No.	Percent
Anaplastic astrocytoma	50	37.6
Glioblastoma	33	24.8
Fibrillary astrocytoma	13	9.8
Oligodendroglioma	12	9.0
Astrocytoma	6	4.5
Gemistocytic astrocytoma	6	4.5
Mixed oligoastrocytoma	5	3.8
Anaplastic oligodendroglioma	3	2.3
Pilocytic astrocytoma	2	1.5
Protoplasmic astrocytoma	2	1.5
Giant cell glioblastoma	1	0.8
Total	133	100

Table 1.9. Incidence of glioma in temporal lobe, Tohoku brain tumor registry (1980–1984)

Finding	Cases	
	No.	Percent
Glioblastoma	32	53.3
Anaplastic astrocytoma	17	28.3
Fibrillary astrocytoma	6	10.0
Astrocytoma	1	1.7
Gemistocytic astrocytoma	1	1.7
Pilocytic astrocytoma	1	1.7
Mixed oligoastrocytoma	1	1.7
Ependymoma	1	1.7
Total	60	100

Table 1.10. Incidence of glioma in parietal lobe, Tohoku brain tumor registry (1980–1984)

Finding	Cases	
	No.	Percent
Glioblastoma	14	46.7
Anaplastic astrocytoma	11	36.7
Fibrillary astrocytoma	2	6.7
Anaplastic oligodendroglioma	2	6.7
Ependymoma	1	3.3
Total	30	100

Table 1.11. Incidence of glioma in occipital lobe, Tohoku brain tumor registry (1980–1984)

Finding	Cases	
	No.	Percent
Glioblastoma	7	53.8
Anaplastic astrocytoma	2	15.4
Astrocytoma	1	7.7
Fibrillary astrocytoma	1	7.7
Oligodendroglioma	1	7.7
Ependymoma	1	7.7
Total	13	100

Table 1.12. Incidence of glioma in cerebellum and fourth ventricle, Tohoku brain tumor registry (1980–1984)

Finding	Cases	
	No.	Percent
Pilocytic astrocytoma	13	26.0
Anaplastic astrocytoma	12	24.0
Medulloblastoma	12	24.0
Ependymoma	4	8.0
Fibrillary astrocytoma	4	8.0
Desmoplastic medulloblastoma	2	4.0
Glioblastoma	1	2.0
Astrocytoma	1	2.0
Protoplasmic astrocytoma	1	2.0
Total	50	100

astrocytoma accounted for 60%–80% of the gliomas in the various lobes of the cerebral hemispheres, followed by fibrillary astrocytoma. A relatively high incidence of oligodendroglioma was characteristic of the frontal lobe. The histological types of the lesions of the cerebellum and fourth ventricle were pilocytic astrocytoma (26%), anaplastic astrocytoma (24%), and medulloblastoma (24%). If desmoplastic medulloblastoma cases are included among the medulloblastoma cases, they account for 28.3% of these lesions and the above three histological types then account for 78% of the gliomas of the cerebellum and fourth ventricle.

Diagnostic Methods

The diagnostic methods used for making the diagnosis are listed in Table 1.13. In the majority of cases, diagnosis was made on the basis of a surgical specimen (69.5%), whereas diagnosis was made at autopsy in 0.5%.

Table 1.13. Diagnostic Methods in glioma cases, Tohoku brain tumor registry (1980–1984)

Method	Cases	
	No.	Percent
Surgical specimen	455	69.5
X-ray, RI, or CT-scan	197	30.0
Autopsy	3	0.5
Total	655	100

CT computed tomography, *RI* radioisotope

Clinical Grade on Admission

Table 1.14 presents the clinical grade of these cases at the time of admission to hospital. A small number of cases (6.0%) had no clinical symptoms whatsoever or had only subjective complaints without accompanying neurological deficits. The largest number (43.8%) had focal neurological signs. There were also a large number (32.4%) with intracranial hypertension and a significant number (17.8%) with disturbances of consciousness or other severe abnormalities of the central nervous system (CNS).

Oncogenesis of Glioma

Several studies on the oncogenesis of glioma have been reported [2, 7, 14, 16, 23]. Among the endogenous factors, a correlation between phacomatosis, as in Reck-linghausen's disease, and glioma is known and, among exogenous factors, the involvement of head trauma, radiotherapy, and viruses has been suggested. No experimental evidence on the involvement of these latter factors, however, has been obtained and all relationships with the genesis of the glioma remain hypothetical. Moreover, it is noteworthy that the brain tumors considered in those reports have usually been neurinoma and meningioma, and little discussion has been made on the causal factors in glioma.

   In the present section, we will briefly discuss those factors which have been suggested in the oncogenesis of the glioma specifically and address the question of the relationship with findings on oncoviruses [10, 12, 21], growth factors, and oncogenes [8, 13, 15, 19, 24] where developments in recent years have been remarkable.

Hereditary Factors

The unambiguous involvement of hereditary factors [2] in the genesis of glioma is known for one of the phacomatosis disorders, Recklinghausen's disease. The majority of such cases develop neurinoma, but some develop meningioma or glioma. With regard to the familial incidence, in a study of 77 glioma cases, Choi et al. [5] found that among 1243 relatives of the glioma patients eight had brain tumors. In contrast, among 1382 relatives of control subjects only one had a brain

Table 1.14. Clinical grade of glioma cases, Tohoku brain tumor registry (1980–1984)

Clinical grade	Cases	
	No.	Percent
No clinical symptoms	18	2.7
Subjective complaints only	22	3.3
Focal signs	289	43.8
Intracranial hypertension	214	32.4
Disturbance of consciousness	102	15.5
Coma	13	2.0
Respiratory impairment	2	0.3
Total	660	100

tumor. The incidence of brain tumors among the relatives of glioma patients was thus some ninefold higher than expected—an incidence which was statistically significant. It must be said, however, that the study of Choi et al. did not distinguish between strictly hereditary factors and factors involving the environment of the families. Studies on the relationship between blood types and glioma have also been made. One reported a high incidence of glioma among patients with type-A blood, but no correlation was found in other studies, thus leaving the question unanswered [18].

Exogenous Factors

There have long been suggestions of a causal relation between head trauma and the development of brain tumors, but most studies have focused on the incidence of meningioma, and little can be said regarding the oncogenesis of glioma. Similarly, many studies have reported on the relationship between irradiation and brain tumors, but they have dealt with the development of meningioma and sarcoma rather than glioma. Again, no conclusions can be drawn with regard to glioma.

Concerning chemical substances, it has previously been demonstrated that glioma can be induced in laboratory animals using agents such as methylcholantren or ethylnitrosourea. The relationship between such chemicals and human glioma cases remains unclear. There has been, however, one noteworthy study by Waxwiler et al. [23], in which they reported a high incidence of glioblastoma among employees in contact with vinyl chloride.

No relationship has yet been established between the incidence of glioma and the factor currently considered the most dangerous oncogenetic factor, tobacco smoke. According to Choi et al. [5], there were no significant differences between a control group and a glioma group.

Racial Factors

Studies concerned with racial factors, such as those by Heshmat et al. [9], have shown that black Americans have a lower incidence of glioma than white Americans. Studies on the Mongoloid races and, specifically, on Japanese, have shown a still lower incidence than among Negroes. These studies, however, did not consider the possible involvement of cultural/environmental factors as the cause for the racial differences.

Oncogenic Viruses and Growth Factors

In 1911, Rous discovered a virus which can give rise to sarcomas in chickens and in 1941 Halbestaedter succeeded in making a cell culture cancerous using the Rous sarcoma virus. Work on oncogenic viruses has been actively pursued ever since, several oncogenes have been discovered in human cancer cells, and such research remains at the basis of many cancer studies.

Oncoviruses can be broadly divided into DNA-type and RNA-type viruses. Most research centers around the retroviruses, which are of the RNA type. Among the genes of the retrovirus are oncogenes, which produce proteins with oncogenetic capabilities. It has been found that among such proteins several have the same structure as the growth factors which are needed for normal human growth, and the relationship between cell growth factor and oncogenes has also been actively pursued. Viewed from a slightly different perspective, it has been said that oncogenes may be essential as growth factors in the process of the evolution of higher animal species, such as man. Amid research on the influences of oncogenes and oncoviruses on human cancers, there have recently been several studies concerned specifically with glioma.

sis-Oncogene and Platelet-Derived Growth Factor

Simian sarcoma virus contains the so-called v-sis oncogene, which codes for the protein called $P28^{V\text{-SIS}}$. It has been found that the amino acid sequence of this protein is nearly identical to that of platelet-derived growth factor (PDGF). The cells which have been found to proliferate in response to PDGF are mesothelium-derived cells, such as fibroblasts and glial cells, whereas epithelial and endothelial cells remain unaffected. Several studies have investigated the relationship between PDGF and the onset and/or proliferation of glioma. Westermark et al. [24] and Nister et al. [15] have demonstrated that in cell lines obtained from glioblastoma patients PDGF-like growth factor is indeed produced.

erb-B Oncogenes and Epidermal Growth Factor

It has been show thàt avian erythroblastosis virus (AEV) can cause cancers of the blood and lymph systems. This virus is now known to contain two oncogenes, v-erb-A and v-erb-B. The protein (gp65$^{erb\text{-}B}$), which is coded for by v-erb-B, has been shown to have a structure similar to that of epidermal growth factor (EGF) receptor, which, among the cell surface receptors responding to EGF, is missing or present in an EGF-combined domain. Libermann et al. [13] have investigated the expression of the EGF receptor in glioma cells and found that in four of ten glioblastoma cases there was EGF receptor gene amplification and in three of ten cases there was a high level of expression of EGF receptors. In light of the fact that a normal level of EGF expression was found in benign tumors, such as low-grade astrocytomas and meningiomas, they concluded that the overexpression of EGF receptor genes in glioblastoma is involved in the development or progression of this kind of tumor.

src-Oncogene

A related study on the relationship between glioma and the v-src oncogene of the Rous sarcoma virus was reported by Takenaka et al. [21]. The src-oncogene was in fact the first oncogene to be discovered and protein it codes for is called pp60^{src}. Using antiserum to the src-gene product, Takenaka et al. studied the response to tumor cells and found that among 44 cases of astrocytoma 27 showed positive responses.

There have as yet been few reports on the relationship between oncogenes (or the related growth factors) and the onset or proliferation of gliomas. It is known that complete surgical resection of glioma is not possible and that satisfactory therapeutic results are not obtainable using externally applied therapies, such as radiotherapy and chemotherapy. Therefore, if the proliferation of glioma tissue is brought about by tumor growth factor, then it is possible that its growth can be prevented by the administration of growth factor antagonists. Further research along those lines in much needed.

References

1. Annegers JF, Schoenberg BS, Okazaki H, Kurland LT (1981) Epidemiologic study of primary intracranial neoplasms. Arch Neurol 38: 217–219
2. Armstrong RM, Hanson CW (1969) Familial gliomas. J Neurol 19: 1061–1063
3. Bailey P, Cushing H (1926) A classification of the tumors of the glioma group on a histologic basis with a correlated study of prognosis. Lippincott, Philadelphia
4. Barker DJP, Weller RO, Garfield JS (1976) Epidemiology of primary tumors of the brain and spinal cord: a regional survey in southern England. J Neurol Neurosurg Psychiat 39: 290–296
5. Choi NW, Schuman LM, Gullen WH (1970) Epidemiology of primary central nervous system neoplasms: II. Case control study. Am J Epidemiol 91: 467–485
6. Dohrmann GJ, Farwell JR, Flannery JT (1985) Astrocytomas in childhood: a population-based study. Surg Neurol 23: 64–68
7. Gold E, Gordis L, Tonascia J, and Sz kho M (1979) Risk factors for brain tumors in children. Am J Epidemiol 109: 309–319
8. Heldin CH, Westermark B (1984) Growth factors: Mechanism of action and relation to oncogenes. Cell 37: 9–20
9. Heshmat MY, Kovi J, Simpson C, Kennedy J, Fank J (1976) Neoplasms of the central nervous system. Incidence and population selectivity in the Washington DC metropolitan area. Cancer 38: 2135–2142
10. Hochberg FH, Miller G, Schooley RT, Mirsch MS, Feorino P, Henle W (1983) Central nervous system lymphoma related to Epstein Barr Virus. N Engl J Med 309: 745–748
11. Kernohan JW, Sayre GP (1952) Tumors of the central nervous system. In: Atlas of tumor pathology, fasc 35. Armed Forces Institute of Pathology, Washington DC
12. Krieg P, Amtmann E, Jonas D, Fischer H, Zang K, Sauer G (1981) Episomal simian virus 40 genomes in human brain tumors. Proc Natl Acad Sci USA 78: 6446–6450
13. Libermann TA, Nusbaum HR, Razon N, Kris R, Lax I, Soreq H, Whittle N, Waterfield M, Ullrich A, Schlessinger J (1985) Amplification and overexpression of the EGF receptor gene in primary human glioblastomas. J Cell Sci Suppl 3: 161–172
14. Musicco M, Filippini G, Bordo BM, Melotto A, Morello G, and Berrino F (1982) Gliomas and occupational exposure to carcinogens: case-control study. Am J Epidemiol 116: 782–790
15. Nister M, Heldin CH, Wasteson A, Westermark B (1984) A glioma-derived analog to platelet-derived growth factor: Demonstration of receptor competing activity and

immunological crossreactivity. Proc Natl Acad Sci USA 81: 926–930

16. Reagan TJ, Freiman IS (1973) Multiple cerebral gliomas in multiple sclerosis. J Neurol Neurosurg Psychiat 36: 523–528

17. Rubinstein LJ (1979) Tumors of the central nervous system. In: Atlas of tumor pathology, 2nd series, fasc 6. Armed Forces Institute of Pathology, Washington DC

18. Schoenberg BS (1978) Epidemiology of primary nervous system neoplasms. Adv Neurol 19: 475–495

19. Shapiro JR (1986) Biology of gliomas: Heterogeneity, oncogenes, growth factors. Seminars in Oncology 13: 4–15

20. Suzuki J, Iwabuchi T, Kanaya H, Kodama N, Kowada M, Nakai A, Tanaka R (1984) Tohoku Brain Tumor Registry, vol. 1 Committee of Tohoku Brain Tumor Registry Sendai Japan

21. Takenaka N, Mikoshiba K, Takamatsu K, Tsukada Y, Ohtani M, Toya S (1985) Immunological detection of the gene product of Rous sarcoma virus in human brain tumors. Brain Research 337: 20–207

22. The committee of brain tumor registry in Japan (1984) Brain Tumor Registry in Japan, vol. 5 The Ministry of Welfare in Japan

23. Waxweiler RJ, Stringer W, Wagoner JK, Jones J, Falk H, Carter C (1976) Neoplastic risk among workers exposed to vinyl chloride. Ann New York Acad Sci 271: 40–48

24. Westermark B, Nister M, Heldin CH (1985) Growth factors and oncogenes in human malignant glioma. Neurol Clinics 3: 785–799

25. Zimmerman HM (1969) Brain tumors: Their incidence and classification in man and their experimental reproduction. Ann New York Acad Sci 159: 337–359

26. Zulch KJ, Wechsler W (1968) Pathology and classification of gliomas. Basel New York (Progr neurol surg, vol. 2, pp 1–84)

27. Zulch KJ (1980) Principles of the new World Health Organization (WHO), classification of brain tumors. Neuroradiol 19: 59–66

Chapter 2

Statistical Considerations of Therapeutic Results in Glioblastoma

K. Mineura

Introduction

Together with recent developments in basic research and reflecting trends in infor-mation technology, there has been a large increase in the number of reports on the most representative of the malignant brain tumors, glioblastoma (GBM). Evalua-tion of the available therapeutic techniques is, however, a wide-ranging task and it is not always a simple matter to obtain an accurate understanding of the current state of GBM therapy. In the present study, we investigated the therapeutic results in GBM cases, as reported in the literature, in relation to the therapeutic methods and the period during which the cases were treated. The study focuses primarily on the survival time and the survival rate of such patients.

Materials and Methods

Study of the literature was undertaken based upon cases which could be traced through the Quarterly Cumulation Index (1916–1956), Current List of Medical Literature (1957–1959), and Cumulated Index Medicus (1960–1983). The data contained in a total of 265 reports were examined and the 4381 cases from 48 reports in which both the histological diagnosis of GBM and the survival time were unambiguously described were used for statistical analysis [1, 3, 8, 11, 15–17, 21, 23–26, 30, 32–35, 38, 39, 43, 47, 50–52, 57, 65, 66, 69–73, 75, 76, 79, 82, 84, 91, 95–98, 100–104]. In addition, 7078 cases from 41 reports in which the survival rate was described were also used [4, 5, 10–13, 16, 19, 20, 28, 32, 34, 37, 38, 45, 46, 53, 55, 61, 62, 64, 67–69, 75–'78, 80–82, 86, 87, 89, 90, 92, 94, 97].

The therapeutic methods were divided into four groups for the purpose of analysis: surgery alone (S), surgery and radiotherapy (S + R), surgery and chemo-therapy (S + C), and surgery, radiotherapy, and chemotherapy (S + R + C). The median survival time (MST) and the postoperative survival rate and their standard deviations were used. The mean value was taken as the group mean of the entire series of cases and no attempt was made to calculate the variability within individual reports. In several studies, mention was made of the "median time to tumor progression," "median progression-free interval," or "median duration of free interval" and these data are designated as such in the tables. There were also reports in which the mean survival rate was noted. In such cases, we have described this value in parentheses after the MST.

Comparisons of MST and SR were also made for two periods of time. The first period is that prior to 1975 when the clinical application of neuroradiological techniques, such as X-ray computed tomography (CT), was not widespread and chemotherapy using anticancer agents and steroids had not yet begun. The second is that after 1975, during which time these techniques have become widely available.

Since several different histological definitions and classifications of GBM have been made [6, 48, 62, 105], their contents differ slightly among different authors. These differences cannot always be determined from the reports themselves, however. Therefore, in this study, we investigated all cases reported as GBM together as a single entity.

Results

Correlation of Prognosis with Therapeutic Methods

Among 1462 cases receiving S, the MST was 4.6 ± 1.6 (7.5 ± 2.2) months. In the majority of cases, a decrease in intracranial pressure was obtained by means of tumor excision (Table 2.1). The MST of 892 cases receiving S + R was 9.3 ± 1.9 (15.0 ± 2.9) months, approximately 5 months longer than those undergoing S (Table 2.2).

Table 2.1. Survival time of glioblastoma patients receiving surgery alone

Author	Year	No. of cases	Survival (months)	
			Median	Mean
Moersch	1941	11[a]		4
Earle	1957	145		6
Tönnis	1959	225	2, 3, 2[d]	
Roth	1960	160		9.8
Grunert	1973	222	6	
Weir	1973	248	6.6	
Walker	1976	20	3.8	
Heiss	1978	16[b]		6.3
Salcman	1980	349	4	
Young	1981	24[c]		3.5[f]
Chin	1981	12	4.8	6.8
		1462	4.6 ± 1.6[e]	7.5 ± 2.2[e]

[a] Age >60 years
[b] Half of cases with radiation therapy
[c] Reoperation
[d] Partial removal, total removal, lobectomy, respectively
[e] Arithmetic mean ± SD, naturally weighted toward the larger study groups
[f] Survival time after reoperation

Table 2.2. Survival time of glioblastoma patients receiving surgery and radiotherapy

Author	Year	No. of cases	Survival (months)	
			Median	Mean
Roth	1960	144		17.4
Edland	1971	17	11.7	
Bloom	1973	35		10.5
Brisman	1976	39	4.2	
Reagan	1976	22	11.6	
Walker	1976	44	6.5	
Weir	1976	15	6.3	8.8
Seiler	1978	32	12.8	
Walker	1978	68	8.7	
Eagan	1979	20	8.8	
Hochberg	1979		5.8	
Reeves	1979	32	9.5	
Cianfriglia	1980	50		13.2
Seiler	1980	16	10[a]	
Walker	1980	94	9	
Chin	1981	25	11.8	14.5
Afra	1983	91	10	
Chang	1983	148	9.9	
		892	9.3 ± 1.9[b]	15.0 ± 2.9[b]

[a] Median progression-free interval
[b] Arithmetic mean $\pm$ SD, naturally weighted toward the larger study groups

Among 521 cases receiving S + C, the MST was 7.0 ± 2.4 months (7.8 ± 2.3). This group included 409 patients who received surgery and chemotherapy with a single drug (S + monoC); their MST was 6.4 ± 1.7 (7.6 ± 2.4) months. The MST in 282 patients treated with nitrosourea, which is an anticancer agent capable of penetrating the blood-brain barrier, was 6.3 ± 1.4 (8.6 ± 1.4) months and that of the remaining 127 cases treated with other anticancer agents was approximately the same—6.5 ± 2.3 months (Table 2.3). The MST of 112 cases receiving surgery and chemotherapy with multiagents (S + polyC) was 9.2 ± 3.0 months, about 2.8 months longer than the S + monoC group and about the same as the S + R group (Table 2.4).

A total of 1506 patients received S + R + C, which resulted in an MST of 11.6 ± 3.0 (12.6 ± 1.5) months, prolonging the survival time in S, S + R, and S + C by more than 7.0, 2.3 and 4.6 months, respectively. Among the S + R + C group of 1506 patients, 442 received S + R + ployC and 1064 received S + R + MonoC. The MST of S + R + polyC was 13.1 ± 3.0 months, which was 2.2 months longer than that of S + R + monoC cases (Tables 2.5, 2.6).

Cases in which survival rates were described were also analyzed according to the therapeutic method. There were 1258 cases of surgical therapy alone reported in eight studies, 2480 cases of S + R reported in 23 studies, 198 cases of S + C reported in five studies, and 1175 cases of S + R + C reported in 13 studies. Among those

Table 2.3. Survival time of glioblastoma patients receiving surgery and single agent chemotherapy

Author	Year	Agent	No. of cases	Survival (months)	
				Median	Mean
Mealey	1962	Vinblastine	9	5	
Dean	1963	Vinblastine	18	8	
Wilson	1964	Vinblastine	19	3	
Aaronson	1963	Thio-TEPA	7	8	
Owens	1965	Vincristine	22	6	
Kennedy	1965	Mithramycin	9	10	
Owens	1966	Mechlorethane	22		3.5
Luyendijk	1966	Methotrexate	12	9.5	
Mahaley	1967	Cyclophophamide	9	5	
			127	6.5 ± 2.3[a]	
Walker	1978	BCNU	51	4.6	
Hochberg	1981	BCNU	11	7	
Greenberg	1981	BCNU	6	8.8	8.3
Chin	1981	BCNU	5	7.5	11.3
Rosenblum	1973	CCNU	13	8.8	11.0
Reagan	1976	CCNU	22	6.6	
Weir	1976	CCNU	13	8.6	8.7
Heiss	1978	CCNU	24		7.0
Cianfriglia	1980	CCNU	27		8.4
Walker	1980	MeCCNU	81	6	
Chin	1981	MeCCNU	9	4	
Gerosa	1981	VM-26	20	8[b]	
			282	6.3 ± 1.4[a]	8.6 ± 1.4[a]
			409	6.4 ± 1.7	7.6 ± 2.4

[a] Arithemetic mean $\pm$ SD, naturally weighted toward the larger study groups
[b] Median progression-free interval

treated with S, the survival rates after 6 months, 1, 2, 3, and 5 years were, respectively, 30% $\pm$ 22%, 7% $\pm$ 2%, 3% $\pm$ 4%, 2% $\pm$ 3%, and 1% $\pm$ 1%; as can be seen, the 1-year survival rate was already less than 10%. Among those receiving S + R, these survival rates were 56% $\pm$ 22%, 30% $\pm$ 11%, 13% $\pm$ 5%, and 5% $\pm$ 3%—longer at each time interval than those receiving S alone. The survival rates after 6 months, 1 year, and 2 years among those receiving S + C were 54% $\pm$ 24%, 23% $\pm$ 13%, and 3% $\pm$ 4%. The survival rates after 6 months and 1 year were longer than those for cases treated with S, but the survival rate after 2 years was the same as with S. Finally, the survival rates among the S + R + C cases after 6 months, and 1 year, and 2 years were, respectively, 82% $\pm$ 11%, 50% $\pm$ 14%, and 20% $\pm$ 6%. These survival rates were longer than those found in any other therapeutic group, but the differences among the groups decreased in proportion to progress from the therapy (Fig. 2.1).

Table 2.4. Survival time of glioblastoma patients receiving surgery and polychemotherapy

Author	Year	Agents	No. of cases	Survival (months)	
				Median	Mean
Pouillart	1976	Adriamycin VM-26 CCNU	43[a]	6	
Heiss	1978	Cyclophoshamide Methylhydrazine 5-Fu 6MP Vinblastine	16		9
Poisson	1979	VM-26 CCNU	28	11	
West	1983	BCNU Vinblastine Procarbazine MeCCNU	25	12.7	
			112	9.2 ± 3.0[b]	

[a] Recurrent or inoperable cases
[b] Arithmetic mean $\pm$ SD, naturally weighted toward the larger study groups

Comparison of Therapeutic Results Before and After 1975

The MST of 2992 cases treated after 1975 was 10.3 ± 2.8 months and that for 1389 cases treated prior to 1975 was 6.6 ± 2.8 months—a difference of 3.7 months (Fig. 2.2). One cause for this prolongation of survival time is the great increase in S + C and S + R + C since 1975.

The survival rates among 3265 cases treated before 1975 were $48\% \pm 20\%$, $21\% \pm 13\%$, $11\% \pm 4\%$, $5\% \pm 4\%$, and $3\% \pm 3\%$ after 6 months, 1, 2, 3, and 5 years, respectively. Those among 3813 cases treated since 1975 were, respectively, $70\% \pm 17\%$, $37\% \pm 17\%$, $13\% \pm 8\%$, $13\% \pm 5\%$, and $3\% \pm 3\%$.

Clearly, the survival rates were longer among the more recently treated patients than among those treated before 1975 except for the 5-year survival rate, but the difference between the two groups decreased in proportion to progress from the therapy (Fig. 2.3).

Discussion

Glioblastoma was first described by Bailey and Cushing [6] as a tumor arising from a hypothetical mother cell, the glioblast. Kernohan et al. [48] considered GBM to be the most anaplastic state of astrocytoma and divided such anaplasia into four grades, grades III and IV corresponding to GBM. In the World Health Organization (WHO) classification, however, GBM is differentiated from anaplastic astrocytoma based upon the degree of anaplasia of the tissue and its microscopic viability [105].

Table 2.5. Survival time of glioblastoma patients receiving surgery, radiotherapy, and monochemotherapy

Author	Year	Therapy		No. of cases	Survival (months)	
					Median	Mean
Ransohoff	1965	Mithramycin	+ RT	14	10	
Walker	1976	Mithramycin	+ RT	52	5.3	
Mahaley	1967	S112	+ RT	11	7	
Edland	1971	5-FU	+ RT	15		11.5
Eagan	1979	DAG	+ RT	22	16.8	
Afra	1983	DBD	+ RT	28	14.3	
Brisman	1976	BCNU, CCNU, MeCCNU	+ RT	23	12	
Walker	1978	BCNU	+ RT	72	8.6	
Levin	1979	BCNU	+ RT	46	7.8[a]	
Walker	1980	BCNU	+ RT	92	12.8	
		MeCCNU	+ RT	81	10.5	
Chin	1981	BCNU	+ RT	26	17.3	
		MeCCNU	+ RT	10	23.0	
Green	1983	BCNU + methyl-predonisolone	+ RT	134	10.3	
		PCZ	+ RT	128	11.8	
Chang	1983	BCNU	+ RT	165	10.0	
Rosenblum	1973	CCNU	+ RT	13	16.0	15.2
Weir	1976	CCNU	+ RT	13	8.4	
Reagan	1976	CCNU	+ RT	19	12	
Cianfriglia	1978	CCNU	+ RT	26		11.9
Hochberg	1979	CCNU	+ RT	74	11.5	
				1064	10.9 ± 2.7[b]	12.6 ± 1.5[b]

DAG dianhydrogalactitol, *DBD* dibromodulcitol, *PCZ* procarbazine
[a] Median time to tumor progression
[b] Arithmetic mean $\pm$ SD, naturally weighted toward the larger study groups

Due to these differences in the definition of GBM, problems remain in considering all reported GBM cases to be the same histological entity. In practice, it is in fact virtually impossible to distinguish the different varieties of GBM solely from the information provided in the reports in the literature.

In reports on Radiation Therapy Oncology Group (RTOG)-Eastern Cooperative Oncology Group (ECOG), comparisons have been made of the therapeutic results in cases of GBM and in cases of astrocytoma with atypical or anaplastic foci (AAF) [62]. Consequently, it was found that the MST of 412 GBM cases (8 months) was much worse than that of 91 AAF cases (28 months; $P < 0.001$). This suggests that the prognosis can be determined by means of careful histological examination and indicates that even today therapeutic results can be heavily influenced by the characteristic features of the tumor.

Factors which influence the therapeutic results include not only the character of the tumor tissue, but also factors of the patient, including age, preoperative condi-

Table 2.6. Survival time of glioblastoma patients receiving surgery, radiotherapy, and polychemotherapy

Author	Year	Therapy	No. of cases	Median survival (months)
Afra	1983	DBD + CCNU + RT	31	12
Levin	1979	BCNU + HU + RT	53	10.5
Chang	1983	MeCCNU + DTIC + RT	136	9.8[b]
Seiler	1978	PCZ + CCNU + BLM + RT	20	14
Poisson	1979	VM-26 + CCNU + RT	46	17
Seiler	1980	VM-26 + CCNU +. RT	15	16.4[b]
EORTC	1981	VM-26 + CCNU + RT + PCZ[a]	61	14.5
		RT + CCNU[a] or VM-26[a] + CCNU	55	15.3
Jacque	1983	VM-26 + CCNU, 5-FU PCZ, DTIC, ADR + RT	25	19
			442	13.1 $\pm$ 3.0[c]

ADR adriamycin, *BLM* bleomycin, *HU* hydroxyurea, *DTIC* imidazole-4 (or 5)carboxamide-5 (or 4)- (3,3-dimethyl-1-trizene)
[a] With recurrence
[b] Median time to tumor progression
[c] Arithmetic mean $\pm$ SD, naturally weighted toward the larger study group

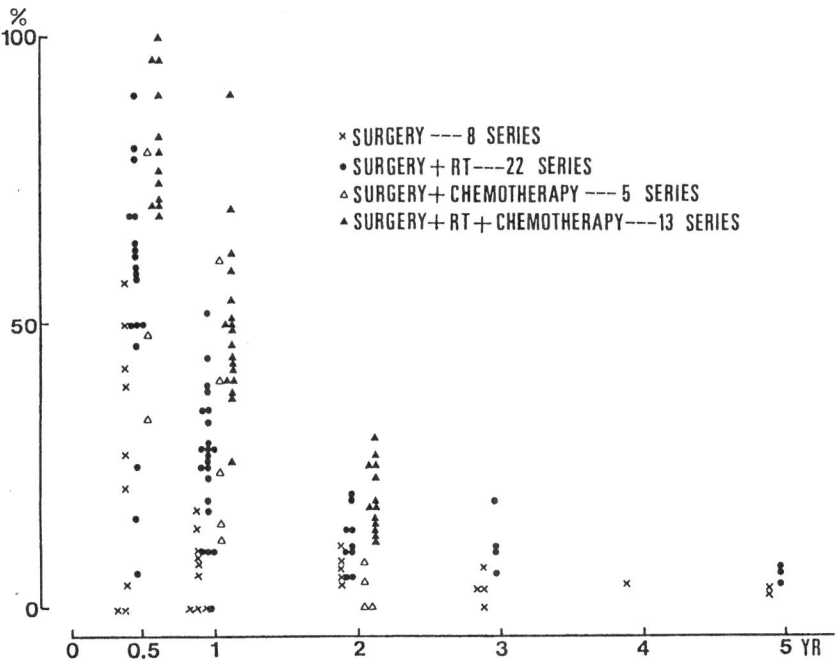

Fig. 2.1. Survival rates in glioblastoma series according to therapeutic modalities

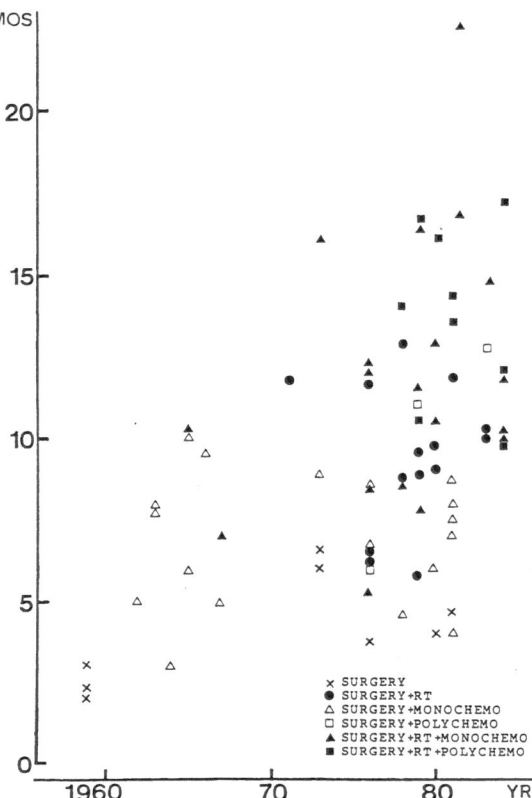

Fig. 2.2. Median survival time of glioblastoma

tion, initial symptoms (Table 2.7). One factor indicative of a favorable outcome is a relatively young age: under 35 years according to some [63], under 50 according to others [100], or upper and lower age limits of 24 and 42 [63] or 30 and 50 years [44]. Unfavorable factors include an extremely young age (less than 10 years [20]) or an age over 40 [19] or 61 [20]. The reason for a poor prognosis among younger patients is the high incidence of infratentorial tumors and a relatively high number of cases with high malignancy levels. Among elderly patients, complications are frequent and responses to adjuvant therapies are low [74]. Moreover, authors often report the absolute survival rate, rather than the relative survival rate, thus indicating a poorer survival for elderly patients than might otherwise be the case.

Favorable factors regarding the preoperative state include no disturbances of consciousness and no paresis or other neurological symptoms [19, 97] and scores on the Karnofsky performance scale in excess of 80 [60]. There have been several studies reporting that favorable outcomes are obtained among patients with convulsive attacks [7, 63, 76, 88, 95], a tendency which is thought to be due to the fact that diagnosis is made at an early period prior to the development of neurological symptoms when the preoperative state is relatively good. There has also been one report suggesting that a relatively long period of convulsions indicates a favorable prognosis (Table 2.7), [88].

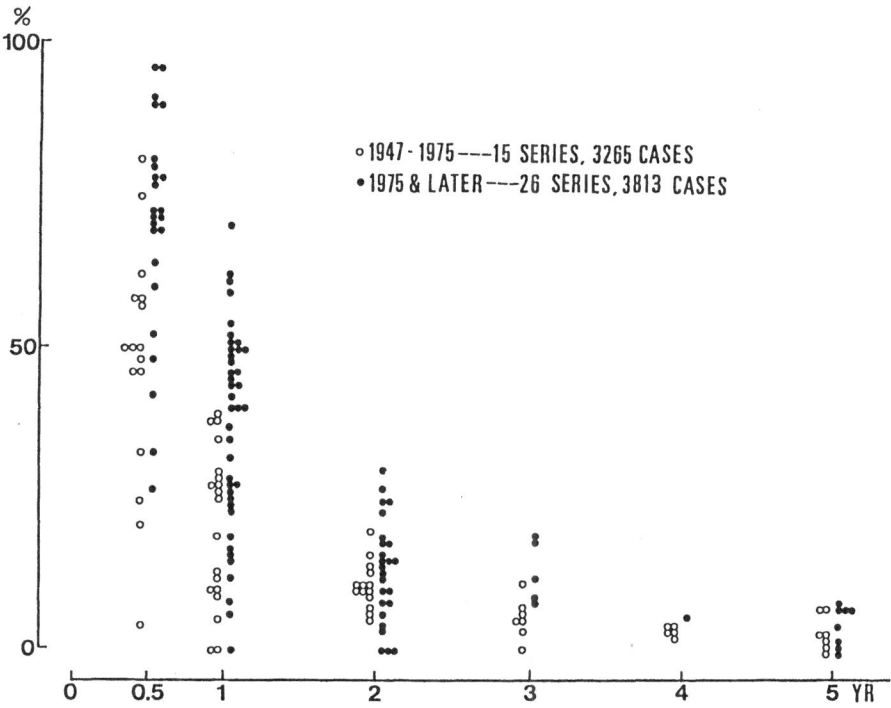

Fig. 2.3. Survival rates in glioblastoma series classified chronologically

Table 2.7. Prognostic factors correlated with postoperative survival of glioblastoma

	No. of references in literature	Positive	Negative
Host factor			
Age	26	24	2
Preoperative state	15	15	
Convulsion	8	8	
Duration of symptom	6	6	
Sex	1	1	
ABO type	1	1	
Tumor factor			
Histology	21	18	3
Location	7	5	2
Extent	3	3	
Therapy			
Radiotherapy	19	19	
Resection	16	16	
Radiation dose	4	4	
Steroid	2	2	
External decompression	1	1	
Radiosensitizer	1	1	

Summarized from 70 references (1926–1983)

The significance of surgical treatment in GBM extends to diagnostic procedures, curative procedures, and palliation [42]. Together with advances in modern techniques such as cerebral angiography, cerebral scintigraphy, cytology, and CT and PET scanning, the importance of surgical diagnostic procedures has diminished. Nevertheless, the rate of definitive diagnoses using stereotaxic operations in deep-seated tumors is reported to be 88% [54] and still higher when used together with CT scanning.

Curative procedures are limited to tumors located at polar sites or superficial regions. In histological research on autopsied brains, invasion to the contralateral hemisphere was found in 64% of cases and an indication for radical resection was reported in less than 20%, except those lying in the dominant hemisphere [56].

Among palliative procedures, a reduction in the volume of the tumor will improve symptoms due to decreased intracranial pressure and improve the general condition. Such procedures, therefore, make it possible to perform radiotherapy or chemotherapy and increase the effectiveness of such therapies by removing hypoxic and necrotic tissue.

The mortality until the 1950s was high at approximately 40% [48] but fell to about 10% by the 1970s. Using echo techniques during surgery, it has recently become possible to determine accurately the extent of the lesion, and usage of the surgical microscope, lasers, and the ultrasonic surgical aspirator has made the resection of such lesions safer and easier.

But, as mentioned above, the MST following S in GBM cases was 4.6 months, whereas the longest survival time was 3 months among nonsurgical cases [13] and 5 months among 30 biopsy cases [28]. Therefore, it can be said that surgical resection prolongs the survival time for less than 2 months.

According to the results of Goldsmith [31], the MST following extensive surgery was 3.9 months, whereas it was 2.3 months following limited surgery. In other words, his patients' lives were prolonged for only 1.6 months. While it cannot be denied that surgical therapy has some positive effects, it is equally certain that adjuvant therapy must also be employed.

Extracranial metastasis in GBM cases is rare and so locally applied radiotherapy is appropriate. Sensitivity to radiation is, however, relatively low and the primary significance of radiotherapy is palliation. The MST of S + R was 9.3 months, which was 5 months longer than S. Many patients receiving postoperative radiotherapy have been in good general condition, thus making evaluation of the therapeutic methods difficult, but several randomized studies [16, 97] have also indicated good results using S + R. Judging from the survival rates in these randomized studies the effectiveness of radiotherapy can be estimated to have extended life for 2–3 years.

With regard to the field of irradiation, one report has noted that among 30 autopsy cases the region of irradiation did not coincide with the tumor in 15 cases [18]. Moreover, the results of follow-up CT studies indicate that recurrence is frequently at sites neighboring the tumor [40]. For these reasons, it is thought important to perform whole-brain irradiation or irradiation of a relatively large field, including the tumor and its surrounding tissues.

With regard to the dose of irradiation, various levels have been proposed, but the maximum dose which does not induce radiation necrosis is said to be most effective, i.e., 50–60 Gy to the whole brain and 20 Gy locally [78], or 40 Gy to the whole brain and 20 Gy locally [86].

Table 2.8. Hypoxic cell sensitizers in radiotherapy of glioblastoma

Author	Year	Sensitizers	No. of cases	Survival (months)	
				Median	Mean
Adams	1976	Metronidazole			
Urtasun	1976	Metronidazole	16	6.5[a]	
Wassermann	1981	Misonidazole		4.8	
Urtasun	1982	Metronidazole	17	4.8	
		Misonidazole	23	6.8	
MRC	1983	Misonidazole	188	8.3	
Nelson DF	1983	Misonidazole	98	10.7	
EORTC	1983		82	7.5[b]	11.1
			424	8.4 ± 1.5[c]	

[a] Significantly longer than conventional group
[b] Median duration of free interval
[c] Arithmetic mean ± SD, naturally weighted toward the larger study groups

Table 2.9. Megavoltage or neutron therapy in treatment of glioblastoma

Author	Year	RT	No. of cases	Survival (months)	
				Median	Mean
Kahr	1978	1 MeV X-ray	40		11.5
Shaw	1978	8 MeV neutron	34	5	
Laramore	1978	8 MeV neutron	26		9.4
		Mixed neutron and photon	10		7.6
Bloom	1982	7.5 MeV neutron	30	(31)[a]	
		6 MeV X-ray	33	(86)[a]	
Herskovic	1982	15 MeV neutron	31	6	
			204	5.5 ± 0.5[a]	10.3 ± 1.4[a]

[a] Recurrence rate
[b] Arithmetic mean ± SD, naturally weighted toward the larger study groups

Regarding the method of irradiation, in addition to the most common technique of postoperative radiotherapy, various alternative techniques and their merits have been reported in the literature. These include preoperative radiotherapy [83], postoperative delayed radiation [69], hyperfractionation [22, 68], brachytherapy [41], and hyperbaric therapy [14]. Recently, radiotherapy has been done using radiosensitizers, but the therapeutic results reported thus far have not indicated significant improvements [27, 59, 60, 94] (Table 2.8). Similarly, megavoltage therapy and treatment with fast neutrons have been attempted, but prolonged survival has not been obtained [9, 36, 46, 85] (Table 2.9). Nevertheless, the results of an autopsy study of 15 cases receiving fast neutron radiation have indicated no recurrences of the tumor in 14 cases (93%) [49], thus demonstrating that fast neutrons may be

Table 2.10. Response of glioblastoma to chemotherapy (1961–1979)

Agents	Cases	Responders (%)
Cyclophoshamide	12	0
Mechlorethamine	22	—
Thio-TEPA	24	54
S112	11[a]	—
MTX	21[a]	33
5-FU	32	—
Mithramycin	45	47
BLM	17	88
VCR	22	32
Vinblastine	46	46
BCNU	75	49
CCNU	152	43
Methyl CCNU	31	26
PCZ	21	48
VM-26	35	37
DTIC	4	50
BCNU + VCR	19	31
Mithramycin + VCR	7	0
BCNU + VCR + PCZ	25	60
MeCCNU + VCR + PCZ	28	32
Total	649	43 ± 13[b]

[a] Including some cases with radiotherapy
[b] Anthmetic mean $\pm$ SD naturally weighted toward the larger study groups. After Walker [98]

effective against tumor tissues.

According to a National Institutes of Health (NIH) report, some 700 000 anti-cancer drugs have been screened since 1955 and about 30 drugs (0.04%) have been brought to clinical use. A number of these drugs have been used in GBM, and in a phase II study an initial response was found in 0%–88%, averaging some 43% [98] (Table 2.10). In GBM, nitrosoureas, cell cycle nonspecific agents, and polychemotherapy are thought appropriate because of penetration of the blood-brain barrier, the existence of anoxic cells, and the heterogeneity of tumor cells. It is noteworthy, however, that the MST following administration of nitrosourea drugs was 6.3 months, which was not significantly different from the MST using other drugs.

Although polychemotherapy is more effective than monochemotherapy, its effectiveness is in fact similar to that of S + R. Chemotherapeutic agents act not only on tumor tissue but also on normal brain tissue. So, in order to enhance the effect for tumor tissue, several chemotherapeutic agents should be used at the same time.

However, the results of clinical studies on polychemotherapy indicate that such enhancement has not yet been attained. The development of new drugs and new techniques for combined therapy is still needed. Moreover, important problems remain with regard to the suppression of side effects and the resistance to various drugs.

Although improvements over S + R and S + C have been small, the best results have been obtained in patients receiving S + R + C. It is noteworthy, however, that the MST of 11.6 months in S + R + C cases was less than the additive effect, since if radiotherapy and chemotherapy worked independently an additive effect of MST of 14.2 months would be expected.

With regard to differences in therapeutic results according to time, it was found that the survival time of the post-1975 cases was 3.7 months longer than that of the pre-1975 cases. In addition, the survival rate was somewhat higher over a period of 6 months to 3 years following therapy. The 5-year survival rates in both groups, however, were the same.

Despite the fact that CT scanning was introduced in 1972, hypoxic cell sensitizers in 1973, fast neutron therapy, BCNU, and CCNU in 1975, and other techniques since then, their effectiveness has been slight and has not produced the expected long-term improvements in the therapy of GBM.

As evident from the above description, various therapeutic methods have their merits, but each has its limitations and the need for new drugs and therapeutic methods is still great. Not only from the approach of clinical therapy, but also from the perspective of basic science, further study is still required to elucidate the biological characteristics of tumor tissue. Only when the nature of tumor growth is better understood will it become possible to develop theoretically sound therapeutic techniques.

Conclusions

A study of the MST in cases of GBM treated with various therapies has shown that surgery alone produces a prolongation of the MST of only 2 months in comparison with nonsurgical cases. The MST among cases treated with S + R, S + C, and S + R + C were 4.7, 2.4, and 7.0 months, respectively. However, prolongation of the MST following S + R + C had a lower than expected additive value. The longest survival times were found following S + R + C, but the effects decreased over several years after treatment and it can be concluded that S + R + C therapy is effective for a period of only about 2 years. In order to obtain further improvement in the clinical application, further study is required, not only regarding therapeutic techniques, but also regarding an understanding of the biological features of tumor tissue and tumor growth.

References

1. Aaronson H, Flanigan S, Mark J (1963) Chemotherapy of malignant brain tumors using regional perfusion: I. Technique and patient selection. Ann Surg 157: 394–399
2. Adams GE, Dische S, Fowler JF, Thomlinson RH (1976) Hypoxic cell sensitizers in radiotherapy. Lancet 7952: 186–188
3. Afra D, Kocsis B, Dobay J, Eckhardt S (1983) Combined radiotherapy and chemotherapy with dibromodulcitol and CCNU in the postoperative treatment of gliomas. J Neurosurg 59: 106–110
4. Anderson AP (1978) Postoperative irradiation of glioblastomas. Results in a randomized series. Acta Radiol Oncol 17: 475–484

5. Avellanosa AW, West CR, Tsukada Y, Higby DJ, Bakshis, Reese PA, Jennings E (1979) Chemotherapy of nonirradiated malignant gliomas. Phase II study of the combination of methyl-CCNU, vincristine, and procarbazine. Cancer 44: 839–846

6. Bailey P, Cushing H (1926) A classification of tumors of the glioma group. Lippincott, Philadelphia

7. Bailey P, Sosman MC, Van Dessel A (1928) Roentgen therapy of glioma of the brain. Am J Roentgenol Radium Ther 19: 203–264

8. Bloom HJG, Peckham MJ, Richardson AE, Alexander P,A, Payne PM (1973) Glioblastoma multiforme: A controlled trial to assess the value of specific active immunotherapy in patients treated by radical surgery and chemotherapy. Br J Cancer 27: 253–267

9. Bloom HJG (1982) Recent results and research concerning the treatment of intracranial tumors. In: Chang CH, Housepian EM (eds) Tumors of the central nervous system. Modern radiotherapy in multidisciplinary management. Masson New York, pp 225–248

10. Bouchard J, Peirce CB (1960) Radiation therapy in the management of neoplasms of the central nervous system, with a special note in regard to children: Twenty years' experience, 1939–1958. Am J Roentgenol Radium Ther Nucl Med 84: 610–627

11. Brisman R, Housepian EM, Chang C, Duffy P, Balis E (1976) Adjuvant nitrosourea therapy for glioblastoma. Arch Neurol 33: 745–750

12. Busch E (1963) Indication for surgery in glioblastomas. Clin Neurosurg 9: 1–17

13. Busch E, Christensen E (1947) The three types of glioblastoma. J Neurosurg 4: 200–220

14. Chang CH (1977) Hyperbaric oxygen and radiation therapy in the management of glioblastoma. Natl Cancer Inst Monogr 46: 163–169

15. Chang CH, Horton J, Schoenfeld D, Salazar O, Perez-Tamayo R, Kramer S, Weinstein A, Nelson JS, Tsukada Y (1983) Comparison of postoperative in the radiotherapy and combined postoperative radiotherapy and chemotherapy in the multidisiplinary management of malignant gliomas. A Joint Radiation Therapy Oncology Group and Eastern Cooperative Oncology Group Study. Cancer 52: 997–1007

16. Chin HW, Young AB, Maruyama Y (1981) Survival response of malignant gliomas to radiotherapy with or without BCNU or methyl-CCNU chemotherapy at the University of Kentucky Medical Center. Cancer Treat Rep 65: 45–51

17. Cianfriglia F, Pompili A, Riccio A, Grassi A (1980) CCNU-chemotherapy of hemispheric supratentorial glioblastoma multiforme. Cancer 45: 1289–1299

18. Concannon JP, Kramer S, Beny R (1960) The extent of intracranial gliomata at autopsy and its relationship to techniques used in radiation therapy of brain tumors. Am J Roentgenol Radium Ther Nucl Med 84: 99–107

19. Cooper JS, Borok TL, Ransohoff J, et al. (1982) Malignant glioma. Results of combined modality therapy. JAMA 248: 62–65

20. Davis L, Martin J, Goldstein SL, Ashkenazy M (1949) A study of 211 patients with verified glioblastoma multiforme. J Neurosurg 6: 33–44

21. Dean M, Newton K, Swann G (1964) Percutaneous intra-arterial chemotherapy in the treatment of intracranial neoplasms: A review of 36 cases. Bar J Radiol 40: 828–833

22. Douglas BG, Worth AJ (1982) Superfractionation in glioblastoma multiforme. Results of a phase II study. Int J Radiat Biol Phys 8: 1787–1794

23. Eagan RT, Childs DS, Layton DD, Laws ER, Bisel HF, Holbrook MA, Fleming TR (1979) Dianhydrogalactitol and radiation therapy. Treatment of supratentorial glioma. JAMA 241: 2046–2050

24. Earle KM, Rentscheer EH, Snodgrass SR (1957) Primary intracranial neoplasms. Prognosis and classification of 153 verified cases. J Neuropath Exp Neurol 16: 321–331

25. Edland RW, Javid M, Ansfield FJ (1971) Glioblastoma multiforme. An analysis of the results of postoperative radiotherapy alone versus radiotherapy and concomitant 5-fluorouracil. Am J Roentgenol Radium Ther Nucl Med 111: 337–342

26. EORTC Brain Tumor Group (1981) Evaluation of CCNU, VM-26 plus CCNU, and procarbazine in supratentorial brain gliomas. J Neurosurg 55: 27–31

27. EORTC (1983) Misonidazole in radiotherapy of supratentorial malignant brain gliomas in adult patients: A randomized double-blind study. Eur J Cancer Clin Oncol 19: 39–42
28. Frankel SA, German WJ (1958) Glioblastoma multiforme. Review of 219 cases with regard to natural history, pathology, diagnostic methods, and treatment. J Neurosurg 15: 489–503
29. Frei E (1982) The National Cancer Chemotherapy Program. Science 217: 600–606
30. Gerosa MA, Stefano ED, Olivi A (1981) VM-26 monochemotherapy trial in the treatment of recurrent supratentorial gliomas: Preliminary report. Surg Neurol 15: 128–134
31. Goldsmith MA (1974) Glioblastoma multiforme—a review of therapy. Cancer Treat Rep 1: 153–165
32. Green SB, Byar DP, Walker MD, Pistenmaa DA, Alexander E, Batzdorf U, Brooks WH, Hunt WE, Mealey J, Odom GL, Paoletti P, Ransohoff J, Robertson JT, Selker RG, Shapiro WR, Smith KR, Wilson CB, Strike TA (1983) Comparisons of carmustine, procarbazeine, and high-dose methylprednisolone as addition to surgery and radiotherapy for the treatment of malignant glioma. Cancer Treat Rep 67: 121–132
33. Greenberg HS, Ensminger WD, Seeger JF, Kindt GW, Chandler WF, Doan K, Dokhil SR (1981) Intra-arterial BCNU chemotherapy for the treatment malignant gliomas of the central nervous system: A preliminary report. Cancer Treat Rep 65: 803–810
34. Grunert V, Jellinger K, Sunder-Plassmann M (1973) Glioblastoma multiforme: A preliminary follow-up study. Mod Aspects Neurosurg 3: 108–115
35. Heiss WD (1978) Chemotherapy of malignant gliomas: Comparison of the effect of polychemo- and CCNU-therapy. Acta Neurochir 42: 109–115
36. Herskovic A, Ornitz RD, Shell M, Rogers CC (1982) Treatment experience. Glioblastoma multiforme treated with 15 MeV fast neutrons. Cancer 49: 2463–2485
37. Hitchcock E, Sato F (1964) Treatment of malignant gliomata. J Neurosurg 21: 497–505
38. Hochberg FH, Linggood R, Wolfson, Baker WK, Kornblith P (1979) Quality and duration of survival in glioblastoma multiforme. Combined surgical, radiation, and lomustine therapy. JAMA 241: 1016–1018
39. Hochberg FH, Pruitt A (1980) Assumptions in the radiotherapy of glioblastoma. Neurology 30: 907–991
40. Hochberg FH, Parker LM, Takvorian T, Canellos GP, Zervas NT (1981) High-dose BCNU with autologous bone marrow rescue for recurrent glioblastoma multiforme. J Neurosurg 54: 454–460
41. Hosobuchi Y, Phillips TL, Stupar TA, Gutin PH (1972) Interstitial brachytherapy of primary brain tumors. Preliminary report. J Neurosurg 53: 613–617
42. Hunt WE (1972) Surgical treatment of adult brain tumors. Pregr Exp Tumor Res 17: 400–407
43. Jacque C, Kujas M, Raoul M, Baumann N, Poisson M (1983) Valeur pronostique du dosage de la prótéine gliofibrillaire dans les gliomes malins traités par chimioet radiothérapie. Sem Hôp Paris 59: 464–467
44. Jelsma R, Bucy PC (1969) Glioblastoma multiforme. Arch Neurol 20: 161–171
45. Jelsma R, Bucy PC (1953) The treatment of glioblastoma multiforme of the brain. J Neurosurg 10: 423–429
46. Kahr E (1978) Megavoltage therapy of glioblastoma multiforme. Acta Neurochir 42: 79–87
47. Kennedy B, Brown J, Yarbo J (1965) Mithramycin (NSC-24559) therapy for primary glioblastomas. Cancer Chemother Rep 48: 59–63
48. Kernohan JW, Mabon RF, Svien HJ, Adson AW (1949) A simplified classification of the glioma. Proc Staff Meet Mayo Clin 24: 71–75
49. Laramore GE, Griffin TW, Gerdes AJ, Parker RG (1978) Fast neutron and mixed (neutron/photon) beam teletherapy for grade III and IV astrocytomas. Cancer 42: 96–103
50. Levin VA, Wilson CB, Davis R, Wara WM, Pisher TL, Irwim L (1979) A phase III comparison of BCNU, hydroxyurea, and radiation therapy to BCNU and radiation

therapy for treatment of primary malignant gliomas. J Neurosurg 51: 526–532

51. Luyendijk W, Beusekom G (1966) Chemotherapy of cerebral gliomas with intracarotid methotrexate-infusion. Acta Neurochir 15: 234–248

52. Mahaley M, Woodhall B (1967) Regional chemotherapeutic perfusion and infusion of brain and face tumors. Ann Surg 166: 266–277

53. Marsa GW, Goffinet DR, Pubinstein LJ, Bagshaw MA (1975) Megavoltage irradiation in the treatment of gliomas of the brain and spinal cord. Cancer 36: 1681–1689

54. Marshall LF, Jennett B, Langfitt TW (1974) Needle biopsy in the diagnosis of malignant glioma. JAMA 228: 1417–1418

55. Marshall LF, Langfitt TW (1977) Needle biopsy, high-dose corticosteroids, and radiotherapy in the treatment of malignant tumors. Natl Cancer Inst Monogr 46: 157–160

56. Matsukado Y, Maccarthy CS, Kernohan JW (1961) The growth of glioblastoma multiforme (astrocytomas, grade 3 and 4) in neurosurgical practice. J Neurosurg 18: 636–644

57. Mealey J (1962) Treatment of malignant cerebral astrocytomas by intraarterial infusion of vinblastine. Cancer Chemother Rep 20: 121–126

58. Moersch FP, Craig WM, Kernohan JW (1941) Tumors of the brain in aged persons. Arch Neurol Psychiat 45: 235–245

59. MRC (Medical Research Council) (1983) A study of the effect of misonidazole in conjunction with radiotherapy for the treatment of grade 3 and 4 astrocytomas. Br J Radiol 56: 678–682

60. Nelson DF, Schoenfeld D, Weinstein AS, Nelson JS, Wasserman T, Goodman RL, Carabell S (1983) A randomized comparison of misonidazole sensitized radiotherapy plus BCNU and radiotherapy plus BCNU for treatment of malignant glioma after surgery; preliminary results of an ROTG study. Int J Radiat Oncol Biol Phys 9: 1143–1151

61. Nelson JS, Schoenfeld D, Tsukada Y, (1982) Histologic criteria with prognostic significance for malignant glioma, In: Chang CH, Housepean EM (eds) Tumors of the central nervous system: Modern radiotherapy in multidisciplinary management. Masson New York, pp 1–4

62. Nelson JS, Tsukada Y, Schoenfeld D, Fulling K, Lamarche J, Peress N (1983) Necrosis as a prognostic criterion in malignant supratentorial, astrocytic gliomas. Cancer 52: 550–554

63. Netsky MG, August B, Fowler W (1950) The longevity of patients with glioblastoma multiforme. J Neurosurg 7: 261–269

64. Onoyama Y, Abe M, Takahashi M, Yabumoto E, Sakamoto T (1976) Radiation therapy in the treatment of glioblastoma. Amer J Roentgenol 126: 481–482

65. Owen G, Javid R, Belmusto L, et al. (1965) Intra-arterial vincristine therapy of primary gliomas. Cancer 18: 756–760

66. Owen G (1966) Infusion chemotherapy. New York J Med 66: 3026–3029

67. Paillas JE, Combalbert A (1964) Évolution compartée des gliomes du orveau. A propos d'une statistigue operatoire de 333 cas observés avec les mênes methodes durant une mêne decennie. Rev Neurol (Paris) 111: 43–60

68. Payne DG, Simpson WJ, Keen C, Platts ME (1982) Malignant astrocytoma. Hyperfractionated and standard radiotherapy with chemotherapy in a randomized prospective clinical trial. Cancer 50: 2301–2306

69. Poisson M, Pouillart P, Bataini JP, Mashaly R, Pertuiset BF, Metzger J (1979) Malignant gliomas treated after surgery by combination chemotherapy and delayed irraddiation: I. Analysis of results. Acta Neurochir 51: 15–25

70. Pouillart P, Mathé G, Poisson M, Buge A, Huguenin P, Gautier H, Morin P, Thy HTH, Lheritier J, Parrot R (1976) Essai de traitement des glioblastomes de I' adulte et des métastases cérébrales par I' association d' adriamycine, de VM-26 et de CCNU. Resultatus d' un essai de type II. Nouv Presse Méd 5: 1571–1575

71. Ransohoff J, Martin BE, Medrek TJ, Harris MN, Golomb FM, Wright JC (1965) Preliminary clinical study of mithramycin (NSC-24559) in primary tumors of the

central nervous system. Cancer Chemother Rep 49: 51–57

72. Reagan TJ, Bisel HF, Childs DS, Layton DD, Rhoton AL Jr, Taylor WF (1976) Controlled study of CCNU and radiation therapy in malignant astrocytoma. J Neurosurg 44: 186–190

73. Reeves GL, Marks JE (1979) Prognostic significance of lesion size for glioblastoma multiforme. Radiology 132: 469–471

74. Rosenblum ML, Gerosa M, Dougherty DV, Wilson CB (1982) Age-related chemosensitivity of stem cells from human malignant brain tumors. Lancet 8277: 885–887

75. Rosenblum ML, Reynolds AF, Smith KA, Rumack. BH, Walker MD (1973) Chloroethyl-cyclo-hexyl-nitrosourea (CCNU) in the treatment of malignant brain tumors. J Neurosurg 39: 306–314

76. Roth JG, Elvidge AR (1960) Glioblastoma multiforme: A clinical survey. J Neurosurg 17: 736–750

77. Sachs E (1954) The treatment of glioblastomas with radium. J. Neurosurg 7: 185–189

78. Salazar OM, Rubin P, McDonald JV, Feldstein ML (1976) Patterns of failure in intracranial astrocytomas after irradiation: Analysis of dose and field factors. AM J Roentgenol 126: 627–637

79. Salcman M (1980) Survival in glioblastoma: Historical perspective. Neurosurgery 7: 435–439

80. Salcman M, Kaplan RS, Montgomery E (1981) Influence of age on survival in glioblastoma patients after combined modality treatment. Neurosurgery 8: 491–492

81. Scanlon PW, Taylor WF (1979) Radiotherapy of intracranial astrocytomas: analysis of 417 cases treated from 1960 through 1969. Neurosurgery 5: 301–308

82. Seiler RW, Greiner RH, Zimmermann A, Markwalder H (1978) Radiotherapy combined with procarbazine, bleomycin, and CCNU in the treatment of high-grade supratentorial astrocytomas. J Neurosurg 48: 861–865

83. Seiler RW, Zimmermann A, Bleher E, Markwalder H (1979) Preoperative radiotherapy and chemotherapy in hypervascular, high-grade supratentorial astrocytomas. Surg Neurol 12: 131–133

84. Seiler RW, Zimmermann A, Markwalder H (1980) Adjuvant therapy with VM-26 and CCNU after operation and radiotherapy of high-grade supratentorial astrocytoma. Surg Neurol 13: 65–68

85. Shaw CM, Sumi M, Alvord EC, Gerdes AJ, Spence A, Parker RG (1978) Fast-neutron irradiation of glioblastoma multiforme. Neuropathological analysis. J Neurosurg 49: 1–12

86. Shehata WM, Meyer RL, Jazy FK (1983) Management of glioblastoma multiforme by irradiation and chemotherapy. Ilinois Med J 163: 30–34

87. Simpson WJ, Platts ME (1976) Fractionation study in the treatment of glioblastoma multiforme. Int J Radiat Oncol Biol Phys 1: 639–644

88. Stage WS, Stein JJ (1974) Treatment of malignant astrocytomas. Am J Roentgenol Radium Ther Nucl Med 120: 7–18

89. Takeuchi K, Hoshino K (1977) Statistical analysis of factors affecting survival after glioblastoma multiforme. Acta Neurochir 37: 57–73

90. Taveras JM, Thompson HG, Pool JL (1962) Should we treat glioblastoma multiforme? Am J Roentgenol Radium Ther Nucl Med 87: 473–479

91. Tönnis W, Walter W (1959) Das Glioblastoma multiforme. Acta Neurochir Supple 6: 40–62

92. Uihlein A, Colby MY, Layton DD, Parsons WR, Carter TL (1966) Comparison of surgery and surgery plus irradiation in the treatment of supratentorial gliomas. Acta Radiol [Ther] (Stockholm) 5: 67–78

93. Urtasun R, Band P, Chapman JD, Feldstein ML (1976) Radiation and high-dose metronidazole in supratentorial glioblastomas. N Engl J Med 294: 1364–1367

94. Urtasun R, Feldstein ML, Partington J, Tanasichuk H, Miller JDR, Russell DB, Agboola O, Mielke B (1982) Radiation and nitroimidazoles in supratentorial high grade gliomas: A second clinical trial. Br J Cancer 46: 101–108

95. Walker MD, Alexander E, Hunt WE, MacCarty CS, Mahaley MS Jr, Mealer J Jr, Norrell HA, Owens G, Ransohoff J, Wilson CB, Gehan EA, Strike TA (1978) Evaluation of BCNU and/or radiotherapy in the treatment of anaplastic gliomas. A cooperative clinical trial. J Neurosurg 49: 333–343

96. Walker MD, Alexander E, Hunt WE (1976) Evaluation of mithramycin in the treatment of anaplastic gliomas. J. Neurosurg 44: 655–667

97. Walker MD, Green SB, Byar DP, Alexander E, Batzderf U, Brooks WH, Hunt WE, MacCarty CS, Mahaley MS Jr, Mealer J Jr, Owens G, Ransohoff J II, Robertson JT, Shapiro WR, Smith K R Jr, Wilson CB, Strike TA (1980) Randomized comparisons of radiotherapy and nitrosoureas for the treatment of malignant gliomas after surgery. N Engl J Med 303: 1323–1329

98. Walker MD (1975) Malignant brain tumors. A synopsis. CA 25: 114–120

99. Wasserman TH, Stetz J, Phillips TL (1981) Radiation therapy oncology group clinical trials with misonidazole. Cancer 47: 2382–2390

100. Weir B (1973) The relative significance of factors affecting postoperative survival in astrocytomas, grade 3 and 4. J Neurosurg 38: 448–452

101. Weir B, Band P, Urtasun R, Blain G, McLean D, Wilson F, Mielke B, Grace M (1976) Radiotherapy and CCNU in the treatment of high-grade supratentorial astrocytomas. J Neurosurg 45: 129–134

102. West CR, Avellanosa AM, Barua NR, Patel A, Hong CI (1983) Intraarterial 1,3-bis(2-chloroethyl)-1-nitrosourea (BCNU) and systemic chemotherapy for malignant glioma: A follow-up study. Neurosurgery 13: 420–426

103. Wilson CB (1964) Chemotherapy of brain tumors by continuous arterial infusion. Surgery 55: 640–653

104. Young B, Old Field EH, Markesbery WR, Haack D, Tibbs RA, McCombs P, Chin HW, Maruyama Y, Meacham WF (1981) Reoperation for glioblastoma. J Neurosurg 55: 917–921

105. Zülch KJ (1980) Principles of the new World Health Organization (WHO) classification of brain tumors. Neuroradiology 19: 59–66

Part II
Basic Studies

Chapter 3

Combined Effects of Radiation, ACNU, and 5-FU on Gliomas: An Experimental Combination Therapy

S. Mashiyama, S. Sugiyama, K. Kuwahara, M. Kitahara,
K. Takahashi, and T. Sasaki

Introduction

Although surgical removal of the tumor is essential for the treatment of malignant glioma, radiotherapy and chemotherapy have also played important roles in recent years. Improvements in therapeutic results obtained by means of combined therapies continue to be reported [50, 55, 56, 60, 85, 98, 99, 101], but there is a need for further experimental research. We consequently undertook several basic studies on the effectiveness of radiotherapy, 1-(4-amino-2-methyl-5-pyrimidinyl)methyl-3-(2-chloroethyl)-3-nitrosourea hydrochloride (ACNU), and 5-fluorouracil (5-FU) either alone or in various combinations and report these results in the present chapter. The possibilities for clinical application of the biological results are also discussed.

Background and Purpose of Experiments

There have been a large number of in vitro, in vivo, and clinical investigations on the effectiveness of combined radio- and chemotherapy in malignant gliomas, and it is well known that while the effectiveness of such therapy on the tumor tissue increases there are simultaneously increases in the damage to normal tissues. Clinically, it is not so rare that the treatment must be discontinued due to side effects, such as myelosuppression or damage to gastrointestinal tissues. Moreover, nitrosourea drugs, which are widely used against malignant brain tumors, are known to be particularly powerful myelosuppressants [1], which limits their usage. It has also been reported that drug-resistant cells may emerge following repeated doses and this is also a significant problem in their therapeutic use.

As a consequence, it is important to study means for enhancing the effectiveness of radiotherapy or chemotherapy and to find more effective means for their combined use. Of special importance in this regard is the need for selective effectiveness for the tumor tissue, while leaving normal tissue relatively unaffected.

The effects of radiotherapy and chemotherapy on brain tumor cells have been analyzed primarily using exponentially growing cells. It is well known, however, that in monolayer cells, many of the characteristics of in vivo solid tumors are absent, including the heterogeneity of cell kinetics, the presence of quiescent and hypoxic cells, the effects of intercellular contact, and the heterogenous nature of the intratumoral pH and nutrient supply. As a result, the effects of chemo- or radio-therapy, which are strongly influenced by these factors, cannot be accurately studied within the framework of an experimental design using monolayer cells. It must be considered that these factors may have influence on the recovery of cells from the damage brought about by radio- or chemothrapy. In contrast, in experiments using in vivo tumor preparations, factors such as the tumor- host relationship and individual differences among hosts greatly hinder the analysis of results. In order to bridge this gap between solid tumors and cultured monolayer cells, it is necessary to use an experimental model which combines some of the in vivo characteristics of solid tumors with the advantages of cultured tumor cell preparations in vitro.

The purpose of the experiments reported here was to clarify the cellular mechanisms of the action of radiation, ACNU, and 5-FU on in vivo gliomas using multicellular spheroids of glioma cells as an experimental tumor model in vitro and to study more refined methods of combination therapy for improving clinical results. Further, some of the results obtained from spheroids were confirmed using subcutaneously transplanted rat gliomas.

Materials and Methods

Monolayer Cultures and Formation of Multicellular Spheroids

The tumor cell lines used were rat glioma cells (RG C-6) [7, 8], induced by N-nitroso-methylurea, and glioblastoma cells (GB A-7) [30], isolated from a human glioblastoma. The cells were maintained in Eagle's Minimum Essential Medium (MEM) Earle's solution containing all essential and nonessential amino acids and 1 mM sodium pyruvate and supplemented with 10% fetal calf serum at 37°C in an atmosphere of 5% CO_2 and 95% air.

The spheroids were constructed as follows: 0.5% Noble Agar (Difco Co. Detroit, USA) containing Eagle's MEM Earle's solution with 10% fetal calf serum was placed on a plastic Petri dish (A/S Nunc, Inc., Roskilde, Denmark, 90 mm diameter). After 10-min quiescence and formation of a gel, it was washed once with the culture medium and 10 ml culture solution, containing 1×10^6 GB A-7 cells or 5×10^5 RG C-6 cells, was placed on the agar surface.

After 24 h, the cell aggregates which had formed were transferred to a 100-ml spinner bottle (Bellco Inc., Vineland, NJ) and a spinner culture was done at 150–200 rpm using a magnetic stirrer (Bellco Inc.) in a CO_2 gas incubator. The culture medium was renewed every other day for the first 6 days of the cultures, and daily thereafter [117].

RG C-6 cell spheroids of 500- to 600-μm diameter and with a central necrosis on the 10th day of the culture were used in the experiments. Similarly, GB A-7 cell shperoids, 450–550 μm diameter, with a necrosis on the 21st day of the culture were used. The volume of the spheroids was calculated from the long (a) and short (b) radii of about 50 spheroids obtained from the spinner bottle every 24 h, using the following formula:

$$V = (4/3) \pi ab^2$$

In the experiments for monolayer cells, the RG C-6 cells were used in their exponential phase, whereas the GB A-7 cells were used in both exponential and plateau phases. Growth curves were obtained from the number of viable cells hourly after placing approximately 10^5 exponential growing cells in a 60-mm Petri dish.

Surviving Fraction of Cells

An appropriate number of spheroids were washed with 0.1% trypsin and incubated for 10–20 min at 37.°C in a 0.1% trypsin solution containing 0.04% Versene. After adding an equal volume of culture medium containing 10% serum, the cells were dispersed using a pipette. In this way, a single cell suspension was obtained. The monolayer cells were similarly dispersed. Unless otherwise stated, the cells from both the spheroids and the monolayer were treated in this way immediately following X-irradiation, 5-FU, or ACNU treatment.

Viable cells, which were not stained with an erythrosine-B solution [73], were counted using an improved Neubauer's hemocytometer. After appropriate dilution, the cells were cultured in 60- or 90-mm petri dishes for 12 days in the case of the RG C-6 cells, or for 16 days in the case of the GB A-7 cells. After staining, the number of colonies of more than 50 intact cells were counted [24] and the surviving fraction was calculated using a colony-forming efficiency of the control group as 100%.

For analysis of the survival curves, the multitarget, single-hit model was used. That is, the surviving fraction was expressed as a function of the radiation dose (D) or the drug concentration (C) [115]:

$$SF = 1 - (1 - e^{-D/D_0 \text{ or } -C/C_0})^n$$

$$D_q \text{ or } C_q = D_0 \ln n \text{ or } C_0 \ln n$$

where SF is the surviving fraction, D the radiation dose, C the drug concentration, and D_q and C_q the quasi-threshold doses obtained by extrapolating from the high-dosage linear portion of the respective curves back to the abscissa where the surviving fraction is 1.0.

The cell-survival curve for cells in spheroids treated with 5-FU showed a biphasic exponential function. This curve was characterized with $_1C_0$ and $_2C_0$, which are the concentrations to reduce the surviving fraction to e^{-1} in each sensitive and resistant cell fraction, respectively.

Autoradiography

Spheroids and monolayer cells cultured on cover glasses were incubated for 1 h in a culture medium containing 2 μCi/ml of [^{3}H-methyl]-thymidine (6.7 Ci/mmol, New England Nuclear Co., USA). After washing three times in ice-cold phosphate buffered salt solution (PBS), they were then fixed in buffered 10% formalin, and the spheroids were embedded in paraffin. After preparing 5 μm-thick sections, the acid-soluble fraction was removed with ice-cold 0.3 N perchloric acid (PCA) and autoradiography was done using the dipping method and a Sakura-NR-M$_2$ emulsion (Konishiroku Co.).

The autoradiograms were developed and stained with hematoxylin-eosin after 30 days' exposure. Following removal of the acid-soluble fraction, autoradiography for monolayer cells was directly performed on a cover glass. Cells containing more than four silver grains were evaluated as labeled cells.

X-Irradiation

For irradiation of the RG C-6 cells, 2 ml of a single-cell suspension obtained from the monolayer cells (culture solution with 10 mM Hepes buffer added) was placed in a 5-ml cryotube (A/S Nunc, Inc.) and irradiated at 37°C with the cryotube in a horizontal position. The GB A-7 cells were irradiated in petri dishes in a culture medium containing 10 mM Hepes buffer.

The RG C-6 spheroids were irradiated at 37°C in polystyrene vials with a bottom surface area of 7.0 cm^2, which contained 5 ml culture medium with 10 mM Hepes buffer. The single-cell suspension obtained from the spheroids was irradiated in a similar fashion. The GB A-7 spheroids were irradiated as follows. The spheroids were transferred to a 100-ml spinner bottle (Bellco Inc.) and after 24 h were irradiated at a constant temperature of 37°C on a magnetic stirrer.

The X-ray equipment was a Shimazu Deep Therapy X-Ray Apparatus (SHT 250M-3), which was operated at 250 kV and 20 mA, with a 0.3-mm Cu and 1-mm Al filter and a focal surface distance (FSD) of 50 cm. The dose rate was 1.05 Gy/min.

Treatment with ACNU and 5-FU

A 25-mg potency of Nimustin hydrochloride (ACNU) or a 50-mg potency of 5-FU was dissolved in 10 ml physiological saline and then diluted with culture medium containing 10% fetal calf serum. The monolayer cells were treated in a culture medium containing these drugs and the spheroids were treated in a similar manner on an agar surface in a Petri dish. After washing three times with Dulbecco's PBS, cells were trypsinized to make a single-cell suspension and plated for colony assay.

Control Probability of Spheroids

Spheroids of similar size using either RG C-6 or GB A-7 cells were X-irradiated at 37°C in a spinner flask. About 20–30 spheroids per dish were directly plated on a Petri dish and incubated for about 3 weeks to determine the spheroid survival. The number of spheroids plated was counted 1 day after plating when the spheroids firmly adhered to the plastic surface. Surviving spheroids were counted as those with an outgrowth of surviving cells on the plastic surface during incubation. The control probability of spheroids was calculated as the ratio of the number of spheroids plated minus those that survived.

Experiments on Subcutaneously Transplanted Rat Gliomas

RG C-6 cells (2 × 10^6 cells) maintained as a monolayer culture were subcutaneously transplanted into both the axillary and inguinal regions of 4-week-old Wistar rats (85–100 g body weight). Ten days after the transplantation, tumors (7–11 mm in diameter) were used for the experiments.

X-irradiation. Irradiation was carried out either on live rats or on dead animals killed by ether 5 min prior to irradiation; the X-rays irradiation (250 kV, 20 mA, filter 0.5-mm Cu and 1.0-mm Al, FSD 60 cm) was given at a dose rate of 0.63 Gy/min. The absorbed dose of the tumor tissue was determined by a subcutaneously transplanted thermoluminescence dosimeter (BeO) (UD-170L, Matsushita Industrial Equipment Co. Ltd., Osaka, Japan) and the thermoluminescence was read with a thermoluminescence dosimetry reader (UD-512p, Matsushita Industrial Equipment Co. Ltd., Osaka, Japan).

Drug injection. Both ACNU and 5-FU were dissolved in physiological saline and 0.2 ml was injected intraperitoneally.

Assay for cell survival. Tumor tissue removed from the surrounding connective tissue was minced with two razor blades. After washing with culture medium and 0.1% trypsin, the minced tumor tissue was incubated with 3 ml of 0.1% trypsin containing 0.04% Versene for 15 min at 37°C in a shaking water bath. An equal volume of 0.001% deoxyribonuclease I from bovine pancreas (Sigma Chemical Co., St. Louis, Mo., USA) solution was added to the tissue in Dulbecco's PBS and then incubated further for 1 min. After vigorous pipetting, the suspension was allowed to stand for 3 min and the supernatant was removed. This procedure was repeated three times. Second and third fractions of cells released from the tumor tissue were pipetted to make a single-cell suspension and the cells were collected by centrifugation. Viable cells unstained with erythrosine-B solution were counted with an improved Neubauer hemocytometer. Colony forming efficiency of the cells was measured by a soft-agar assay [18]. Namely, a cell suspension previously diluted to an appropriate concentration in 0.3% Noble agar (Difco) containing 10% FBS was plated onto a 0.5% agar layer containing 10% FBS in a Petri dish (60 mm diameter). After 21 days of incubation in a CO_2 incubator, colonies larger than 0.2 mm in diameter were counted under a dissecting microscope. The surviving fraction of cells was expressed as the mean and the standard error of three tumors.

Results

Structure and Growth of Spheroids: Validity of Experimental Model

Due to the limited supply of oxygen and nutrients to the tumor cells in solid tumor tissue, those which are located close to blood vessels actively proliferate, whereas those located further away receive a weaker supply and often show necrosis. Tumors can consequently be considered as having a basic cord structure centering around blood vessels—what Thomlinson and Gray termed a "tumor cord structure" [106]. Hypoxic cells, thought to be located near the necrotic zone, are known to be relatively radio-resistant [77, 94, 103] and drugs administered via the blood vessels are, therefore, thought not to penetrate to such regions. These factors are believed to be important in the treatment of tumors.

The autoradiography of the RG C-6 spheroids (diameter 500–600 μm) following ^{3}H-thymidine labeling on the 10th day of culture indicated that the cells were labeled only in the external four to five layers from the surface and were not labeled in the layers close to the center of the spheroids. When PCA treatment was not done, silver grains were also seen in the necrotic region. The labeling index was found to be 40% over the external five layers and 5.6% over the inner layers, giving a mean labeling index of 9.1% for the cells obtained from the entire spheroids. The labeling of monolayer cells in the exponential phase was found to be 50.8%.

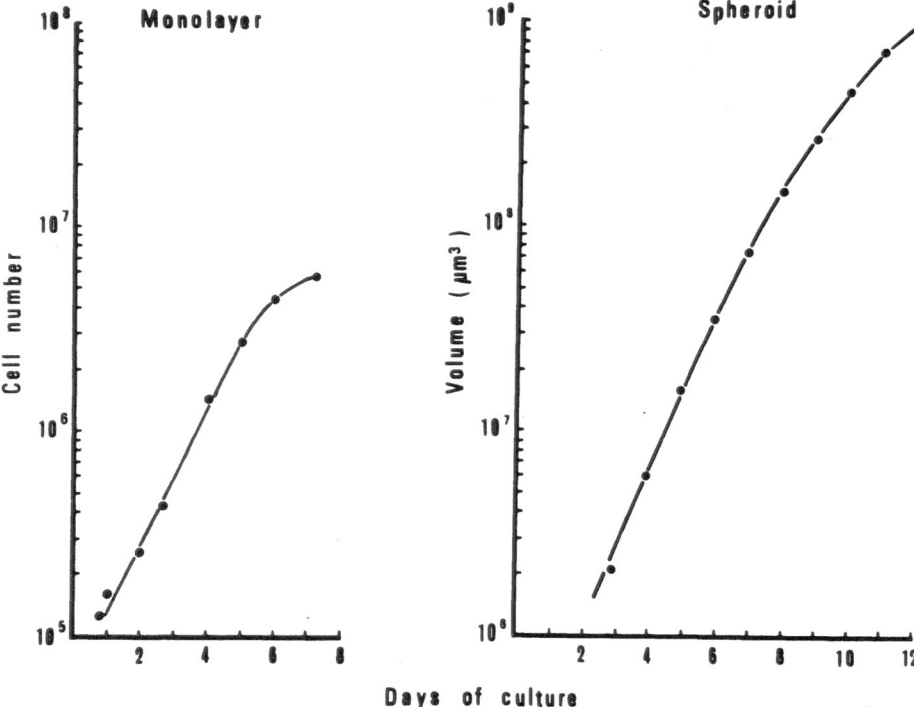

Fig. 3.1. Growth curve of RG C-6 cells in the number of cells per dish grown as monolayer and in spheroid volume versus days of culture

Hoshino [38] reported that the labeling index in human malignant gliomas was 5%–10% for glioblastomas and less than 1% for astrocytomas. Moreover, Sasaki et al. [82] reported that the labeling index for human gliomas averaged 3.6%, which was significantly lower than the 6.9% found in all solid malignant tumors. The labeling index for in vivo solid tumors has been found [79] to be closely related to the growth fraction, which is calculated as the ratio of proliferating cells (P) to the sum of P cells and quiescent cells (Q).

The growth curves for the spheroids and the monolayer cells using RG C-6 and GB A-7 cells are shown in Figs. 3.1 and 3.2 respectively. In both cell lines, the exponential phase for the monolayer cells continued over the first 120 h of the culture, after which a plateau was reached. The doubling time (Td) in the exponential phase was found to be 22 h for the RG C-6 and 28 h for the GB A-7 cells. The volume of the spheroids increased exponentially during the early stages of the culture but increased more slowly thereafter. The Td of the RG C-6 spheroids was about 24 h during the early stages and about 37 h after 10 days of cultivation. The Td of the GB A-7 spheroids was also 24 h during the early stages, but increased gradually to more than 50 h after the 8th day of culture.

In the growth curve for the spheroids, a larger Td than that for the monolayer cells in exponential growth was found. This suggests that even in the early phase of

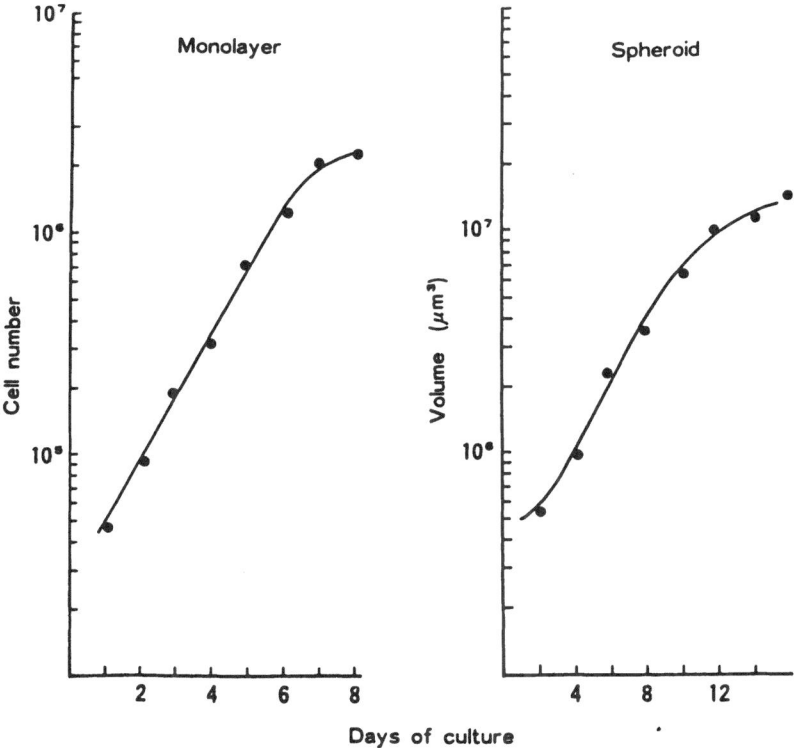

Fig. 3.2. Growth curve of GB A-7 cells in the number of cells per dish grown as monolayer and in spheroid volume versus days of culture

growth the rate of cellular proliferation in the spheroids is less than unified. Together with increases in the number of days of cultivation, the cell loss factor in the region of the central necrosis became larger, and as a result the Td for the spheroid volume was increased. These growth curves closely resemble those found for many animal tumor tissues [89]. Durand [21] reported that the growth fraction for spheroids of V-79 cells was 0.93 on the 1st day of culture, but 0.39 on the 25th day. Sasaki and Sakka [81] and Sasaki et al. [82] analyzed 700 human cases of solid tumors and found that the main difference in the Td of the various histological types was due to differences in the growth fraction.

In light of the above findings, we conclude that while the spheroids are in fact an in vitro tumor model, as cellular aggregates of similar size, they display the fundamental characteristics of in vivo solid tumors and at the same time do not involve the many difficulties associated with the tumor-host relationship and individual differences among hosts [40, 41, 84, 95]. As a consequence, this model has several technical and theoretical advantages not found in monolayer cultures and is, therefore, thought suitable as an experimental solid glioma model [92]. Spheroids of GB A-7 cells and their histological appearance are shown in Figs. 3.3 and 3.4.

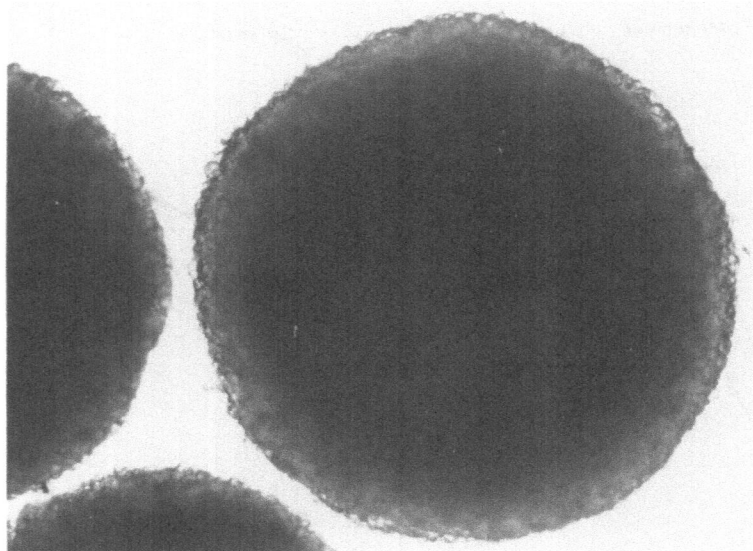

Fig. 3.3. Phase-microscopic view of the multicellular spheroids of GB A-7 cells

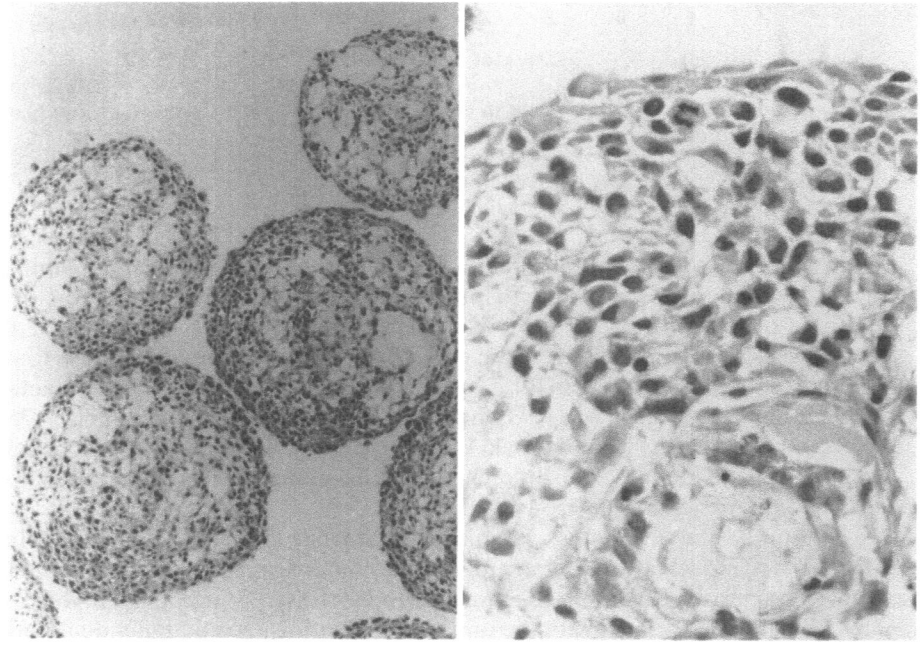

Fig. 3.4a, b. Histological findings of multicellular spheroid of GB A-7 cells

Effects of X-Irradiation

Dose-Survival Curves

RG C-6 cells. The X-ray dose-survival curves are shown in Fig. 3.5 and the related parameters (D_0, D_q, and n) for each survival curve are listed in Table 3.1. The survival curve for cells from X-irradiated spheroids showed the greatest radioresistance. Above 10 Gy, a biphasic curve was seen and the inverse value of the final slope (D_0) was 4.31 Gy. Moreover, in the survival curve when the cell suspension from the spheroids was irradiated, the radio-resistant fractin disappeared, resulting in $D_0 = 1.45$ Gy, $D_q = 3.85$ Gy, and $n = 14.3$. Since it is thought that the cells in suspension from the spheroids remained virtually unchanged in the distribution of the cells in the cell cycle after trypsin treatment, the large D_0 in the spheroid cell population is considered not to be due to the cell cycle phase distribution but to the

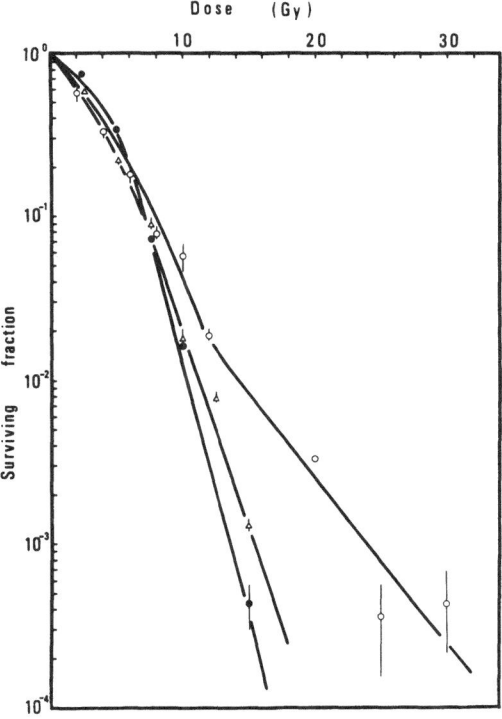

Fig. 3.5. The X-ray dose-survival curves for exponentially growing monolayer cells (△), cells in large spheroids (○), and cells in single-cell suspension from the same batch of spheroids (●). RG C-6

Table 3.1. Parameters of the dose survival curve of RG C-6 cells for X-rays

	D_0 (Gy)	D_q (Gy)	n	D_0 ratio
Large spheroids	4.31		0.3	2.9
Single cells from large spheroids	1.45	3.85	14.3	1.0
Exponentially growing cells	1.84	3.0	5.1	

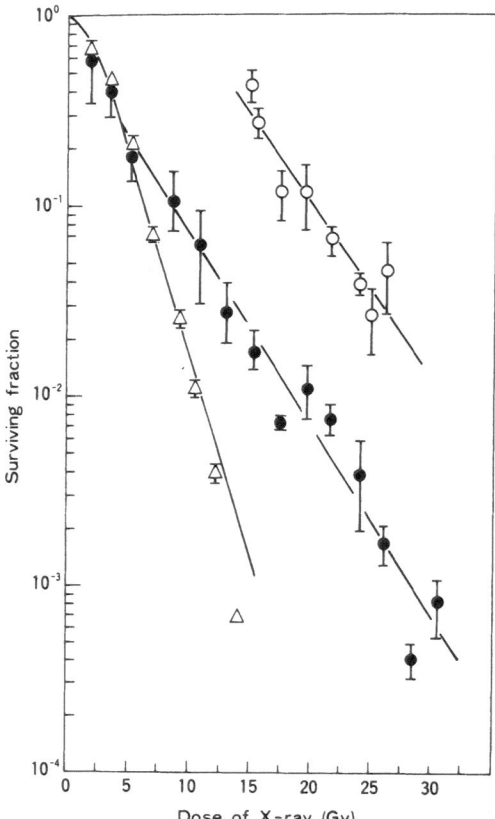

Fig. 3.6. Dose-survival curves of subcutaneously transplanted RG C-6 cells. ● live rat, ○ fully anoxic condition (dead rat), △ cell suspension from the same transplanted tumor

microenvironment around the cells when they were in the spheroids in situ.

The D_0 value for the spheroids was threefold greater than that for the fully oxygenated cell suspension—the ratio of the D_0 values similar to that previously reported for the oxygen enhancement ratio [76].

In light of the above findings, we conclude that the cells near the necrotic region within the large RG C-6 spheroids irradiated in a plastic vial were hypoxic. Moreover, since such cells have the capacity for colony formation (regeneration), the presence of hypoxic cells must be considered when undertaking radiotherapy. It should be noted that although studies on the survival curve following the irradiation of spheroids (from 9-L stock cultured rat glioma cells) have not indicated the presence of hypoxic cells [19], other studies using 9-L rat glioma have shown the presence of such cells when experimental subcutaneous tumors were used [63].

In order to confirm the presence of hypoxic cells in glioma in vivo, subcutaneously transplanted rat gliomas of RG C-6 cells were also X-irradiated. Cell survival immediately after X-irradiation was measured by the soft-agar assay, as described above. The results shown in Fig. 3.6 indicate that an apparent radioresistant cell fraction was present in tumors irradiated in live rats. The final portion of the curve was almost parallel to that of the curve obtained from tumors made fully anoxic in previously killed rats. The evidence of a two-component survival curve in tumors

Table 3.2. Survival parameters for RG C-6 cells in subcutaneously transplanted rat gliomas immediately after X-irradiation

	D_0 (Gy)	D_q (Gy)	n	OER
Tumors irradiated in live rats	4.28	—	0.76	2.15
Tumors irradiated in ether-killed rats	4.73	9.32	7.16	2.38
Cell suspension	1.99	1.89	2.58	1.0

OER oxygen enhancement ratio, expressed as D_0 ratio

Table 3.3. Parameters of the dose-survival curves of GB A-7 cells for X-rays alone and X-ray irradiation after ACNU administration

	D_0 (Gy)	D_q (Gy)	n
Exponentially growing cells			
X-ray alone	1.6	2.2	4.0
X-ray + ACNU	1.1	2.3	8.1
Plateau phase cells			
X-ray alone	1.2	2.6	8.7
X-ray + ACNU	1.1	2.2	7.4

from live rats indicates that there is a significant fraction of hypoxic cells in glioma in vivo. The hypoxic cell fraction was estimated as the ratio of the surviving fraction of tumors and was 7.0%–7.3% at 15–20 Gy. The single-cell suspension obtained from unirradiated tumors was irradiated in a petri dish and the cell survival curve is also shown in Fig. 3.6. The survival curve for the cells in suspension was identical to the sensitive component at the dose below 5 Gy of the survival curve obtained from tumors irradiated in live rats. Since the cells in suspension are fully oxygenated, the oxygen enhancement ratio (OER) was calculated as the isoeffect dose ratio in the survival curve of the cell suspension to that of fully anoxic tumors. The OER was 3.03 at the surviving fraction of 0.05 and 2.38 as the final D_0 ratio. The parameters of these survival curves from in vivo glioma are summarized in Table 3.2.

GB A-7 cells. The survival curves following irradiation of GB A-7 cells in both exponential and plateau phases are shown in Fig. 3.7 and the respective parameters (D_0, D_q, and n) are shown in Table 3.3. Although similar surviving fractions were seen for both the exponential and plateau phase cells, which had been trypsinized and dispersed immediately following irradiation, in the plateau phase cells, there was an increase in the survival when 6 or 24 h elapsed between the time of cell dispersion and the irradiation. This is interpreted as being due to the recovery from potentially lethal damage (PLD) incurred in the plateau phase cells. Such PLD recovery was not seen in the exponential phase cells.

The X-ray dose-survival curves for the large and small spheroids are shown in Fig. 3.8. The sensitivity of small spheroids to the radiation was similar to that of the monolayer cells, but radiation doses only up to 16 Gy were used for large spheroids, so that a curve with a inflection point such as that found for the spheroids of RG C-6 cells was not obtained. The surviving fraction increased when the spheroids were dispersed 24 h after irradiation for both the small and large spheroids, indicating that there was some recovery from potentially lethal damage.

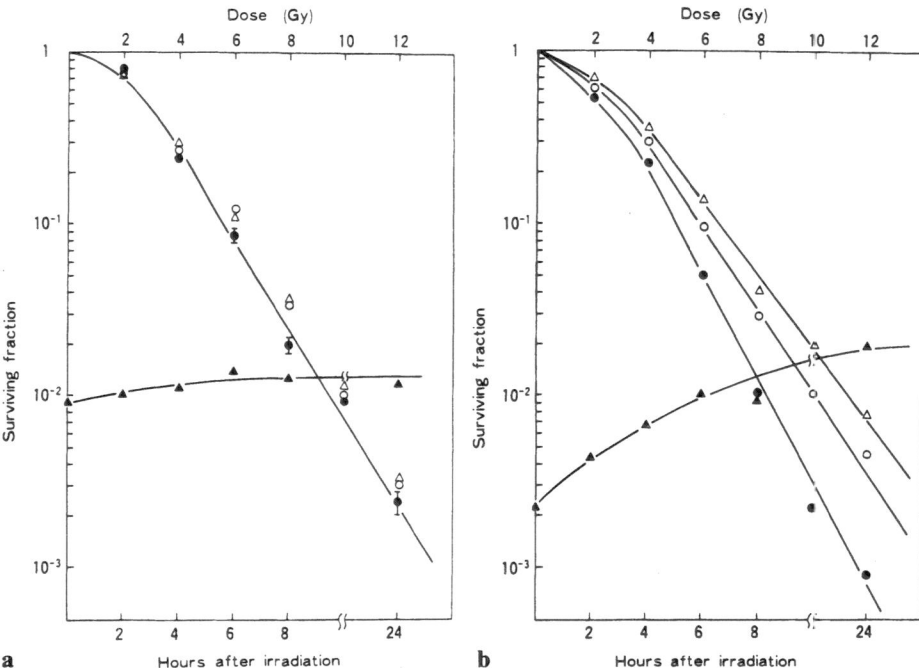

Fig. 3.7a, b. X-ray dose-survival curves 0 (●), 6 (○), 24 (△) h after irradiation, and the time-survival curve (▲) after irradiation of 10 Gy. **a** GB A-7, exponential phase. **b** GB A-7, plateau phase

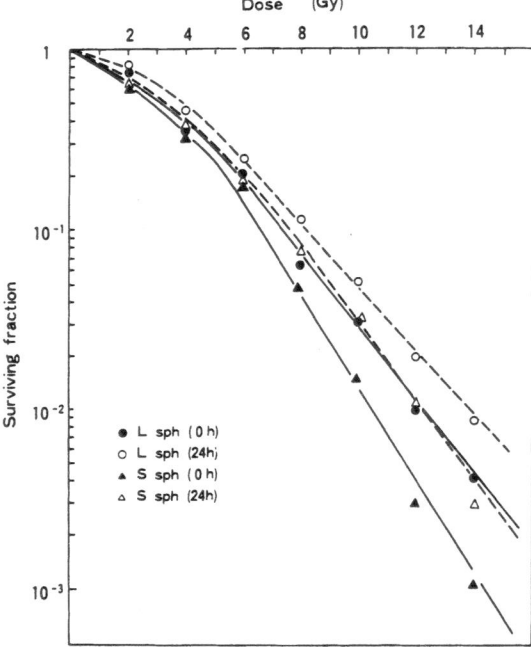

Fig. 3.8. Dose-survival curves of GB A-7 cells in small (▲, △) and large (●, ○) spheroids immediately or 24 h after X-irradiation

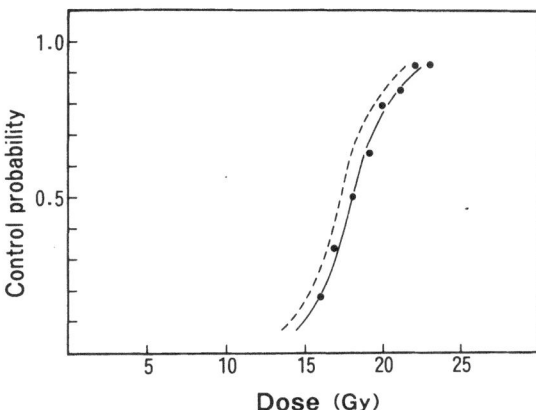

Fig. 3.9. Control probability of small spheroids as a function of dose. The *broken line* indicates the probability expected from cell-survival curve 24 h after X-irradiation; the *solid line* shows the observed findings. GB A-7

Dose-Control Probability of Spheroids

The control probability curve for irradiated small spheroids of GB A-7 cells (diameter about 200 μm), which were plated directly onto a petri dish without cell dispersion, is shown in Fig. 3.9. When the dose was large enough compared with the D_0 value, the relationship between the cell-surviving fraction (SF) and the dose (D) with parameters of D_0 and n (calculated from the survival curve for the spheroid cells in the same batch) could be approximated as:

$$SF = n \cdot e^{-D/D_0}$$

The expected value, $CD_{0.5(exp)}$, of the dose at which 50% control probability of the spheroids was expected from the cell-survival curve can be expressed as:

$$CD_{0.5(exp)} = -D_0 \cdot \ln(-\ln 0.5/N_0 \cdot E \cdot n)$$

where N_0 = cells/spheroid and E is the plating efficiency.

The expected control probability curve based upon this formula is shown as a broken line in Fig. 3.10. The experimentally observed control probability curves for spheroids of both the GB A-7 and RG C-6 (data not shown) cells were almost identical to those expected from cell-survival curves. The mean $CD_{0.5} \pm$ SD from seven experiments was 17.9 $\pm$ 1.2 Gy and the corresponding $CD_{0.5(exp)}$ expected from cell-survival curves was 16.7 $\pm$ 2.2 Gy. Since the expected value, $CD_{0.5(exp)}$, is based upon data obtained after PLD recovery, it is thought that no further PLD recovery would have occurred in the spheroids in situ 24 h after irradiation.

Effects of ACNU

The lipid-soluble nitrosourea anticancer drug ACNU is already in clinical use and its effectiveness is under clinical evaluation [61, 62]. The principal action of ACNU is known to be the alkylation of DNA and the carbamoylation of proteins, but it has also been reported to damage DNA-protein complexes, break DNA strands into smaller molecules, and to inhibit DNA and RNA synthesis [36, 42, 67]. When stored under ice-cold, 4°C dark conditions, ACNU is virtually 100% stable for at least 24 h, but it has been found to lose about 50% of its activity after about 20 min when

S. Mashiyama, et al.

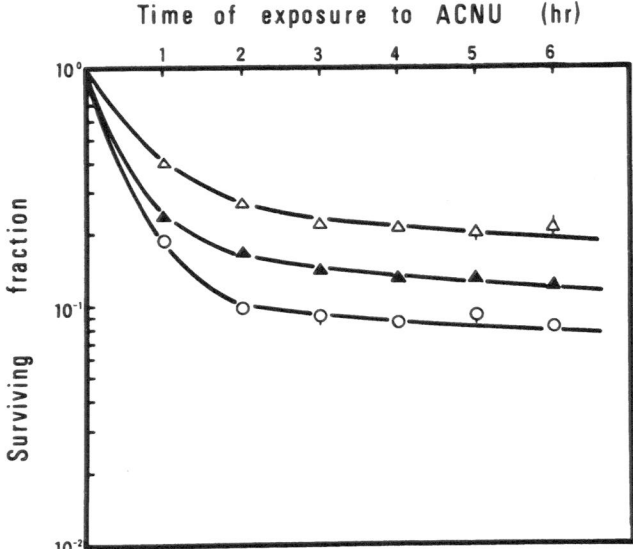

Fig. 3.10. Time-survival curves for cells grown as a monolayer without trypsinization after ACNU treatment (△), grown as a monolayer trypsinized after ACNU treatment (▲), and grown in spheroids (○). The duration of ACNU treatment (40 μg/ml) is shown in the *abscissa.* RG C-6

kept at 37°C and pH 7.4 [66]. When kept at a pH of below about 6.0 [65], however, it is relatively stable. ACNU was dissolved in distilled water immediately prior to use and stored in a light-shielded contaminer at 0°C during the experiment.

Time-Survival Curves

Experiments were done using the RG C-6 cells. Comparisons were made between the spheroids and monolayer cells. Monolayer cells were either trypsinized after ACNU treatment or were plated 6 h before and then treated with ACNU without trypsinization. The final concentration of ACNU was fixed at 40 μg/ml and the cell-surviving fraction was obtained hourly for 6 h.

The results are shown in Fig. 3.10. In all three curves, there was a marked decrease in survival 2 h after treatment, after which there was a gentle exponential decrease. The effectiveness of ACNU was greatest for the spheroids, followed by the mono-layer cells treated with ACNU and then trypsinized. It was smallest for the mono-layer cells treated with ACNU but without trypsinization.

Concentration-Survival Curves

The RG C-6 cells were treated for 2 h at various final ACNU concentrations up to 100 μg/ml, whereas the GB A-7 cells were treated for 2 h at final concentrations up to 10.0 μg/ml.

RG C-6 Cells. The various survival curves are shown in Fig. 3.11 and the related parameters (C_0, C_q, and n) are listed in Table 3.4. All the curves can be seen to have

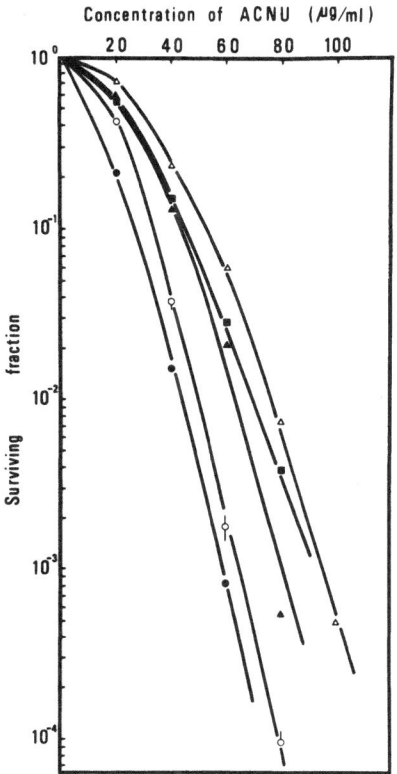

Concentration of ACNU ($\mu g/ml$)

Fig. 3.11. Survival curves for cells grown as monolayer without trypsinization after ACNU treatment ($\triangle$), for cells grown as monolayer trypsinized after ACNU treatment ($\blacktriangle$), in large spheroids (o), in small spheroids ($\blacksquare$), in a single-cell suspension from large spheroids ($\bullet$). All cells were treated with a graded concentration of ACNU for 2 h. RG C-6

Table 3.4. Parameters of survival curves of RG C-6 cells after ACNU treatment

	C_0 ($\mu g/ml$)	C_q ($\mu g/ml$)	n
Large spheroids with necrosis	6.8	17.6	13.6
Small spheroids without necrosis	10.9	19.9	6.3
Single cells from large spheroids	6.7	12.1	6.2
Exponentially growing cells trypsinized after ACNU	7.3	27.2	41.6
Exponentially growing cells without trypsinization	8.4	37.2	84.5

shoulders at low concentrations, while at higher concentrations there were exponential decreases. The C_q value for the spheroids was smaller than that for the monolayer cells, indicating that the effect of ACNU was greater in the spheroids. When the cells dispersed from the spheroids were treated with ACNU immediately following trypsinization, the effect was only marginally greater than that for the spheroids in situ. The effects of ACNU for spheroids without a central necrosis were smaller than those for large spheroids with a central necrosis. In monolayer cells, it was found that the effect was larger after the ACNU treatment when trypsinization was done than when it was not done, but it was smaller than with the spheroids.

One reason for the greater effects in the spheroids with a necrotic layer is that the pH within the necrotic layer is low, thereby leading to greater stability of the ACNU itself. In studies where direct measurements of in vivo tumor pH have been made, values between 5.8 and 7.2 have been reported [111]. Moreover, in spheroids made of human glioma cells, it has been reported that the pH is low and dependent upon the glucose concentration in the culture solution [1].

Since the growth fraction of cells has been reported to correlate with the labeling index by ^{3}H-thymidine and the doubling time [81, 82], the nonproliferating Q-cell fraction (the majority of which became quiescent in the G_1 phase) was considered largest in the large spheroids, followed by the small spheroids, and smallest in the monolayer cells in the exponential phase.

Using cultured mouse L cells in the exponential phase, Asamura et al. [4] reported that the cells most sensitive to ACNU were those between the G_1 and S phases. In flow cytometric studies of the DNA distribution in glioma 9L cell spheroids, it has also been found that a majority of the cells have DNA in the G_1 phase [19], the majority of which are thought to be quiescent. Therefore, the fact that the effect of ACNU was greater in the spheroids with a necrotic layer may be due in part to a difference in the number of Q cells. In fact, even when the cells dispersed from the spheroids were treated with ACNU, the effectiveness of the ACNU was greater than that in the monolayer cells, indicating that the cells comprising the large spheroids were intrinsically more sensitive to the ACNU.

A survival curve for cells in subcutaneously transplanted RG C-6 cell gliomas was also obtained 2 h after ACNU injection and the results are shown in Fig. 3.12. The survival parameters of $C_0 = 17$ mg/kg and $C_q = 11$ mg/kg are comparable with those obtained from large spheroids. The evidence indicates that there was no significant fraction of cells in these gliomas in vivo which was resistant to ACNU.

GB A-7 cells. The survival curves of the GB A-7 cells are shown in Fig. 3.13 and the related parameters are shown in Table 3.5. The sensitivity of these cells to ACNU was much greater than that of the RG C-6 cells. The C_0 value for the RG C-6 cells in the exponential phase was 8.4 μg/ml, whereas it was 1.4 for the GB A-7 cells. Moreover, there were no increases in survival even when the GB A-7 cells were dispersed with trypsin after 6 or 24 h, regardless of whether they were in the exponential or plateau phase. This finding indicates that there was no PLD recovery such as that observed in the X-ray experiments.

It was also found that the plateau phase cells were more sensitive to the ACNU than the exponential phase cells, but this is thought to be due to the presence of Q cells. Moreover, it has been reported that among CHO cells, those in the plateau phase are more sensitive to BCNU than those in the exponential phase [6, 107].

Effects of 5-FU

The effects of 5-FU were analyzed using RG C-6 monolayer cells and spheroids.

Time-survival curves. In the monolayer cells, when cells were either trypsinized or not following 5-FU (5 μg/ml) administration, a decrease in survival was observed for 5-FU treatment longer than about 12 h (Fig. 3.14). The effect was particularly large when trypsinization was done after 5-FU treatment, suggesting the occurrence

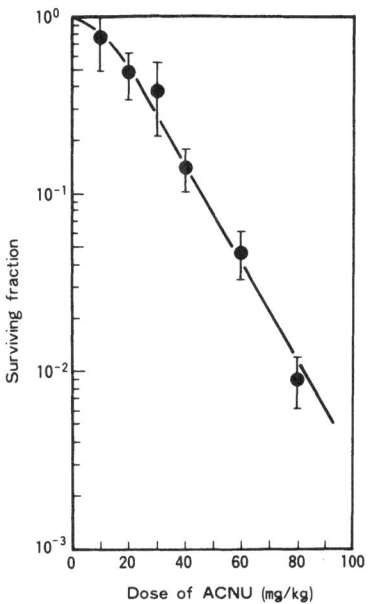

Fig. 3.12. Concentration-survival curve of subcutaneously transplanted RG C-6 cells for ACNU

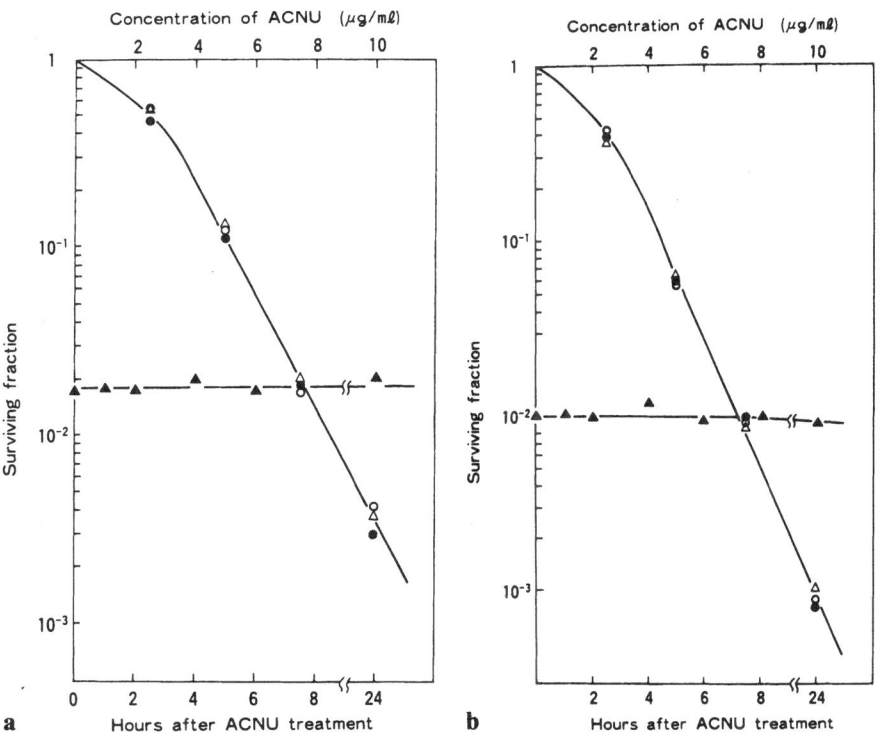

Fig. 3.13a, b. Cell survival and time-survival curves after treatment with ACNU. **a** GB A-7, exponential phase. **b** GB A-7, plateau phase

Table 3.5. Parameters of survival curves of GB A-7 cells for ACNU alone and ACNU administration before X-ray irradiation

	C_0 (μg/ml)	C_q (μg/ml)	n
Exponentially growing cells			
ACNU alone	1.4	2.2	4.8
ACNU + X-ray	0.95	2.5	13.9
Plateau phase cells			
ACNU alone	1.2	2.3	6.8
ACNU + X-ray	1.0	2.3	10.0

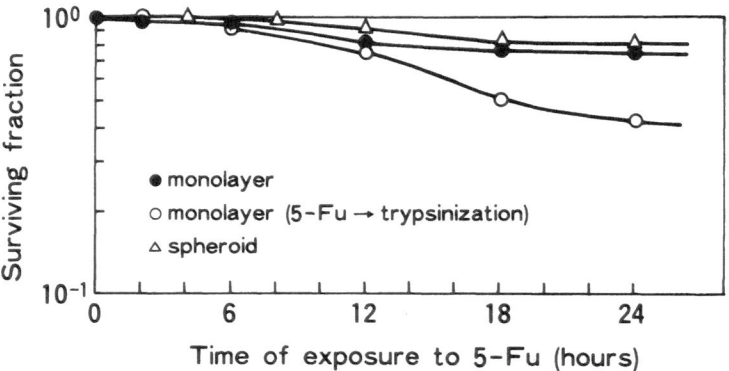

Fig. 3.14. Time-survival curves for 5-FU (5 μg/ml)

of PLD recovery following administration. In the spheroids, a gradual decrease in survival occurred after 12 h of 5-FU (5 μg/ml) treatment.

Dose-survival curves. In the monolayer cells, a small shoulder in the dose-survival curve was found, and with increasing concentrations there was an exponential decrease in cell survival (Fig. 3.15). Here the C_0 value was 7.45 μg/ml and the C_q value was 12.1 μg/ml.

In the spheroids, a biphasic curve without a shoulder was obtained. That is, when the concentration of 5-FU was below 50 μg/ml, the slope [$_1C_0 = 14.5$ μg/ml] was relatively steep, whereas above 50 μg/ml it [$_2C_0 = 124$ μg/ml] was gentle.

It is known that the rate of diffusion of 5-FU into glioma spheroids is rapid, with a homogenous distribution being reached within 15 min [69]. The biphasic survival curve is thus thought to reflect the presence of 5-FU-resistant cells. The fraction of 5-FU-resistant cells, the resistant fraction (RF), is expressed as the surviving fraction obtained by extrapolating back from the slope of the second phase to the ordinate; it was 0.8, indicating that about 80% of the cells were resistant to 5-FU.

Biphasic survival curves were also obtained from subcutaneously transplanted RG C-6 cell gliomas [33]. In this experiment, rats bearing gliomas were killed at either 2, 6, or 24 h after 5-FU injection. Cell-survival curves for cells from these gliomas are shown in Fig. 3.16. The effects of 5-FU increased with time after injection from 2 to 6 h, but decreased at 24 h. The increase in the surviving fraction

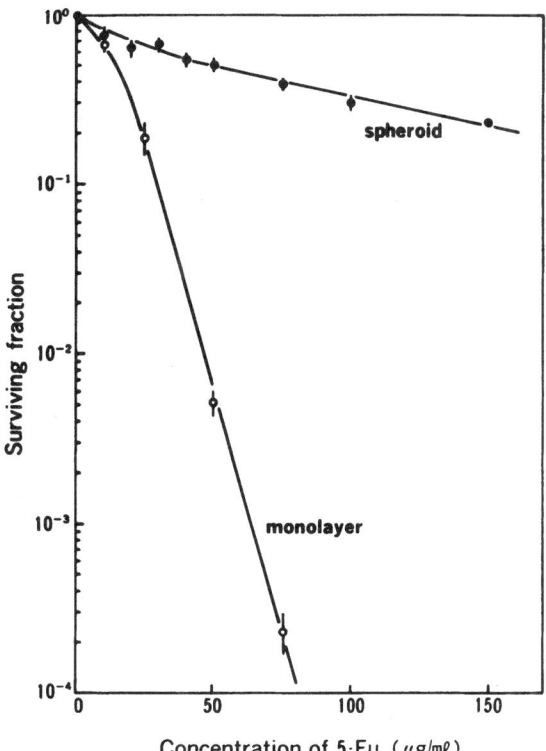

Fig. 3.15. Dose-survival curves of RG C-6 cells for 5-FU

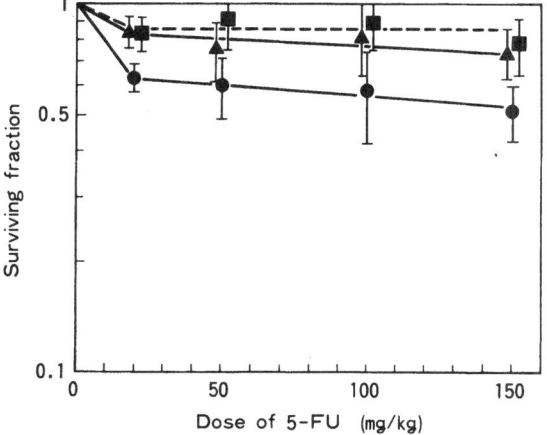

Fig. 3.16. Concentration-survival curves of subcutaneously transplanted RG C-6 cells. The cells were treated with 5-FU for 2 h (■), 6h (●), and 24 h (▲)

is considered to have been due to recovery from 5-FU-induced PLD, as described below. The inflection point in the curve was at about 20 mg/kg, which was comparable with that obtained in the survival curve for cells in large spheroids expressed as 5 µg/ml.

Effects of Combined X-Ray and ACNU Treatment

Timing of Combinations

RG C-6 cells.

Monolayer cells. The relationship between the surviving fraction and the interval between X-irradiation and ACNU administration is shown in Fig. 3.17. The abscissa shows the time interval between the addition of the ACNU and irradiation; the duration of the ACNU treatment was 2 h in all cases. When irradiation was done 2–24 h after the start of ACNU treatment, the surviving fraction was significantly lower than the additive range, i.e., the surviving fraction expected from simple addition of the independent activities of irradiation and ACNU. The largest effect was found when the irradiation was done 4–12 h after ACNU treatment. Significant improvements beyond the additive range were not found when ACNU was administered at the same time as or after irradiation.

Spheroids. The results using cell spheroids are illustrated in Fig. 3.18. Significant effects beyond the additive range were obtained when ACNU was administered simultaneously or prior to X-irradiation, whereas the effects were in the additive range when the ACNU was administered 4 h or more after irradiation. The greatest

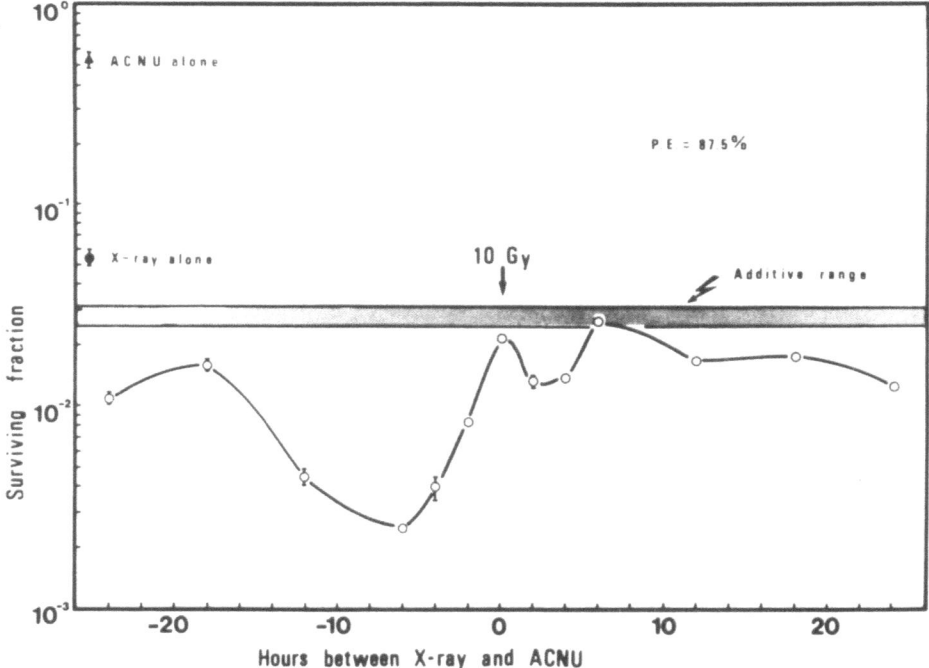

Fig. 3.17. Effects of ACNU (20 μg/ml) combined with 10-Gy X-irradiation on RG C-6 cells in monolayer. The surviving fraction is plotted versus the time interval between X-irradiation and the addition of ACNU to the medium

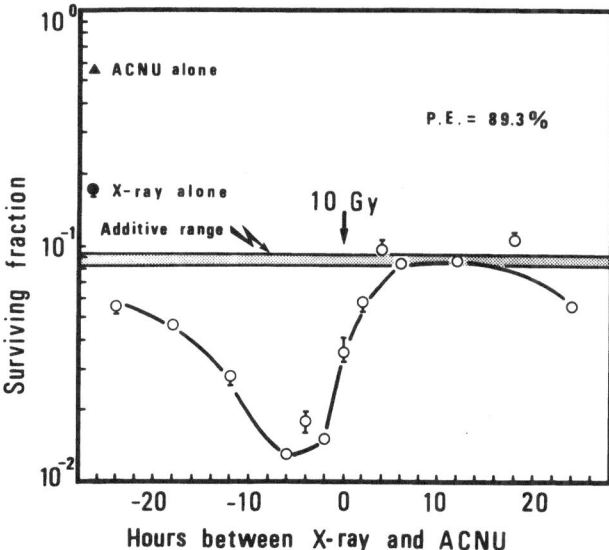

Fig. 3.18. Effects of ACNU (20 μg/ml) combined with 10-Gy X-irradiation on RG C-6 cells in spheroids. The surviving fraction was plotted versus the time interval between X-irradiation and the addition of ACNU to the medium

combined effects were obtained when the ACNU was administered 2–6 h prior to the X-rays.

GB A-7 cells

Monolayer cells in exponential phase. The results on the interval between X-rays and ACNU treatment are shown in Fig. 3.19. A pattern similar to that in the RG C-6 cells was seen. The lowest surviving fraction was found when ACNU was added to the culture medium 2–8 h prior to irradiation.

Monolayer cells in plateau phase. The results on the cells in the plateau phase are shown in Fig. 3.20. Effects greater than the additive range were obtained when the ACNU was given at the same time or prior to irradiation. When the ACNU was given 4 h or more after radiotherapy, the surviving fraction was in the additive range. The strongest combined effects were obtained when the ACNU was given 1–4 h prior to irradiation.

The fact that simultaneous treatment with a large dose of ACNU and a large dose of irradiation in both the RG C-6 and GB A-7 monolayer cells in the exponential phase did not show effects beyond the expected additive range is thought to indicate that the simultaneous combined use of X-rays and ACNU produces essentially additive effects. It is noteworthy, however, that effects greater than the expected additive range were obtained even for the simultaneous combined use of these treatments for the large spheroids of the RG C-6 cells and the GB A-7 cells in the plateau phase. These facts clearly indicate that the presence of a necrotic layer of cells or Q cells has a significant influence on the effectiveness of the combined therapy.

S. Mashiyama, et al.

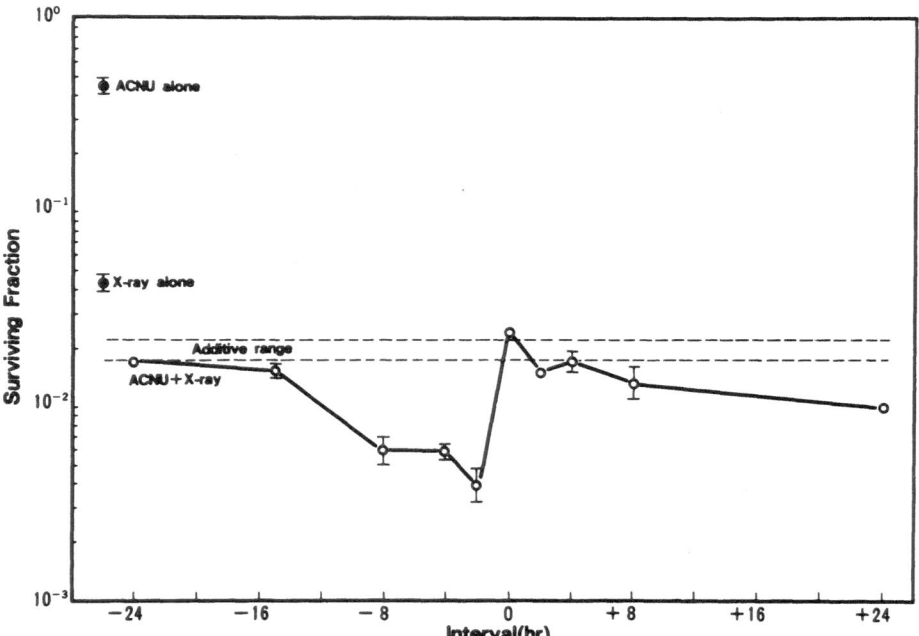

Fig. 3.19. Effects of ACNU (3 μg/ml) combined with 10-Gy X-irradiation on GB A-7 cells in monolayer, exponential phase

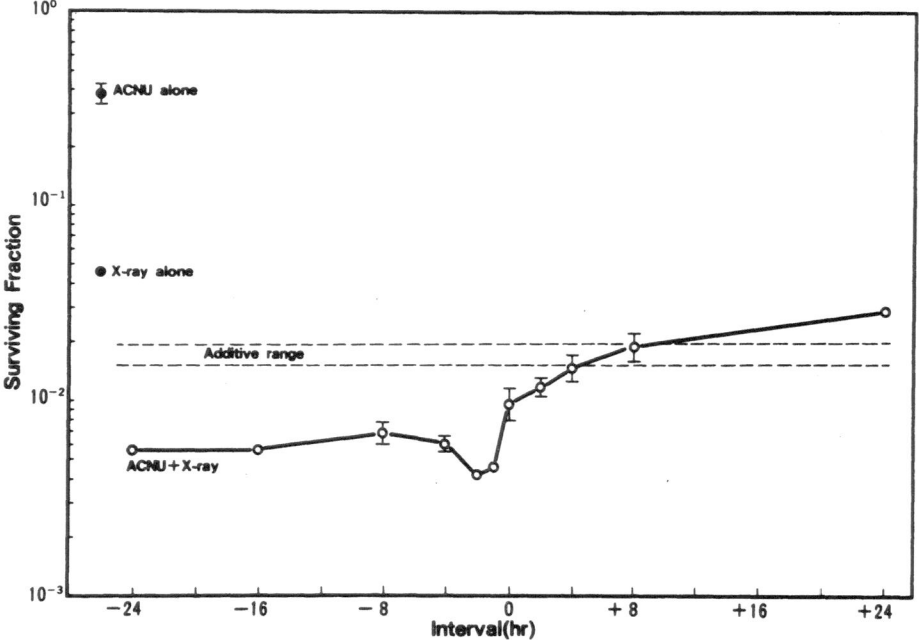

Fig. 3.20. Effects of ACNU (3 μg/ml) combined with 10-Gy X-irradiation on GB A-7 cells in monolayer, plateau phase

Kanazawa and Miyamoto [42] reported that there was a marked prolongation of the G_2 phase when G_1 phase HeLa S3 cells were treated with ACNU; 10 h were required to cause the G_2 accumulation. In addition using RG C-6 cells, Takakura et al. [100] and Shitara et al. (87) found that 30% were in the G_2-M phase within 24 h, whereas 47.2% were in that phase after 72 h. Although it is true that the time when G_2 accumulation occurs due to partial synchronization differs according to the generation time of the particular cell line, we believe that a similar phenomenon was observed in our experiments with RG C-6 and GB A-7 cells.

Nevertheless, it does not suffice to argue that the X-irradiation effects in the early period following ACNU treatment were due solely to accumulation of G_2-M phase cells. Leenhouts and Chakwick [54] reported that there was additive interaction between X-rays and BCNU or CCNU at the DNA level. Namely, if there are double-strand breaks in cellular DNA due to X-irradiation, the cell will die, but if there is only a single-strand break, the cell will survive. As a consequence, when a single-strand break due to BCNU or CCNU and one due to X-rays are brought about on an identical complementary DNA molecule, the cell will be killed. They also reported that the strongest synergistic effects were obtained when BCNU was given 5 h before irradiation or when CCNU was given 1 h before irradiation.

In an experiment by Kaneko et al. [44] using rats, it was found that if ACNU was given 1 h before irradiation, there was longer survival of the animals. In our experiments as well, we found that the most effective timing of irradiation was within several hours of the start of the ACNU treatment, regardless of whether the cells were monolayer cells in the exponential or plateau plase or were spheroids.

X-Ray Dose-Survival Curves Combined with ACNU

RG C-6 cells

Monolayer cells. The dose survival curve for the monolayer cells receiving irradiation only and that for the cells receiving irradiation 2 h after administration of ACNU are shown in Fig. 3.21. The related parameters are shown in Table 3.6. Due to the combined treatment with X-rays and ACNU, the D_0 was reduced to $1/1.7$ ($P < 0.05$), and when the dose of irradiation was large the effects were beyond those of the additive range. It is possible that one of the reasons why the D_0 value was smaller is that the ACNU brings about a partial synchronization of the cells and the cells in the G_2 phase had increased sensitivity to X-rays. Again, however, the accumulation of G_2 phase cells alone is not sufficient to explain the increased X-ray sensitivity in the relatively early period following ACNU treatment. The interaction of ACNU and X-rays discussed above must also be considered.

Table 3.6. Parameters of the dose-survival curves of RG C-6 cells in the monolayer for X-rays alone and ACNU administration after X-ray irradiation

	D_0 (Gy)	D_q (Gy)	n
X-ray alone	2.0	2.7	3.8
X-ray + ACNU	1.2	3.4	17.8

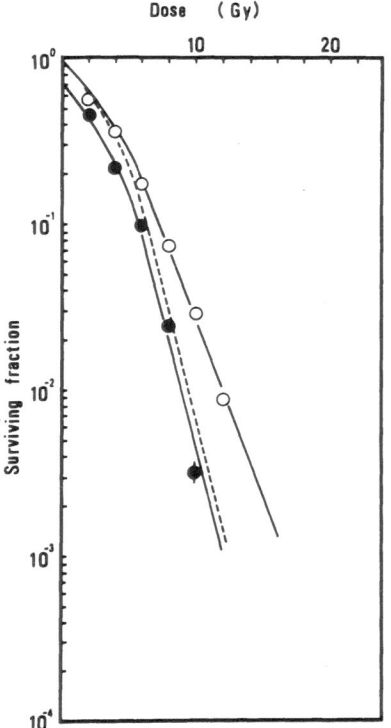

Dose (Gy)

Fig. 3.21. Dose-survival curves for RG C-6 cells in monolayer treated by X-rays alone (○) and ACNU prior to X-irradiation (●). The *broken line* represents the curve of combined treatment when the surviving fraction by ACNU alone is normalized to 1.0

Spheroids. Figure 3.22 shows the dose-survival curve for three conditions: (a) spheroids treated with X-rays alone, (b) spheroids treated with X-rays after ACNU administration, and (c) cells from the spheroids in single-cell suspension treated with X-rays alone. When X-ray treatment alone was done, there was a change in the slope of the curve at about 10 Gy and the final D_0 was 4.3 Gy. When ACNU pretreatment was also employed, however, the X-ray resistant portion above 10 Gy disappeared. The results are similar to those obtained when the cell suspension from the spheroids was treated with X-rays. A comparison of the various survival parameters is shown in Table 3.7, where it can be seen that the D_0 value with combined ACNU treatment had significantly decreased ($P < 0.001$). The broken line in Fig. 3.19 is the survival curve of combined treatment when the surviving fraction for ACNU treatment alone is normalized to 1.0. Therapeutic effects greater than the expected additive effects were obtained for all radiation doses greater than 2 Gy, with the effects being larger when the X-ray dose was increased.

The biphasic survival curve for the spheroids, obtained when only X-irradiation was done, lost its characteristic biphasic nature due to ACNU pretreatment and the D_0 value was similar to that obtained when the (fully oxygenated) single-cell suspension from the spheroids was treated only with irradiation. This is thought to indicate that there was a reduction in the hypoxic fraction that is X-ray resistant as a result of ACNU administration. In this regard, it is of interest that Wharam et al. [113] also found that BCNU treatment 2 h before irradiation eliminates the biphasic

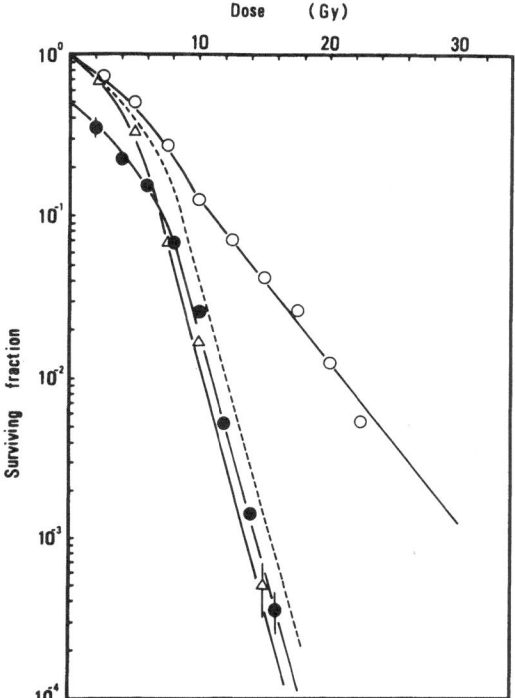

Fig. 3.22. Dose-survival curves for RG C-6 cells in spheroids treated by X-rays alone (o) or X-rays after ACNU administration (•) and for cells in single-cell suspension from the spheroids treated by X-rays alone (△). The *broken line* represents the curve of combined treatment when the surviving fraction by ACNU alone is normalized to 1.0

Table 3.7. Parameters of dose-survival curves of RG C-6 cells of large spheroids for X-rays

	D_0 (Gy)	D_q (Gy)	n
Large spheroids	1.5	5.3	35.1
Single cells from large spheroids	1.5	3.9	14.3

survival curve seen when only X-irradiation was given to EMT-6 mouse tumor cells; the number hypoxic cells is likewise decreased.

GB A-7 cells

Monolayer cells in exponential phase. The dose-survival curves when irradiation was given 2 h after the start of ACNU treatment and when X-rays alone were used are shown in Fig. 3.23. Related parameters are shown in Table 3.3. Following the combined therapy with ACNU and X-rays, the D_0 value was reduced to 1/1.5 ($P < 0.05$). When a large X-ray dose was used, effects slightly greater than the additive range were obtained—a tendency similar to that seen with the RG C-6 cells.

Monolayer cells in the plateau phase. Figure 3.24 shows the dose-survival curves for cells treated with X-rays alone and those treated with ACNU, followed 2 h later by X-irradiation. Related parameters are shown in Table 3.3. A slight decrease in the

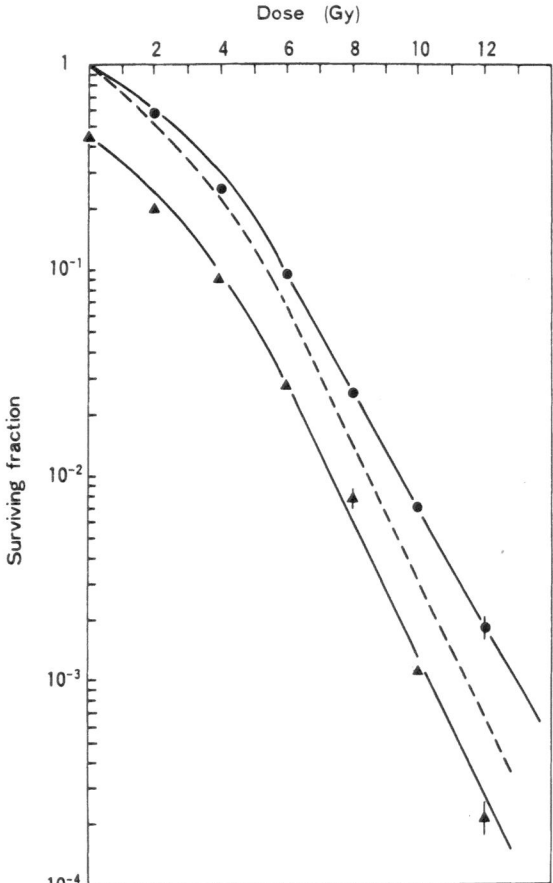

Fig. 3.23. Dose-survival curves for exponentially growing GB A-7 cells in monolayer treated by X-rays alone (●) or ACNU prior to X-irradiation (▲). The *broken line* represents the curve of combined treatment when the surviving fraction by ACNU alone is normalized to 1.0

D_0 value was seen due to the combined therapy, but this was not statistically significant and needs to be confirmed.

ACNU Concentration-Survival Curves Combined with X-Rays

RG C-6 cells

Monolayer cells. The concentration-survival curves for ACNU treatment alone and various doses of ACNU followed 2 h later by X-irradiation are shown in Fig. 3.25. All of the curves are seen to have shoulders and, at higher concentrations of ACNU, to have a surviving fraction which decreased exponentially. The parameters for the various curves are shown in Table 3.8. The C_0 value showed little change with the addition of X-ray treatment, but the C_q values decreased by half. The combined effect was more than additive for all concentrations of ACNU. This effect of the X-ray treatment is thought to be due to an apparent decrease in the accumulation capacity of sublethal damage (SLD) to cells caused by the ACNU.

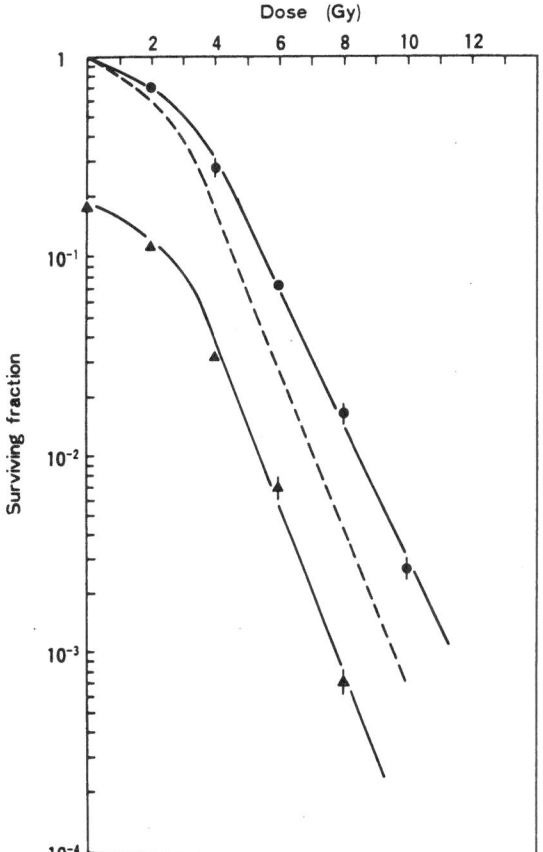

Fig. 3.24. Dose-survival curves for GB A-7 cells in the plateau phase. *Symbols* are the same as in Fig. 3.23

Spheroids. The concentration-survival curves are shown in Fig. 3.26 and the related parameters in Table 3.9. Both the C_0 and the C_q values were found to decrease ($P < 0.01$) when combined therapy with 10 Gy irradiation was done. A large effect beyond the expected additive range was found over the entire range of ACNU concentrations when 10 Gy irradiation was used.

In order to determine whether or not the combined therapy with ACNU in spheroids was in fact supra-additive, analysis was made following the isobologram method advocated by Steel [90] and Steel and Pekham [91]. That is, based upon the results of combined treatment with X-rays and ACNU in doses required to obtain isoeffects, a combination of more than 10 Gy X-rays with 16–19 μg/ml ACNU showed supra-additive effects for the isoeffect level of the surviving fraction of 10^{-2}. For the isoeffect level of the surviving fraction of 10^{-3}, a combination of X-rays with 18–27 μg/ml ACNU showed supra-additive effects.

GB A-7 cells

Figures 3.27 and 3.28 show the concentration-survival curve for, respectively, exponential and plateau phase cells which were treated with ACNU alone or various

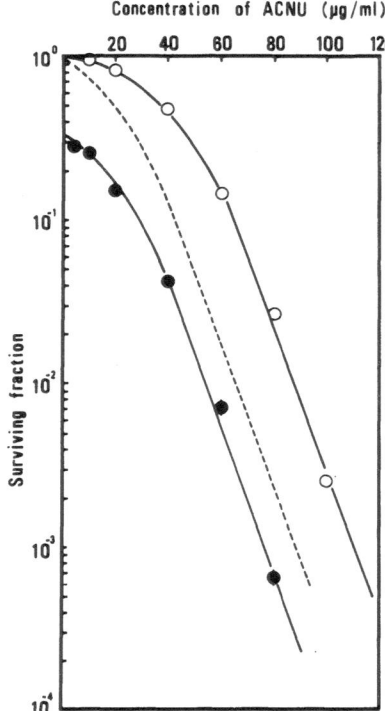

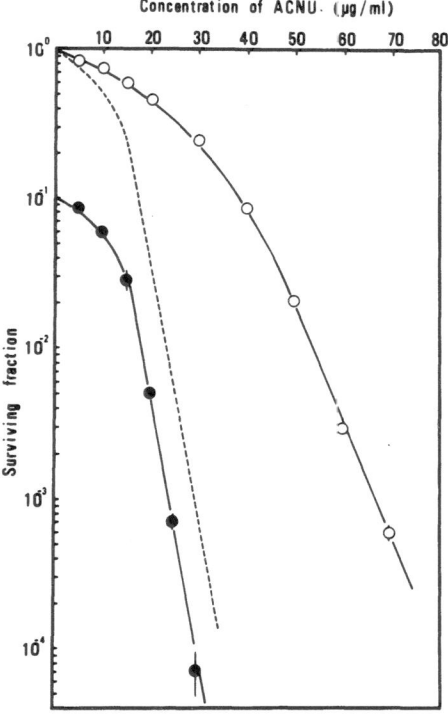

Fig. 3.25. Concentration-survival curves for RG C-6 cells in monolayer treated by ACNU alone (o) or X-rays after ACNU administration (●). The *broken line* represents the curve of combined treatment when the surviving fraction by X-rays alone is normalized to 1.0

Fig. 3.26. Concentration-survival curves for RG C-6 cells in spheroids treated by ACNU alone (o) or X-rays after ACNU administration (●). The *broken line* represents the curve of combined treatment when the surviving fraction by X-rays alone is normalized to 1.0

Table 3.8. Parameters of the survival curves of RG C-6 cells in monolayer for ACNU

	C_0 (μg/ml)	C_q (μg/ml)	n
ACNU alone	9.9	42.2	71.8
ACNU + X-ray	9.6	20.9	8.8

Table 3.9. Parameters of the survival curves of RG C-6 cells in spheroids for ACNU

	C_0 (μg/ml)	C_q (μg/ml)	n
ACNU alone	5.6	27.9	144.6
ACNU + X-ray	2.5	19.7	127.9

concentrations of ACNU followed 2 h later by 4 Gy X-irradiation. The related parameters are shown in Table 3.5. There were slight decreases in the C_0 and n values when combined X-ray treatment was performed, but there were no changes in C_q. At all concentrations of ACNU, the effect was more than additive when combined with 4 Gy X-rays.

Optimal Dose of ACNU and X-Rays

In order to facilitate the determination of the optimal dose of X-rays and ACNU, a comparison was made between the enhancement ratio (ER) in the monolayer cells and that in the spheroids [93]. The ER was defined as the ratio of the dose of radiation (or ACNU) alone for a given level of the surviving fraction to the dose of radiation (or ACNU) combined with ACNU (or X-ray) that would give the same surviving fraction. Analysis of the relationship between the radiation dose and tumor control probability showed that in order to increase the probability of tumor control from 10% to 90%, theoretically the required radiation dose needed to be increased only 20%, and this value was virtually unchanged even with slight

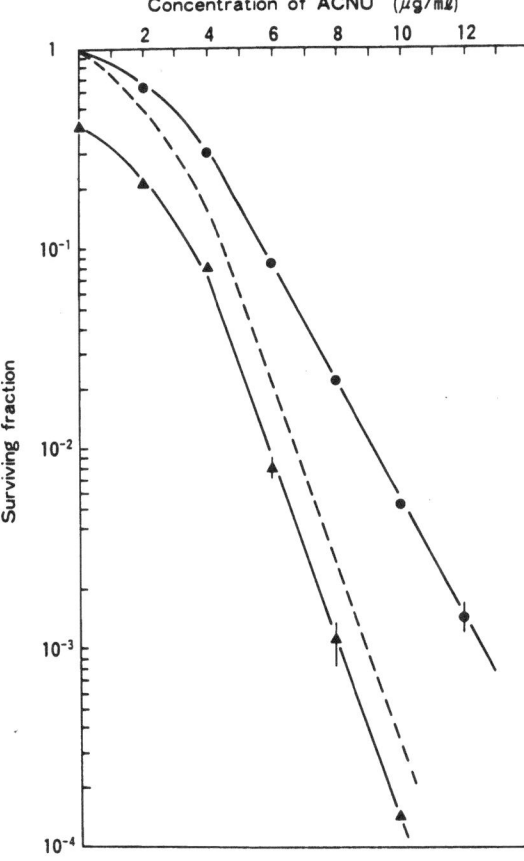

Fig. 3.27. Concentration-survival curves for exponentially growing GB A-7 cells in monolayer treated by ACNU alone (●) or X-rays (4 Gy) after ACNU treatment (▲). The *broken line* represents the curve of combined treatment when the surviving fraction by X-rays alone is normalized to 1.0

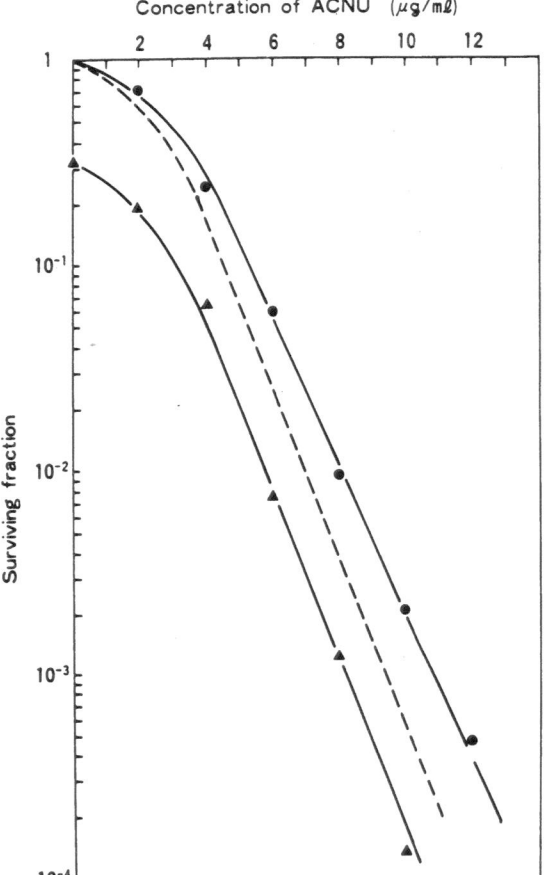

Fig. 3.28. Concentration-survival curves for GB A-7 cells in the plateau phase. *Symbols* are the same as in Fig. 3.27

differences in the cell-survival curves. Indeed, a wide variety of experimental and clinical data support these findings [80]. This fact implies that good therapeutic effects can be expected when the ER of the radiation combined with ACNU is greater than 1.2.

Although it is true that the most important factor in combined therapy is the effect on the tumor tissue, there is also a need to consider the so-called therapeutic ratio [72], in which the possible damage to normal tissue is considered. Among exponential phase cells, there are few hypoxic cells or Q cells, and from the perspective of cellular proliferation there are many similarities between exponential phase cells and actively proliferating tissues, such as intestinal and bone marrow tissues, which are susceptible to acute damage [80]. In this sense, it is desirable that the effects due to combined therapy on the spheroids as a tumor model exceed the effects on the exponential phase cells. Taking this into consideration, Fig. 3.29 shows the ER obtained from the X-ray survival curves. At all levels of the surviving fraction, the ER for the spheroids was found to be greater than 1.2 and greater than that for monolayer cells.

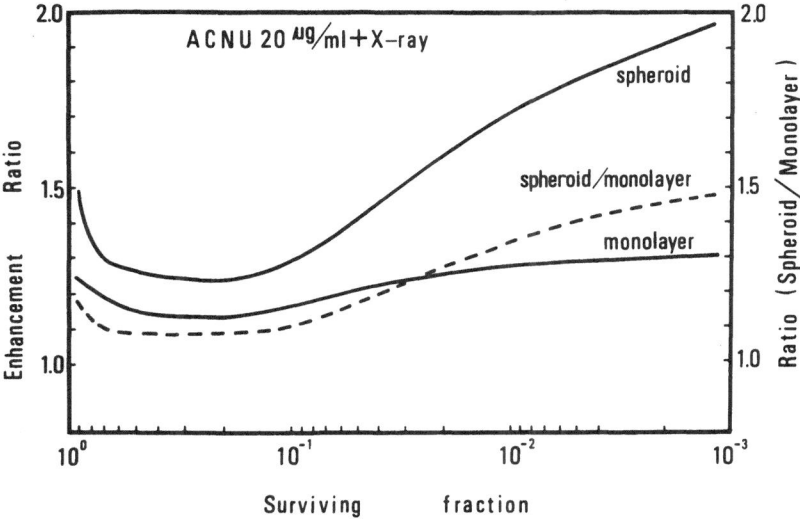

Fig. 3.29. Enhancement ratio in the treatment by X-rays combined with ACNU for RG C-6 cells in monolayer and in spheroids

The fact that ACNU is more effective against Q cells and hypoxic cells than X-rays and also has a similar cytocidal effect on P cells is considered to be the reason why in combined X-ray and ACNU therapy the effects are greater against spheroids than against monolayer cells. The fact that the ER was large even at high levels for the surviving fraction (i.e., at low X-ray doses) is thought to reflect the fact that the D_q value is smaller with combined X-ray-ACNU therapy than with X-ray therapy alone, and subsequent accumulation of sublethal damage is small.

When the surviving fraction is less than 4×10^{-2}, the ER ratio (spheroids/ monolayer cells) becomes larger than 1.2, which corresponds to an X-ray dose of more than 15 Gy. Similar results for the ER ratio obtained from the ACNU concentration-surviving fraction curve are shown in Fig. 3.30. The ER for the spheroids was again found to be greater than 1.2 at all levels of the surviving fraction. It was greater than that for monolayer cells at surviving fractions less than 0.4. The region where the ER was greater than 1.2 corresponded to an ACNU concentration greater than 24 μg/ml when the surviving fraction was less than 0.2.

The X-ray dose which is currently in common clinical usage is 2–5 Gy per fraction, whereas that for ACNU is 2 mg/kg i.v., thus producing a blood concentration of 5 μg/ml 5 min after injection [61]. However, the results obtained from the RG C-6 experiments indicate that quite large doses of radiation and ACNU were needed to obtain supra-additive effects. In contrast, the sensitivity to ACNU of the GB A-7 cells was extremely high and, depending upon the nature of the tumor tissue, it seems possible to reduce greatly the ACNU dose.

With regard to X-rays, Tamura et al. [102] reported that twice weekly doses of 5 Gy X-rays produced no acute side effects. Moreover, Kapp et al. [45] used a single X-ray dose of 6 Gy in combination with metronidazole and found no acute deficits

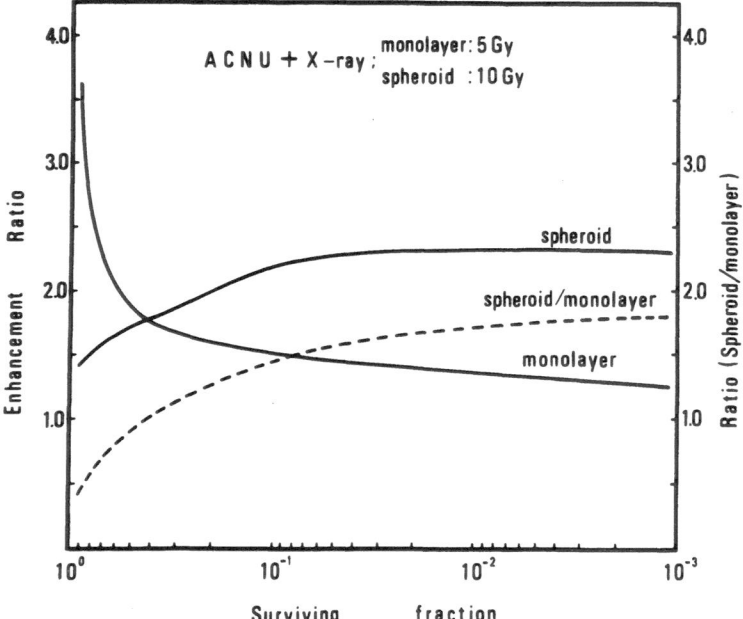

Fig. 3.30. Enhancement ratio in the treatment by ACNU combined with X-rays for RG C-6 cells in monolayer and spheroids

due to the radiation. Finally, Kogelnik et al. [51] reported no side effects following a single 4-Gy dose of radiation in combination with misonidazole. In the light of reports of various techniques for increasing the local concentration of ACNU, such as intra-arterial administration, direct injection into the tumor tissue, or by means of induced hypertension [98], it is thought to be entirely feasible to administer relatively large doses of ACNU to tumor tissue.

Dose-Control Probability of Spheroids Treated with X-Rays Combined with ACNU

GB A-7 cells. A typical example of the relationship between the dose of X-rays and the control probability of small spheroids (about 200 μm in diameter) of GB A-7 cells which had been treated with either X-rays alone or ACNU (3 μg/ml) for 2 h followed by X-rays and then plated immediately without trypsinization is shown in Fig. 3.31. The mean value and the standard deviation of the 50% control dose ($CD_{0.5}$) thus obtained from seven experiments was 17.9 ± 1.2 Gy for X-rays alone and that from three experiments for ACNU combined with X-rays was 12.3 ± 1.2 Gy. The dose ER with ACNU was $17.9/12.3 = 1.46 \pm 0.17$. The dose-survival curve for cells in the same batch of spheroids used in Fig. 3.31 is shown in Fig. 3.32. The surviving fraction of cells from spheroids treated with X-rays alone increased during the 24 h after X-irradiation when the spheroids were trypsinized ($P < 0.05$). The increase in the surviving fraction seen for spheroids with X-rays alone was inhibited by pretreatment with ACNU and the survival curve was almost unchanged

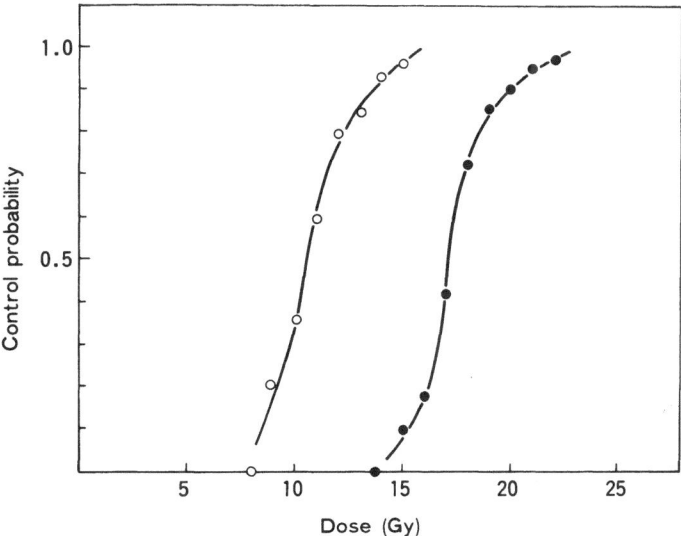

Fig. 3.31. Control probability of small spheroids of GB A-7. X-rays alone (●) and X-ray irradiation after 3 μg/ml ACNU treatment (o)

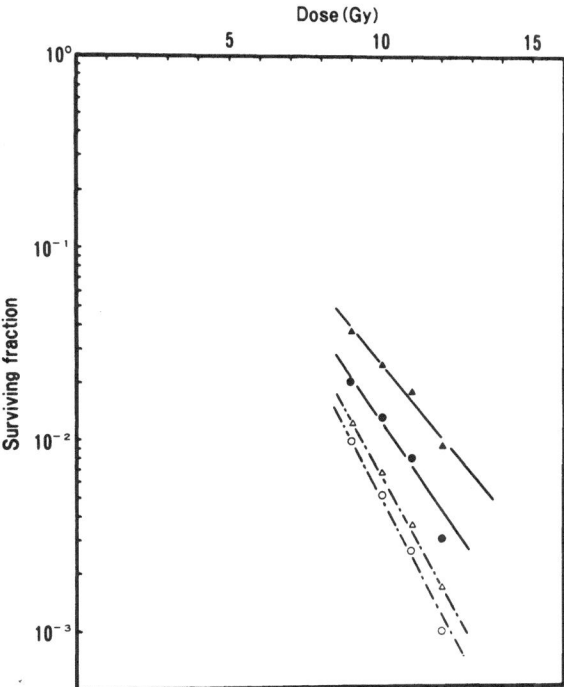

Fig. 3.32. Dose-survival curves of GB A-7 cells in small spheroids. Cells were irradiated with X-rays alone and assayed immediately (●) or 24 h after irradiation (▲). ACNU treatment combined prior to X-ray irradiation and assayed immediately (o) or 24 h after irradiation (Δ)

with a common D_0 of 1.3 Gy. This evidence indicates that the PLD recovery which occurred during 24 h in spheroids with X-rays alone was inhibited by pretreatment with ACNU. The isoeffect dose and the standard deviation for the surviving fraction of 10^{-2} was estimated after PLD recovery as 13.0 ± 1.2 and 9.2 ± 2.2 Gy, respectively, for spheroids treated with X-rays alone and for those with ACNU combined with X-rays. The corresponding ER with ACNU was 1.41 ± 0.36 which was identical to that (1.46) estimated from the control probability curves of spheroids.

As previously described, the expected values of $CD_{0.5}$, $[CD_{0.5 \text{ (exp)}}]$, can be calculated from the values of D_0, n, the viable cell number per spheroid, and the plating efficiency of cells. $CD_{0.5 \text{ (exp)}}$ was estimated as 16.7 ± 2.2 and 9.6 ± 1.2 Gy, respectively, for spheroids treated by X-rays alone and for those treated by ACNU combined with X-rays. These values are identical to those actually observed in the spheroid-control curves. The evidence indicates that the spheroid-control curve can be estimated from the cell-surival curves for both X-rays alone and X-rays combined with ACNU.

RG C-6 cells. Small spheroids (about 200 μm in diameter) of RG C-6 cells were treated in the same manner as those of GB A-7 cells, as described in the previous section, except that a concentration of ACNU of 30 μg/ml was used. The spheroid-control curves thus obtained are shown in Fig. 3.33. $CD_{0.5}$ was 18.6 ± 1.9 and 14.1 Gy, respectively, for the spheroids treated with X-rays alone (three experiments) and for those treated with the combined ACNU and X-rays (one experiment). The ER with ACNU was 1.32 ± 0.13. Cell-survival curves obtained from the same batch of spheroids shown in Fig. 3.34 indicate that a slight PLD recovery seen for X-rays alone was again inhibited by the combined treatment. The isoeffect dose for the surviving fraction at 10^{-2} after PLD recovery was 13.8 ± 2.2 and 8.3 Gy, respectively, for spheroids treated with X-rays alone and for those with the combined treatment. The ER was 1.66 ± 0.27, which was slightly larger than that obtained from spheroid-control curves. $CD_{0.5(\text{exp})}$ was 20.3 ± 3.0 and 15.5 Gy, respectively, for spheroids treated with X-rays alone and for those with the combined treatment.

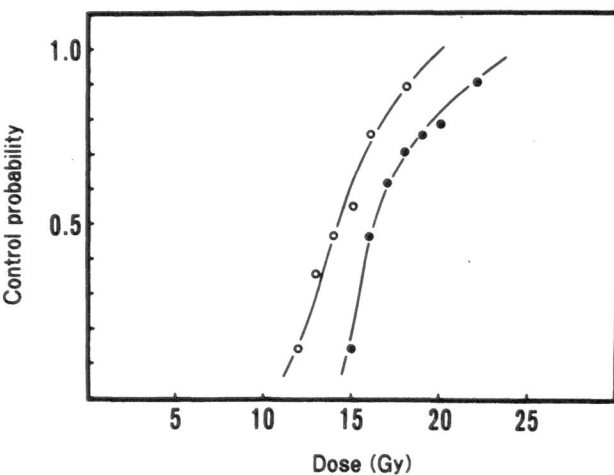

Fig. 3.33. Control probability of small spheroids of RG C-6. X-rays alone (●) or X-ray irradiation after 30 μg/ml ACNU administration (△)

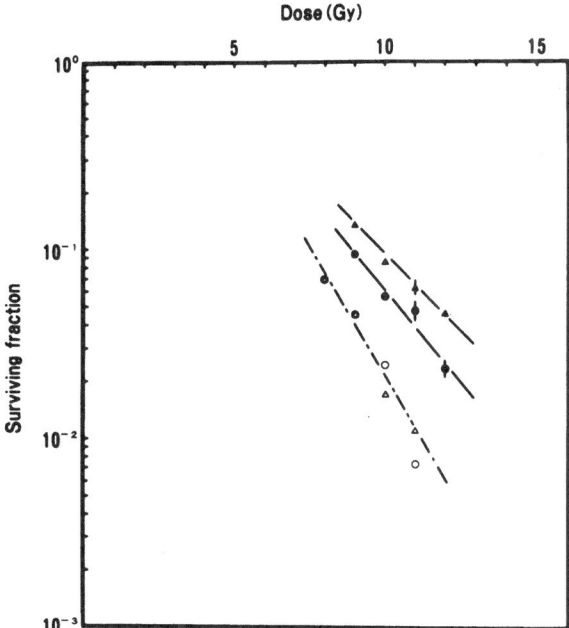

Fig. 3.34. Surviving fraction of RG C-6 cells in small spheroids. X-rays alone assayed immediately after irradiation (●) or 24 h after irradiation (▲). ACNU was added before X-ray irradiation, assayed immediately after irradiation (○) or 24 h after (△)

The expected ER was 1.31 ± 0.19. The difference was not statistically significant for either the $CD_{0.5}$ or ER.

A similar experiment for larger spheroids (about 500 μm in diameter) was performed except that a concentration of ACNU of 20 μg/ml was used. The spheroid-control curves thus obtained are shown in Fig. 3.35, and the cell survival curves shown in Fig. 3.36. Again, the PLD recovery seen for spheroids treated with X-rays alone was inhibited by the pretreatment with ACNU (Fig. 3.34). The $CD_{0.5}$ of 33.1 Gy for spheroids treated with the X-rays alone was reduced to 22.1 Gy for spheroids with the combined treatment. The corresponding ER with ACNU was 1.50, which was larger than that for small spheroids. The evidence is comparable with our finding that ACNU was more effective for cells in larger spheroids than in smaller ones. However, the value of $CD_{0.5(exp)}$ estimated from cell-survival curves after PLD recovery was 26.7 ± 1.4 Gy which was apparently smaller than the $CD_{0.5}$ of 33.1 Gy actually observed. Further, the D_0 value calculated as the value of the difference of $CD_{0.9}$ and $CD_{0.1}$ divided by 3.0 [27] from the spheroid-control curve was 3.35 Gy, but that actually observed in the cell-survival curve after PLD recovery was 1.79 Gy. The discrepancy may be due to the possibility that radioresistant hypoxic cells undetectable in the cell-survival curve are actually responsible for the survival of spheroids. In order to clarify this possibility, spheroids were irradiated in a medium containing a hypoxic radiosensitizer, misonidazole [86] 1-(2-nito-1-imidazolyl)-3-methoxy-2-propanol; a gift from Nippon Roche KK, Tokyo, added 15 min prior to X-irradiation at a concentration of 1 mmol/l. The results are shown in Figs. 3.37 and 3.38. In the presence of misonidazole, the cell-survival curve was unchanged, but the spheroid-control curve was shifted to the left. Correspondingly,

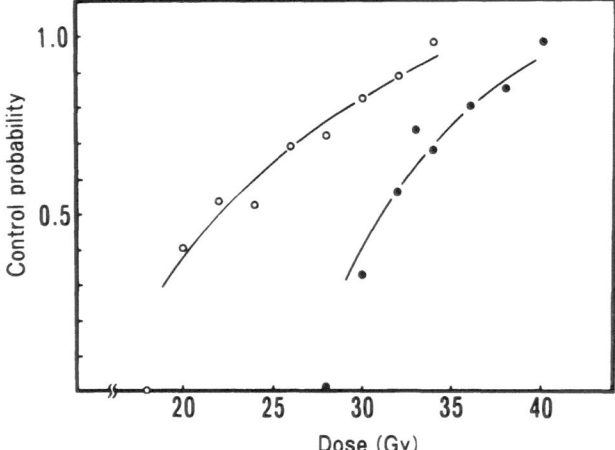

Fig. 3.35. Control probability of large spheroids of RG C-6 cells. X-rays alone (●) or X-ray irradiation after 20 μg/ml ACNU administration (○)

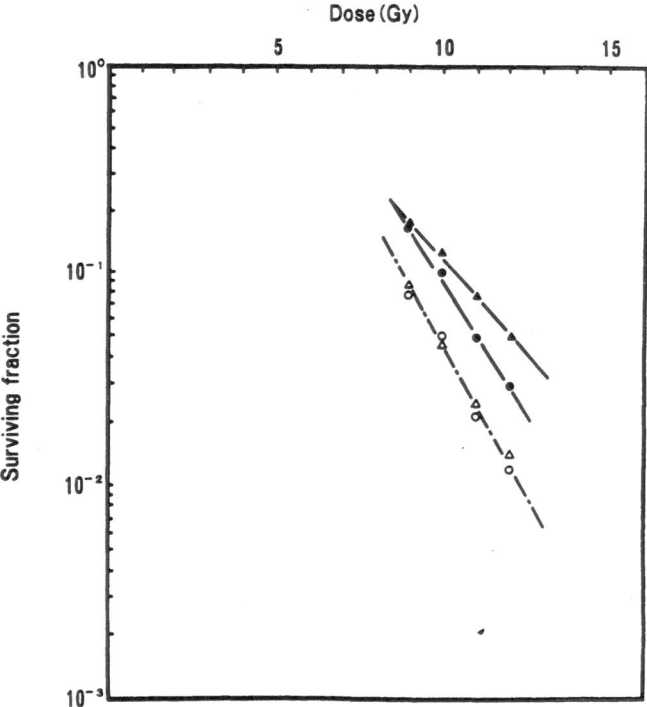

Fig. 3.36. Surviving fraction of RG C-6 cells in large spheroids. X-rays alone assayed immediately after irradiation (●) or 24 h after irradiation (▲). ACNU was added before X-ray irradiation, assayed immediately after irradiation (○) or 24 h after (△)

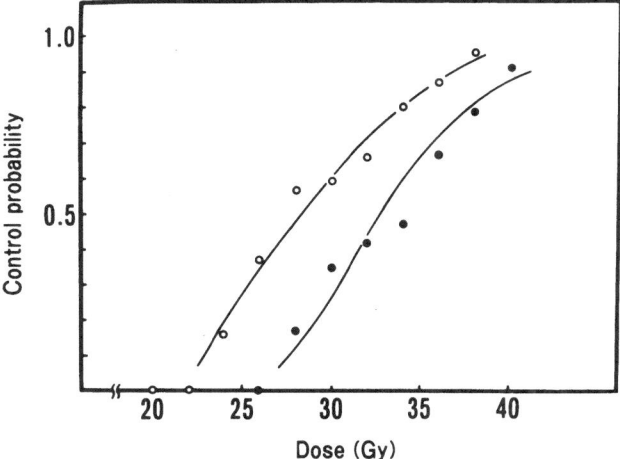

Fig. 3.37. Control probability of large spheroids of RG C-6 cells. X-rays alone (●) or X-ray irradiation after misonidazole administration (o)

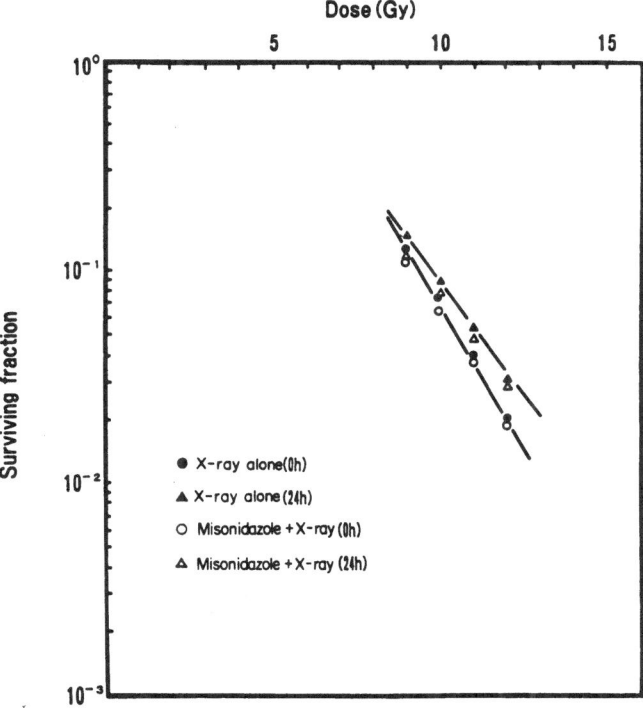

Fig. 3.38. Surviving fraction of RG C-6 cells in large spheroids. PLD recovery was not inhibited in the presence of misonidazole

$CD_{0.5}$ was reduced from 33.0 to 28.0 Gy in the presence of misonidazole. These results clearly showed that hypoxic cells, which are sensitized to X-rays by misonidazole, were responsible for the survival of the spheroids, but the presence of these cells was not detected in the cell-survival curve. $CD_{0.5(exp)}$ was reduced by the combined treatment with ACNU from 26.6 to 23.1 Gy and the expected ER was 1.16. This contrasted with the ER actually observed (1.50). These results are also supported by our finding described below (Fig. 3.71) that ACNU has preferential effects on cells in the deeper layers of large spheroids.

The results of the experiments described thus far, where spheroids were irradiated in a spinner flask, are somewhat different from those obtained in previous experiments where spheroids in a medium under static conditions were irradiated in a plastic vial. In the latter experiments, an apparent hypoxic cell fraction was observed in the cell-survival curves. These hypoxic cells may have been caused by the medium under static conditions since the stirring of the medium in a spinner flask tends to result in a more efficient oxygen supply. The difference in the condition of the medium may have also influenced the extent of the PLD recovery, since little PLD recovery was observed when spheroids were irradiated in a vial. Although the extent of oxygenation in the microenvironment of cells in situ in the gliomas of patients is not yet precisely known, it has been reported from animal experiments that both chronically hypoxic cells and acutely hypoxic cells may be present in solid tumors [13, 16].

Effects of Combined Treatment with X-Rays and 5-FU

Effects of combined treatment with X-rays and 5-FU described below were analyzed using RG C-6 cells in the monolayer and spheroids.

X-Ray Treatment Following 5-FU

Monolayer cells. In the X-ray dose-survival curves, there was a shoulder in the curve for X-rays alone extending as far as $D_q = 2.3$ Gy, after which there was an exponential decrease in the survival with increasing X-ray doses and a D_0 value of 1.7 Gy. In combined therapy with 5-FU, there was a marked reduction in D_q and the effect was more than the additive one of the individual therapies acting independently (Fig. 3.39; Table 3.10).

In the 5-FU concentration-survival curves, there was a shoulder extending as far as $C_q = 2.1$ μg/ml, after which there was an exponential decrease in the survival curves and a C_0 value of 13.5 μg/ml. When combined therapy with X-rays was done, there were decreases in both C_q and C_0, with effects in excess of the additive range (Fig. 3.40; Table 3.11).

The time-survival curve for 5-FU showed a decrease in the surviving fraction 12 h after treatment with 5-FU (25 μg/ml) alone. When combined with 5 Gy X-irradiation, there was a sharp decrease in the survival rate following 12 h of 5-FU therapy in comparison with the effects of X-rays alone, and the effect became greater thereafter (Fig. 3.41).

From the above findings, it can be seen that combined 5-FU treatment and irradiation produced effects which were truely supra-additive. This conclusion can be drawn from the isobologram analysis (Fig. 3.42), as advocated by Steel [90]. In the analysis, the isobologram was constructed using the single-agent curves for the

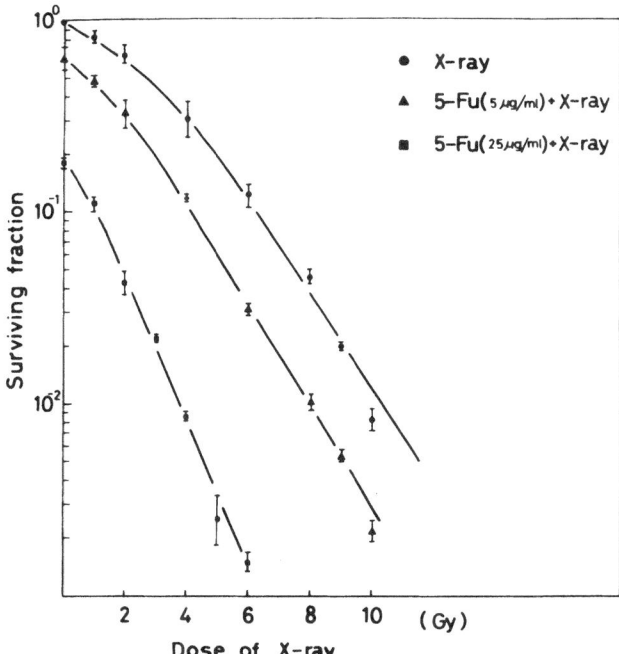

Fig. 3.39. Survival curves of RG C-6 cells in monolayer X-irradiated after treatment with a fixed concentration of 5-FU (0, 5, 25 μg/ml). C_q was decreased by the combined treatment, while C_0 was essentially unchanged

Table 3.10. Survival parameters of RG C-6 cells for graded doses of X-rays

	Monolayer		Spheroid	
	D_0 (Gy)	D_q (Gy)	Terminal D_0 (Gy)	HF
X-rays alone	1.7 (1.0)	2.3 (1.0)	4.2 (1.0)	0.44 (1.0)
5-FU (5 μg/ml) + X-rays	1.6 (0.94)	1.0 (0.48)	4.3 (1.0)	0.19 (0.43)
5-FU (25 μg/ml) + X-rays	1.1 (0.65)	0.46 (0.20)*	3.7 (0.88)	0.054 (0.12)*
X-rays alone				
Immediately	1.7 (1.0)	2.2 (1.0)	4.3 (1.0)	0.42 (1.0)
After 24 h	1.8 (1.0)	2.1 (0.95)	4.5 (1.0)	0.36 (0.86)
X-rays + 5-FU (5 μg/ml)	1.8 (1.0)	1.9 (0.86)		
X-rays + 5-FU (25 μg/ml)	1.4 (0.82)	2.5 (1.1)	5.2 (1.2)	0.34 (0.81)

HF hypoxic fraction
Figures in parentheses show relative values for X-rays alone
Difference from X-rays alone was statistically significant at $P < 0.05$*

isoeffect levels of the surviving fraction at 0.01 and 0.1. The results shown in Fig. 3.42 indicate that the effect of two agents combined was below the "envelope of additivity," where the lower curve was drawn as an additive interaction of the two agents. The radiation dose-survival curve when 5-FU was also employed showed a decrease in the D_q value. This has been interpreted as reflecting a decrease in the accumulation of SLD [23] as a result of the 5-FU treatment. Two main causes must

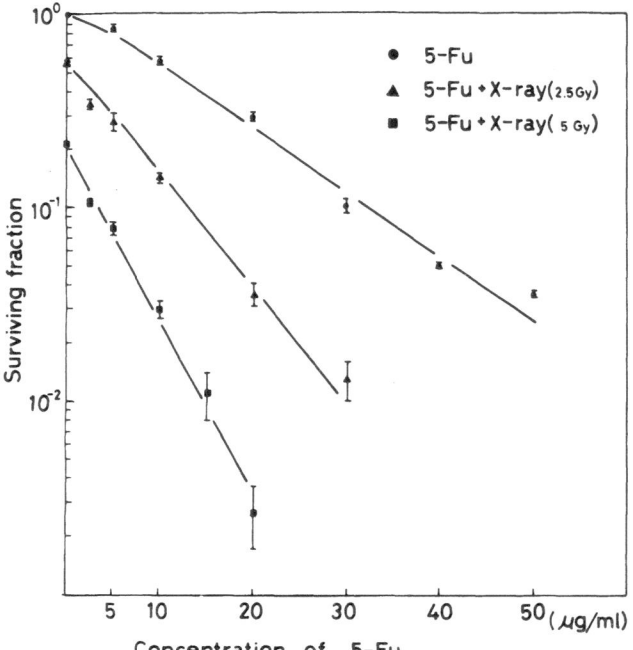

Fig. 3.40. Survival curves of RG C-6 cells in monolayer treated with 5-FU before a fixed dose of X-irradiation (0, 2.5, 5 Gy). Both C_q and C_0 were decreased by the combined treatment

Table 3.11. Survival parameters of RG C-6 cells for graded concentrations of 5-FU

	Monolayer		Spheroid		
	C_q (μg/ml)	C_0 (μg/ml)	$_1C_0$ (μg/ml)	$_2C_0$ (μg/ml)	RF
5-FU alone	2.1 (1.0)	13.5 (1.0)		59.6 (1.0)	0.84–1.1 (1.0)
5-FU + 2.5 Gy	0.86 (0.4)	8.0 (0.60)**			
5-FU + 5.0 Gy	0.02 (0.0)	4.8 (0.36)**	7.4	28.1 (0.47)*	0.72 (0.72)
5-FU + 10 Gy			3.1	32.8 (0.55)*	0.37 (0.37)
5-FU alone	4.9 (1.0)	14.9 (1.0)	8.3 (1.0)	56.9 (1.0)	0.84 (1.0)
2.5 Gy + 5-FU	3.7 (0.76)	12.0 (0.81)			
5.0 Gy + 5-FU	4.6 (0.94)	9.9 (0.66)	8.4 (1.0)	45.1 (0.79)	0.90 (1.1)
10.0 Gy + 5-FU			8.8 (1.1)	55.9 (0.98)	0.97 (1.2)

Figures in parentheses show relative values to 5-FU alone
Difference from 5-FU alone was statistically significant at $P < 0.05$* and $P < 0.01$**

be considered for this. The first is interaction between the damage incurred by X-rays and that by 5-FU. This is not considered to be a strong possibility [78] for the following reasons: (a) In the 5-FU dose-survival curve, a small C_q value was found, but the extrapolation number (*n*) at $C_q = C_0 \times \ln n$ was actually 1.0, suggesting that there was almost no SLD due to 5-FU treatment. (b) As discussed below (and shown in Figs. 3.48–3.50, when 5-FU treatment was done following irradiation

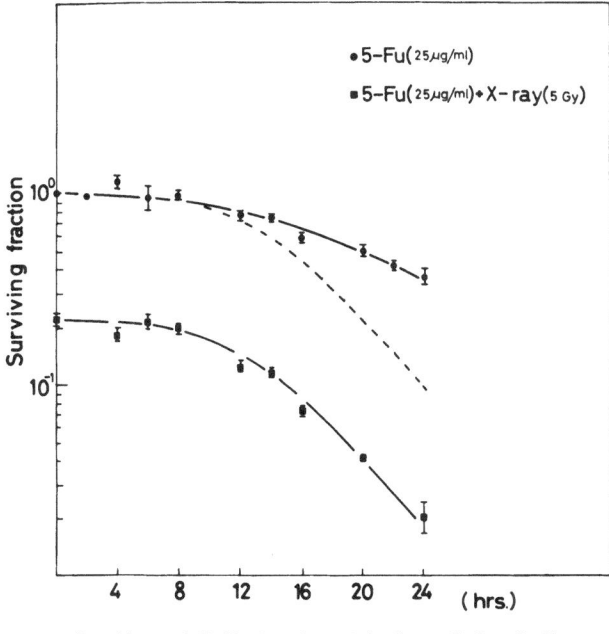

Fig. 3.41. Surviving fraction of RG C-6 cells in monolayer as a function of the duration of 5-FU treatment before X-irradiation (0, 5 Gy). The *broken line* represents the curve from which the surviving fraction by X-irradiation alone was normalized to 1.0. The effect was more than additive and both agents acted independently when cells were treated with 5-FU longer than 12 h

there was no decrease in the D_q value. The second possibility concerns the partial synchronization of the cells in the cell cycle due to prolonged 5-FU treatment. It has previously been reported that using human cancer cells there is partial synchronization of cells at the G_1/S border [10, 113], while cells are most radiosensitive at the G_1/S border and in the G_2 and M phases [104]. For these reasons and based on the fact that the supra-additive effects were first seen when 5-FU treatment preceded the irradiation by 12 h, we believe that the most likely mechanism for the supra-additive effects of 5-FU and X-rays in the monolayer culture cells is that the 5-FU treatment did in fact cause a partial synchronization of the cell cycle at the G_1/S border.

Spheroids. In the X-ray dose-survival curve, a biphasic curve with a reflection point at 10 Gy was found. The ratio of D_0 in the second phase of the curve ($= 4.2$ Gy) to that in the curve for monolayer ($= 1.7$ Gy) was 2.5—a value which is in agreement with the oxygen enhancement ratio usually reported [31]. For this reason, the biphasic curve of the spheroids is thought to indicate the presence of hypoxic cells. If the back-extrapolated value to the ordinate of the second phase is, for convenience, used as a measure of the hypoxic fraction (HF) [63], an HF value of 0.44 was found, indicating that some 40% of the cell population of the spheroids were

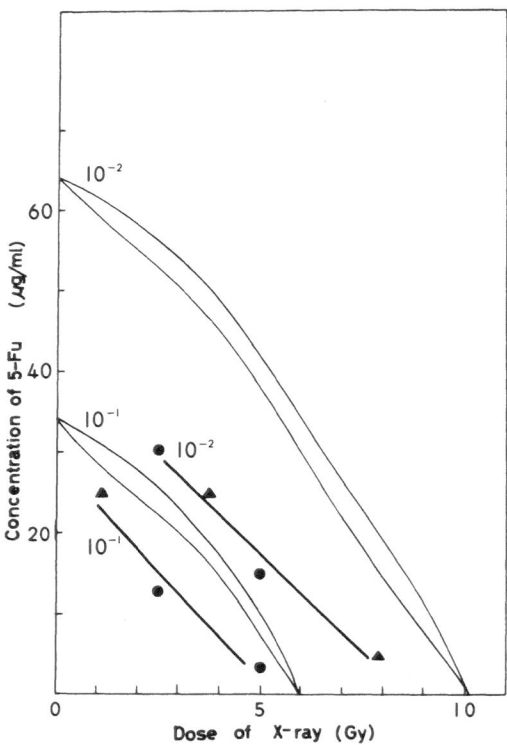

Fig. 3.42. Isobolograms of RG C-6 cells in monolayer for X-ray irradiation at 24 h after 5-FU treatment were constructed from Figs. 3.39 and 3.40 for isoeffect levels of the surviving fraction at 0.01 and 0.1, where the additive envelope was surrounded by the curves of independent action and of additive interaction of the two agents. Data of combined treatment represented by ▲ are from Fig. 3.39, and ● are from Fig. 3.40

hypoxic. In contrast to the unchanged final D_0 value when 5-FU was combined with X-rays, the HF value then decreased and combined effects greater than the additive value were obtained (Fig. 3.43; Table 3.10).

In the 5-FU concentration-survival curves, a gentle, exponential decrease in the survival curve was seen when 5-FU alone was administered. The C_0 value was 59.6 μg/ml and the ratio with the C_0 from the monolayer cells (13.5 μg/ml) was 4.4, thus indicating that in comparison with the monolayer cells the spheroids had a greater resistance to 5-FU. When irradiation was combined, there were decreases in the $_1C_0$, $_2C_0$, and RF values and the combined effects were also found to be more than the additive effect of the two agents acting independently (Fig. 3.44; Table 3.11).

In the 5-FU time-survival curves, there was only a slight decrease in the surviving fraction at 16 h treatment with 25μg/ml 5-FU alone. When, however, 8-Gy irradiation was also employed at various times during 5-FU treatment, there was a mild decrease in the surviving fraction. The maximal effect was obtained after 8 h of 5-FU treatment, subsequent to which there were no further increases (Fig. 3.45). The combined effect was apparently more than the additive effect of the two agents acting independently.

From the above experimental findings, it is concluded that supra-additive effects on the spheroids were also obtained by the combined use of 5-FU and X-rays. It is evident that this conclusion can also be drawn from the supra-additive effects obtained in the isobologram analysis (Fig. 3.46).

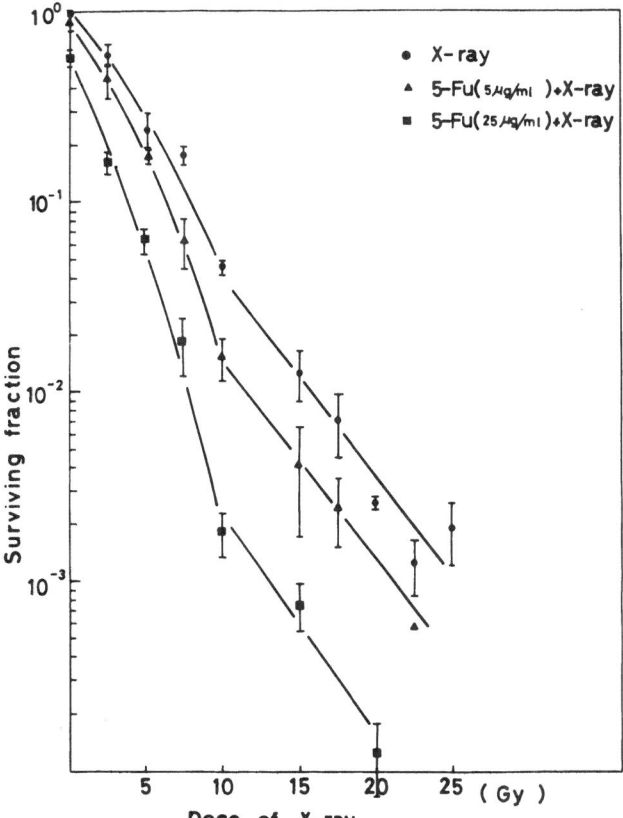

Fig. 3.43. Survival curves of RG C-6 cells in spheroids X-irradiated after treatment with a fixed concentration of 5-FU (0, 5, 25 μg/ml). The fraction of cells resistant to X-rays decreased by the combined treatment while the C_0 of the resistant phase was unchanged

In the high-dose region of the X-ray dose-survival curve when combined 5-FU and X-rays were used, a decrease in the fraction of X-ray-resistant cells was seen, indicating that reoxygenation of the previously hypoxic cells in the deep layers of the spheroids had occurred [21].

In the light of various experimental results, it is thought that the actions of 5-FU are confined to the actively proliferating outer layers of the spheroids [14, 49, 58]. The mechanism by which the hypoxic cells of the deep layers of the spheroids are reoxygenated may, therefore, be as follows [64]. Following 5-FU treatment, there is a decrease in the oxygen consumption by the cells at the spheroid surface per unit volume and, as a consequence, oxygen then diffuses into the deeper layers. It is of course known that several drugs, such as rotenon and antimycin A, bring about a reduction in cellular respiratory activity [22, 46]. Further, it is established that a reduction in oxygen consumption occurs within 2–15 min and, in regions of low O_2 concentration, only a small increase in the PaO_2 is required to bring about a marked increase in cellular sensitivity to radiation [31].

In the 5-FU concentration-survival curves, a reduction in the fraction of the 5-FU-resistant cells and a reduction in the C_0 values were observed in both the first and second phases. The cell cycle synchronization effects of 5-FU seem to be limited

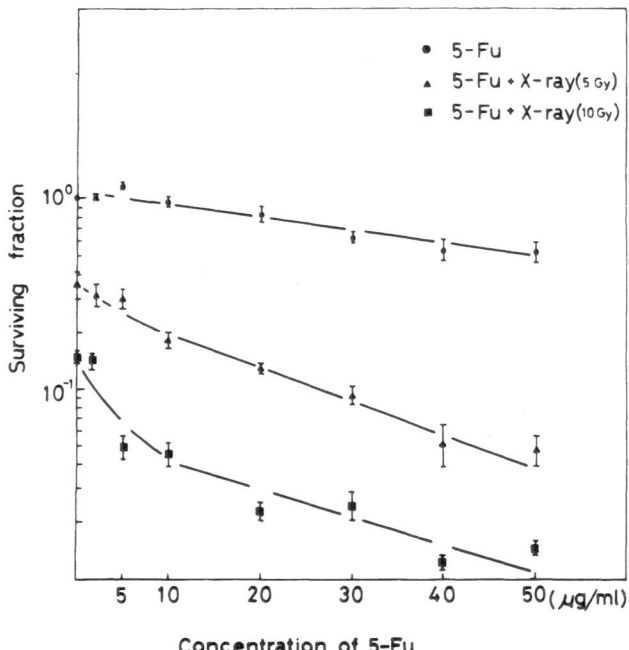

Fig. 3.44. Survival curves of RG C-6 cells in spheroids treated with 5-FU before a fixed dose of X-irradiation (0, 5, 10 Gy). The C_0 of both sensitive and resistant phases were decreased by the combined treatment

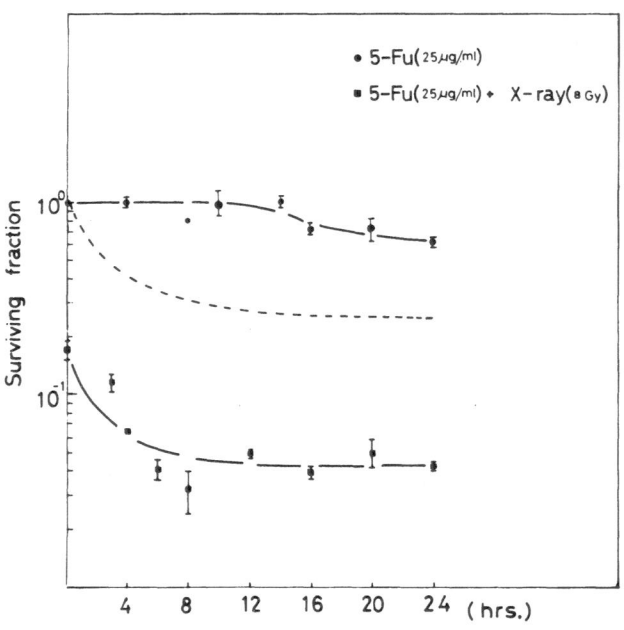

Fig. 3.45. Surviving fraction of RG C-6 cells in spheroids as a function of the duration of 5-FU treatment before X-irradiation (0, 8 Gy). The *broken line* represents the normalized curve. The effect of the combined treatment was more than additive at 3 h and saturated at around 8 h

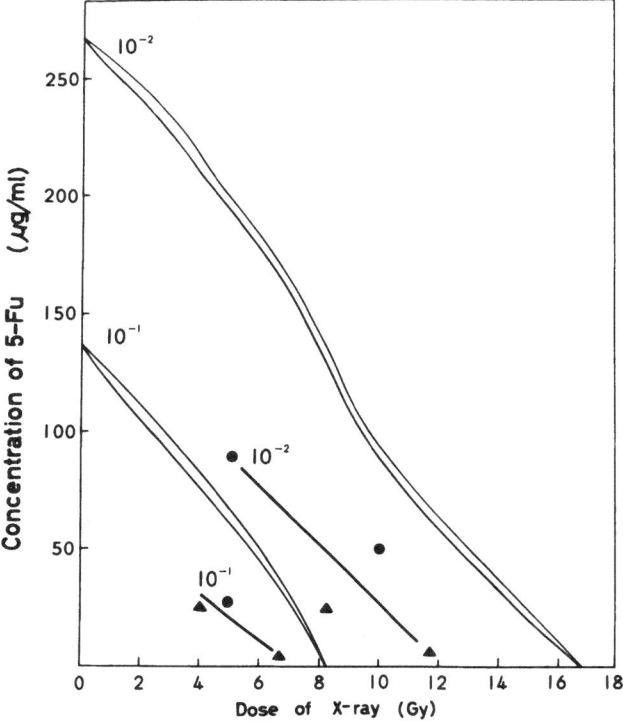

Fig. 3.46. Isobolograms of RG C-6 cells in spheroids for X-ray irradiation at 24 h after 5-FU treatment were constructed from Figs. 3.44 and 3.45 for the isoeffect levels of the surviving fraction at 0.01 and 0.1, where the additive envelope was surrounded by curves of independent action and of additive interaction of the two agents. Data of combined treatment represented by ▲ are from Fig. 3.44 and by ● are from Fig. 3.45

to the actively proliferating cells at the outer layers of the spheroids and the reduction in C_0 in the first phase is thought to reflect this effect. In contrast, the 5-FU-resistant fraction was greater than 84% and is thought to include hypoxic cells.

In light of the reoxygenation phenomenon discussed above, we believe that a portion of the hypoxic cells included in the 5-FU-resistant fraction are reoxygenated and then become radiosensitive. As a consequence, there was an apparent, rather than actual, reduction in the size of the 5-FU-resistant cell fraction (Fig. 3.47).

As discussed above, in both the monolayer cells and the spheroids, supra-additive effects were obtained by means of X-ray treatment following 5-FU treatment, but a comparison of the effects of X-rays and 5-FU showed differences between them: In the X-ray dose-survival curves, there was a decrease in D_q in the monolayer cells and a decrease in the number of hypoxic cells in the spheroids due to the combined treatment. In contrast, in the 5-FU concentration-survival curves, there were decreases in both C_q and C_0 in the monolayer cells and a reduction in the number of 5-FU-resistant cells due to the combined treatment.

Before 5-Fu treatment

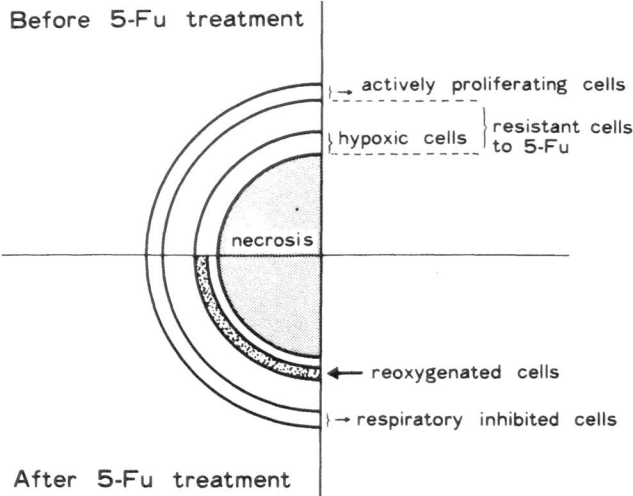

Fig. 3.47. Relationship between the effect of 5-FU and tumor cord structure

These differences are thought to indicate that the mechanisms in the action of combined therapy in the monolayer cells and the spheroids are dissimilar. Namely, in the monolayer cells, cells are partially synchronized as a result of the 5-FU treatment at the G_1/S border, where cells are known to be highly radiosensitive. In the spheroids, a decrease in the oxygen consumption per unit volume of the actively proliferating cells occurs and, as a consequence, oxygen can diffuse into the deeper layers, thereby reoxygenating hypoxic cells. In contrast, when 5-FU treatment is given after X-irradiation, essentially no supra-additive effects are obtained either in the monolayer cells or the spheroids, as discussed below.

5-FU Treatment Following X-Irradiation

Monolayer cells. The X-ray dose-survival curve, when cells were trypsinized immediately after irradiation, was virtually the same as the dose-survival curve when X-rays alone were given without trypsinization, as shown in Fig. 3.39. When trypsinization was done after 24 h of cultivation following X-irradiation, a similar curve was obtained and there were no signs of recovery from PLD [74]. The addition of 5-FU therapy did not alter the D_q and D_0 values, and essentially additive effect was obtained (Fig. 3.48; Table 3.10).

The 5-FU concentration-survival curve was virtually identical to that shown in Fig. 3.40, where 5-FU alone was administered. There was only an additive effect when combined therapy with X-rays was used (Fig. 3.49; Table 3.11). In the 5-FU time-survival curve, there was a decrease in the surviving fraction about 16 h after the addition of 25 μg/ml 5-FU, and combined X-ray treatment even after 48 h produced only an additive effect (Fig. 3.50).

Spheroids. The X-ray dose-survival curve when trypsinization was done immediately following the irradiation was similar to that when X-ray treatment alone was

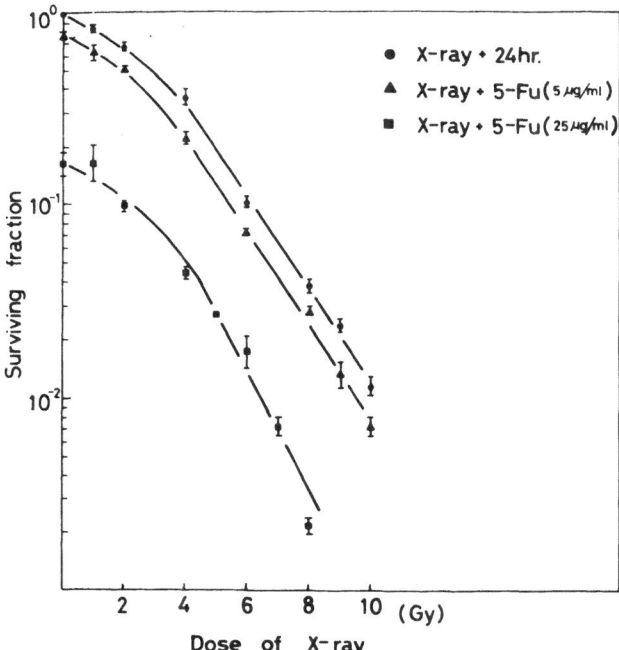

Fig. 3.48. Survival curves of RG C-6 cells in monolayer X-irradiated before treatment with a fixed concentration of 5-FU (0, 5, 25 μg/ml). C_0 and C_q were unchanged by the combined treatment

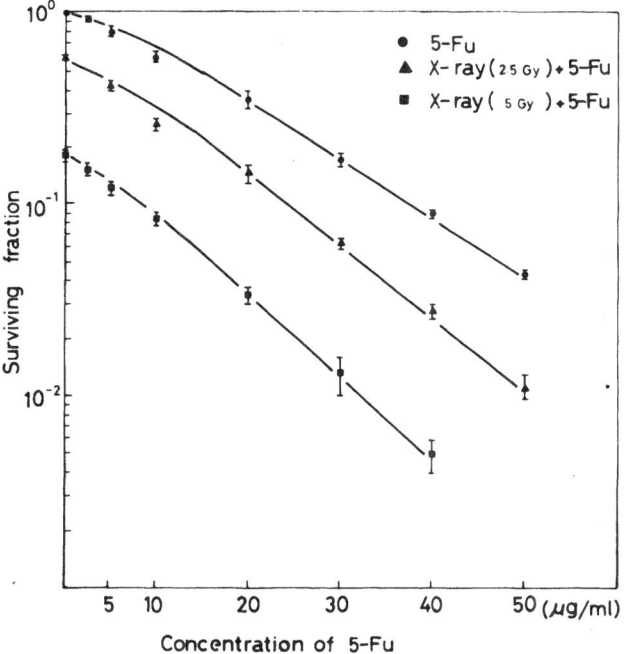

Fig. 3.49. Survival curves of RG C-6 cells in monolayer treated with 5-FU after a fixed dose of X-irradiation (0, 2.5, 5 Gy). Both C_q and C_0 were unchanged by the combined treatment

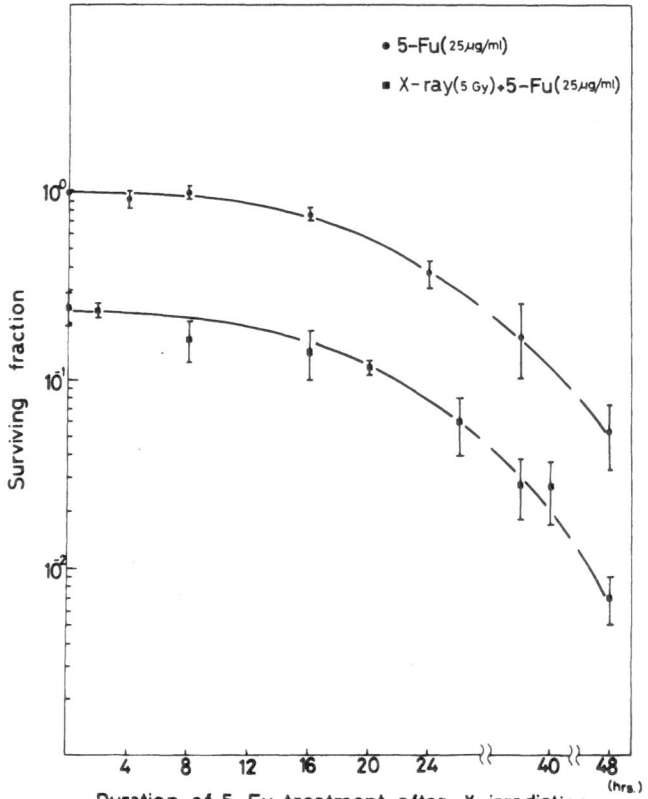

Fig. 3.50. Surviving fraction of RG C-6 cells in monolayer as a function of the duration of 5-FU treatment after X-irradiation (0, 5 Gy). The two *curves* are parallel

done as in Fig. 3.43 and again a similar curve was obtained when trypsinization was done 24 h after X-irradiation. No indication of recovery from PLD was found during 24 h incubation in a Petri dish (Fig. 3.51; Table 3.10). In the 5-FU concentration-survival curve, a biphasic curve with a change of slope at a 5-FU dose of 10 µg/ml was found. Combined therapy with X-rays produced only additive effects (Fig. 3.52; Table 3.11).

In the 5-FU time-survival curve, the effect was additive when 5-FU was combined with 8-Gy X-ray therapy (Fig. 3.53). Note that the curves obtained from Figs. 3.45 and 3.53 were obtained in experiments performed simultaneously, and the 5-FU time-survival curves are virtually identical.

Several studies have been reported concerning the effects of combined X-rays and 5-FU therapy. In experiments using mouse L-5 cells, Nakajima et al. [68] found the combined effect to be greater than the additive effect due to a decrease in D_q when 5-FU treatment either preceded or followed X-irradiation. They argued that when X-rays followed 5-FU treatment, there was a decrease in the accumulation of SLD, whereas when irradiation preceded 5-FU treatment, there was an interaction between the X-irradiation and the drug treatment. There have also been reports in which a decrease in D_0 but not in D_q was found; these experiments, however, used human cancer cells, such as HeLa cells [9, 15], and the only combination of treat-

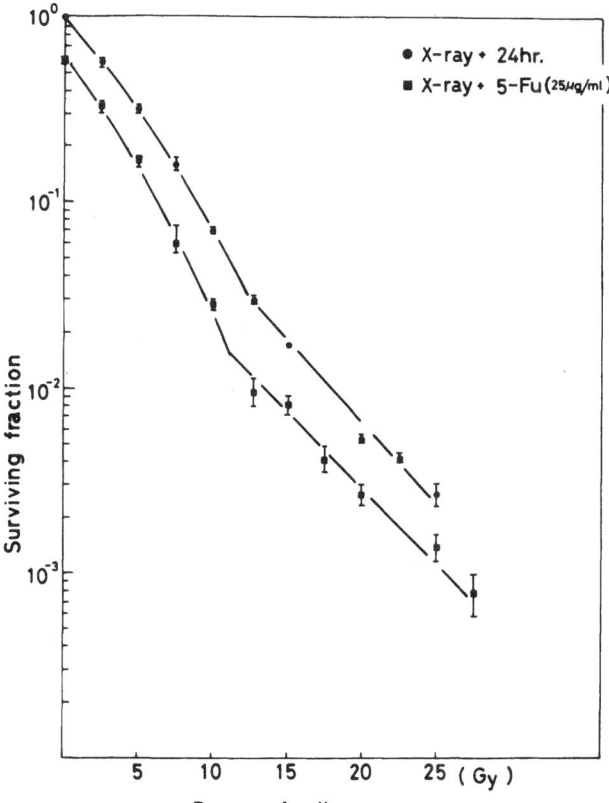

Fig. 3.51. Survival curves of RG C-6 cells in spheroids X-irradiated before treatment with a fixed concentration of 5-FU (0, 25 μg/ml). The fraction of cells resistant to X-rays and the D_0 of the resistant phase were unchanged by the combined treatment

ments which was studied was 5-FU treatment immediately following irradiation. In animal experiments using lymphomas, it has been reported that effects greater than the additive effect were obtained either when X-irradiation was performed 14–24 h after 5-FU treatment or when 5-FU treatment was done within 8 h after the irradiation; with the latter the effect was, however, significantly stronger [112]. Finally, there was one report of synergistic effects when 5-FU therapy either preceded or succeeded the X-irradiation by 12 h [52].

These differences which have been reported in the literature are thought to have been due primarily to differences in the experimental system. In any case, no studies prior to our own have appeared which have made any attempt to obtain a unified understanding of such therapies by contrasting the results obtained in exponentially growing cells, such as monolayer cells and spheroids. Sasaki [80] proposed an experimental method for estimating combined effects in order to confirm that more damage is done to tumor tissue than normal tissue. He proposed a method involved the comparison of the degree of increased effects due to X-irradiation for combined therapy using monolayer cells in the exponential phase (which resemble the cell proliferation and microenvironment of rapidly proliferating normal tissues, such as bone marrow and intestinal cells) as a standard model and spheroids with a central necrotic layer as a solid tumor model.

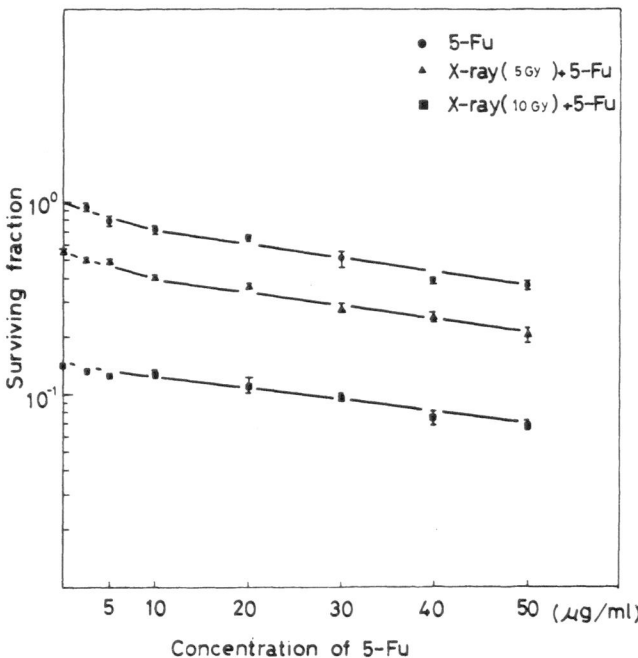

Fig. 3.52. Survival curves of RG C-6 cells in spheroids treated with 5-FU after a fixed dose of X-irradiation (0, 5, 10 Gy). The C_0 of the sensitive and resistant phases to 5-FU were unchanged by the combined treatment

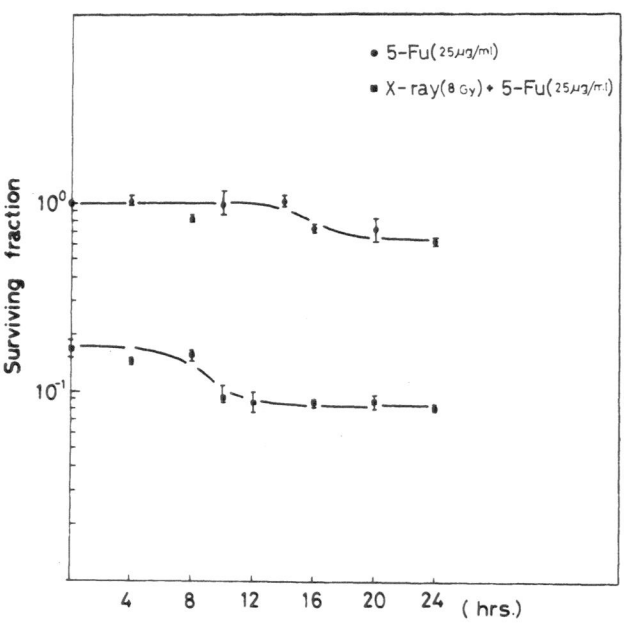

Fig. 3.53. Surviving fraction of RG C-6 cells in spheroids as a function of the duration of 5-FU treatment after X-irradiation (0, 8 Gy). The two *curves* are almost parallel

In the present experiments, combined therapy with 5-FU preceding X-ray treatment by 24 h did not produce results in which the spheroids (as a solid tumor model) were damaged to an extent greater than the monolayer cells (as a normal tissue model). The following results, however, are of considerable interest: In the 5-FU time-survival curves for monolayer cells (Fig. 3.41), a supra-additive effect was obtained when X-irradiation was done 12 h after 5-FU treatment, and the subsequent effect continued to increase. In contrast, in the spheroids (Fig. 3.45), X-irradiation 3 h after 5-FU treatment already showed an effect greater than the additive and the enhancement became greater for X-irradiation after 8 h treatment with 5-FU. These findings suggest that the greatest antitumor effects can be expected from X-ray therapy several hours after 5-FU therapy, while acute damage to normal tissue is at a minimum [35].

In recent years, the in vivo intratumoral state of tegaful has been greatly clarified and tegaful is now known to be converted into 5-FU even within tumor cells. Due to the low level of 5-FU degradation in tumor cells, 5-FU accumulates there [71, 108] and reaches a high concentration compared with that in normal tissues [3]. These findings also suggest that the combined therapy of X-rays and 5-FU should be effective.

Combined Effects of ACNU and 5-FU

RG C-6 cells were used in these experiments as described below.

Concentration-Survival Curves for 5-FU Combined with a Fixed Concentration of ACNU

Treatment with 5-FU after ACNU. In the monolayer cells, the effects of pretreatment with 30 or 60 μg/ml ACNU (Fig. 3.54) followed by 5-FU treatment were analyzed. In all cases, shoulders were found up to a dose of 20 μg/ml 5-FU and thereafter exponential decreases in the surviving fraction (SF) were found with increasing doses. Comparison of the C_0 and C_q ratios for 30 and 60 μg/ml ACNU pretreatment showed C_0 ratios of 0.76 and 0.56 and C_q ratios of 1.12 and 0.84, respectively. Thus, the combined treatment showed an enhanced effect mainly due to the decrease in the C_0 following the ACNU pretreatment (Table 3.12).

In the spheroids, the effects of 5-FU and of 20 and 40 μg/ml ACNU pretreatment prior to 5-FU treatment were analyzed (Fig. 3.55). In both cases, a biphasic survival curve was obtained. The initial slope $_1C_0$ ratio for 5-FU treatment alone was 0.78 for 20 μg/ml ACNU pretreatment and 0.52 for 40 μg/ml. The second slope $_2C_0$ ratios were 0.32 and 0.29, respectively, the decrease in the C_0 value of the second slope due to ACNU pretreatment was the more marked. Comparison of the RF values showed that there was a decrease in the 5-FU-resistant fraction from 0.80 when 5-FU alone was administered to 0.69 and 0.23 when 20 and 40 μg/ml ACNU, respectively, were given (Table 3.13).

Treatment with 5-FU before ACNU. In the monolayer cells, the effects of 5-FU alone and of posttreatment with 30 and 60 μg/ml ACNU following 5-FU treatment were analyzed (Fig. 3.56). In all cases, a shoulder was found to extend to 10–20 μg/ml 5-FU, and from there exponential decreases in the SF were seen with further increases in the 5-FU concentration. The C_0 ratio for 5-FU treatment with com-

S. Mashiyama, et al.

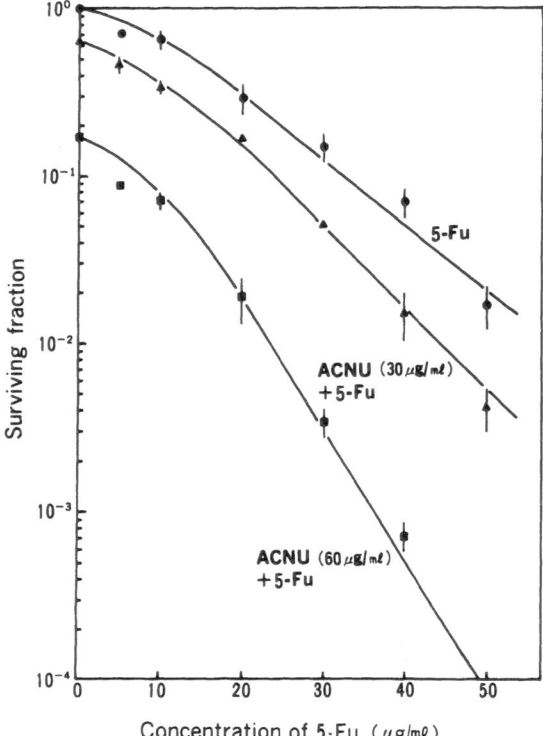

Fig. 3.54. Survival curves of RG C-6 cells in the monolayer for 5-FU combined with a fixed concentration of ACNU (0.3 μg/ml, 60 μg/ml). C_0 was decreased by the combined treatment, while C_q was not

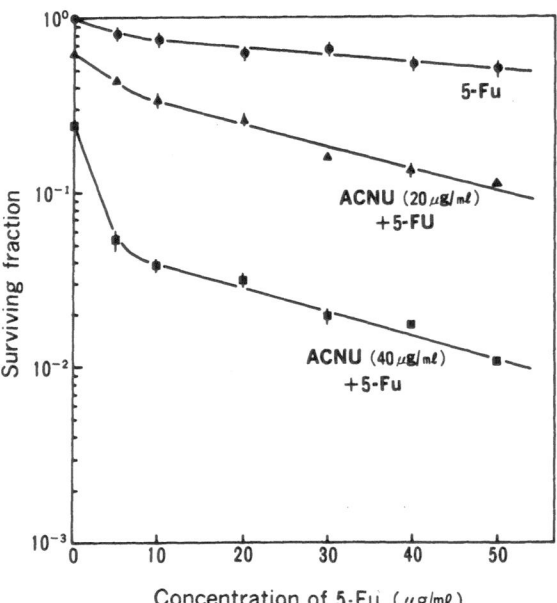

Fig. 3.55. Survival curves of RG C-6 cells in spheroids for 5-FU combined with a fixed concentration of ACNU (0.20 μg/ml, 40 μg/ml). The C_0 of both the sensitive and resistant phases was decreased by the combined treatment. The fraction of cells resistant to 5-FU was also decreased by combined treatment with ACNU

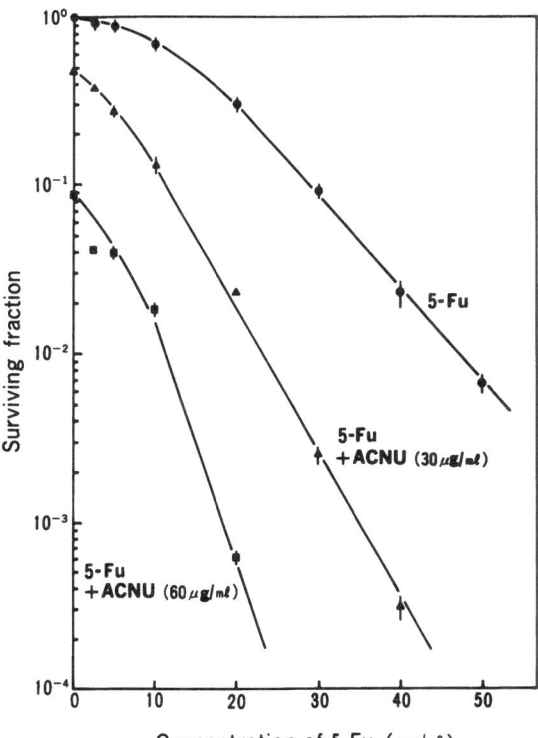

Fig. 3.56. Survival curves of RG C-6 cells in monolayer for 5-FU followed by treatment with a fixed concentration of ACNU (0.3 μg/ml, 60 μg/ml). The decrease in C_0 and C_q with combined treatment was larger than with ACNU + 5-FU

bined ACNU was 0.60 with 30 μg/ml ACNU posttreatment and 0.39 with 60 μg/ml; the respective C_q ratios were 0.52 and 0.45. Both the C_q and C_0 ratios showed marked decreases due to the ACNU posttreatment (Table 3.12).

In the spheroids in which 20 or 40 μg/ml ACNU posttreatment was done (Fig. 3.57), in both cases biphasic survival curves were seen, as was the case with ACNU pretreatment. When 20 μg/ml ACNU posttreatment was carried out, the $_1C_0$ ratio with respect to treatment with 5-FU alone was 1.79; it was 0.89 with 40 μg/ml ACNU posttreatment. The $_2C_0$ ratios were 1.09 and 0.44, respectively. The RF values were 0.75 when 5-FU alone was used, 0.38 when there was 20 μg/ml ACNU posttreatment, and 0.23 with 40 μg/ml ACNU posttreatment (Table 3.13).

Concentration-Survival Curves for ACNU Combined with a Fixed Concentration of 5-FU

Treatment with ACNU before 5-FU. Study was made of the effects of ACNU treatment alone and ACNU combined with 5 or 25 μg/ml 5-FU posttreatment in monolayer cells (Fig. 3.58). In both cases, a shoulder extended up to 30–40 μg/ml ACNU, after which there were exponential decreases in the SF together with increasing ACNU concentrations. With regard to the C_0 ratios relative to treatment with ACNU alone, it was found that posttreatment with 5 or 25 μg/ml 5-FU gave C_0 ratios of 0.87 and 0.67, respectively. C_q ratios were 0.98 and 0.63. In other words,

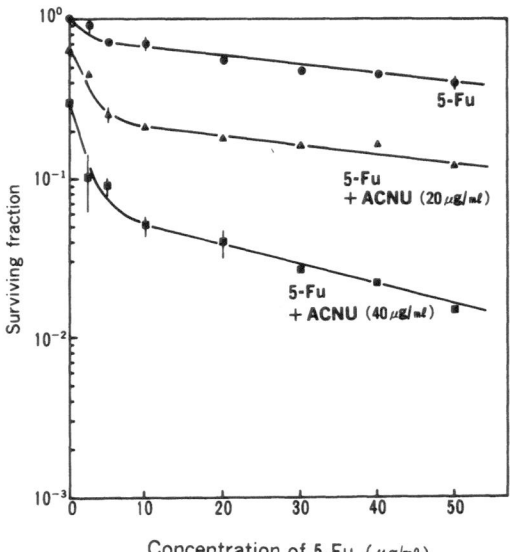

Fig. 3.57. Survival curves of RG C-6 cells in spheroids for 5-FU followed by treatment with a fixed concentration of ACNU (0.2 μg/ml, 40 μg/ml). The C_0 of the sensitive and resistant phases was decreased by combined treatment

Table 3.12. Survival parameters with graded concentrations of 5-FU for RG C-6 monolayer cells

	C_0 (μg/ml)	C_q (μg/ml)
5-FU alone	11.1 (1.0)	7.2 (1.0)
ACNU (30 μg/ml) + 5-FU	8.4 (0.76)	8.0 (1.12)
ACNU (60 μg/ml) + 5-FU	6.2 (0.56)*	6.0 (0.83)
5-FU alone	7.8 (1.0)	11.0 (1.0)
5-FU + ACNU (30 μg/ml)	4.7 (0.60)**	5.7 (0.52)*
5-FU + ACNU (60 μg/ml)	3.0 (0.39)**	5.0 (0.45)*

Figures in parentheses show relative values to 5-FU alone
Difference from 5-FU alone was significant at $P < 0.05$* and $P < 0.01$**

Table 3.13. Survival parameters with graded concentrations of 5-FU for RG C-6 cells in spheroids

	$_1C_0$ (μg/ml)	$_2C_0$ (μg/ml)	RF
5-FU alone	4.9 (1.0)	109.0 (1.0)	0.8
ACNU (20 μg/ml) + 5-FU	3.8 (0.78)	34.6 (0.32)*	0.69
ACNU (40 μg/ml) + 5-FU	2.5 (0.52)	31.5 (0.29)*	0.23*
5-FU alone	1.4 (1.0)	75.8 (1.0)	0.75
5-FU + ACNU (20 μg/ml)	2.5 (1.79)	82.6 (1.09)	0.38*
5-FU + ACNU (40 μg/ml)	1.3 (0.89)	33.3 (0.44)*	0.23*

Figures in parentheses show relative values to 5-FU alone
Difference from 5-FU alone was significant at $P < 0.05$*

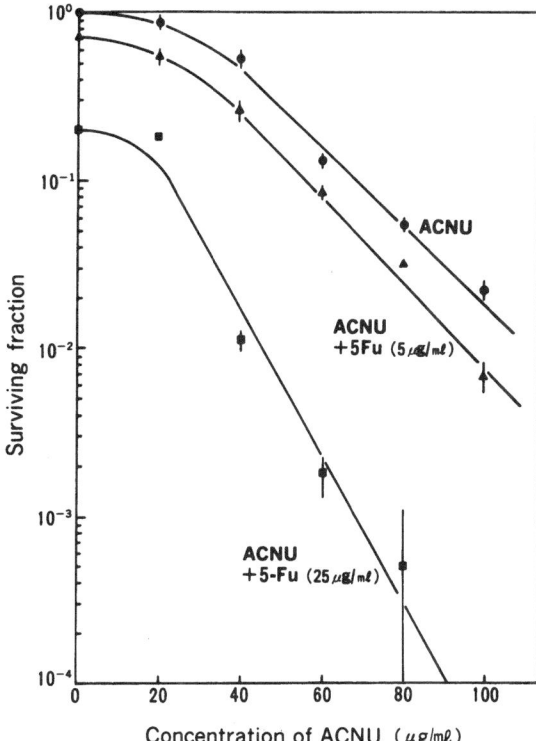

Fig. 3.58. Survival curves of RG C-6 cells in monolayer for ACNU followed by a fixed concentration of 5-FU (0.5 μg/ml, 25 μg/ml). The C_0 and C_q were decreased by combined treatment with 25 μg/ml of 5-FU but were unchanged for cells in the monolayer by combination with 5 μg/ml 5-FU

there were decreases in both C_0 values and C_q values due to the 5-FU posttreatment (Table 3.14).

Study was also made of the effects of 5 or 25 μg/ml 5-FU posttreatment in the spheroids (Fig. 3.59). In both cases, a shoulder extended up to the ACNU concentrations of 20–30 μg/ml, after which there were exponential decreases in SF values with increasing ACNU concentrations. The C_0 values relative to ACNU treatment alone were found to be 1.06 for 5 μg/ml 5-FU posttreatment and 0.91 for 25 μg/ml. The C_q ratios were 0.55 and 0.52, respectively. In other words, much stronger effects were obtained on C_q values than on C_0 values due to 5-FU posttreatment (Table 3.14).

Treatment with ACNU after 5-FU. In the monolayer cells, study was made of the effects of pretreatment with 5 μg/ml 5-FU, followed by ACNU (Fig. 3.60). The C_0 and C_q ratios relative to treatment with ACNU alone were 0.30 and 1.18, respectively. The decrease in the C_0 value due to 5-FU pretreatment was remarkable and was a larger decrease than when 5-FU posttreatment was employed (Table 3.14).

A similar study was made on the effects of 5 μg/ml 5-FU pretreatment on the spheroids (Fig. 3.61). The C_0 and C_q ratios of combined ACNU and 5-FU treatment, relative to those of ACNU alone, were 0.82 and 0.56, respectively. As is evident from these findings, in both the monolayer cells and the spheroids the effects of combined ACNU and 5 μg/ml 5-FU treatment were stronger when 5-FU was given before ACNU (Table 3.14).

Table 3.14. Survival parameters for graded concentration of ACNU for RG C-6 cells

	Monolayer		Spheroid	
	C_0 (μg/ml)	C_q (μg/ml)	C_0 (μg/ml)	C_q (μg/ml)
ACNU alone	19.2 (1.0)	24.9 (1.0)	14.0 (1.0)	12.0 (1.0)
ACNU + 5-FU (5 μg/ml)	16.7 (0.87)	24.5 (0.98)	14.9 (1.06)	6.6 (0.55)
ACNU + 5-FU (25 μg/ml)	12.9 (0.67)*	15.4 (0.63)*	12.7 (0.91)	6.2 (0.52)
ACNU alone	22.5 (1.0)	11.0 (1.0)	14.0 (1.0)	12.0 (1.0)
5-FU (5 μg/ml) + ACNU	8.2 (0.36)**	12.5 (1.18)	11.5 (0.82)	6.7 (0.56)

Figures in parentheses show relative values to 5-FU alone
Difference from ACNU alone was significant at $P < 0.05$* and $P < 0.01$**

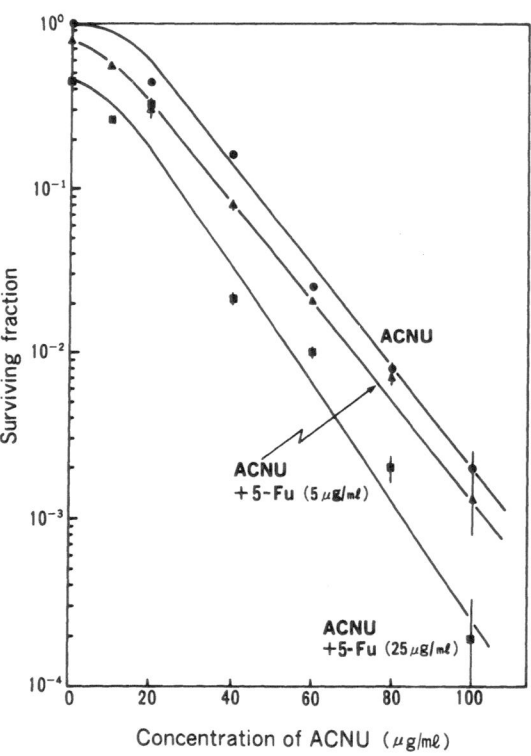

Fig. 3.59. Survival curves of RG C-6 cells in spheroids for ACNU followed by a fixed concentration of 5-FU (0.5 μg/ml, 25 μg/ml)

From the point of view of the cell kinetics, which is responsible for the combined effects, two mechanisms of action of ACNU and 5-FU are considered to be of possible relevance. The first is that there is an accumulation of proliferating cells at the G_1/S boundary as a of result of 5-FU treatment [10, 28, 114] and the second is that there are greater cell killing effects of ACNU during the interval between the G_1 phase and the early S phase [5, 43]. Combined administration of these drugs is, therefore, thought likely to lead to increased cell killing. This hypothesis is also

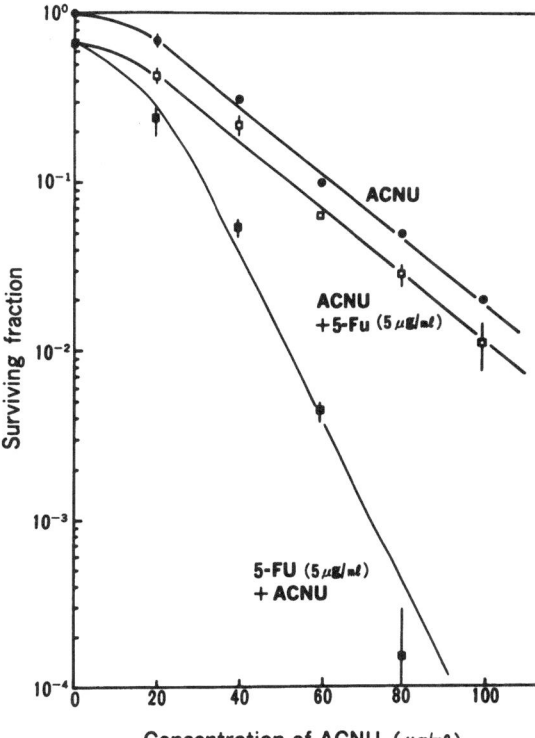

Fig. 3.60. Survival curves of RG C-6 cells in monolayer for ACNU with combined treatment by a fixed concentration of 5-FU (5 μg/ml). The C_0 for cells in the monolayer was decreased by the combined treatment by 5-FU before ACNU

supported by the fact that higher concentrations of these drugs in exponentially growing monolayer cells (where quiescent cells are not present) have greater killing effects. There is also the possibility that the ACNU inhibits the repair of the 5-FU-induced damage; in any event, these questions require further study. When ACNU pretreatment is carried out, there is a clear increase in the cell-killing effects with higher 5-FU concentrations. The possible mechanisms of action for these effects are thought to be as follows: ACNU blocks the transition of the cell cycle from the S phase to the G_2 phase [5, 43] and there is a high concentration of lethal effects on cells in the S phase [11, 12, 88].

In the 5-FU concentration-survival curve, two phases were always observed, regardless of the order of ACNU and 5-FU administration. Comparison of the RF values from these survival curves shows that there were marked decreases in RF values due to ACNU combined treatment, regardless of which drug was given first. These findings are thought to indicate the possibility that ACNU has lethal effects even on 5-FU-resistant cells lying in the deep layers of spheroids (i.e., quiescent cells). The fact that the effects of ACNU are stronger in the deeper layers than in the surface layers of spheroids [48] is evidence of the validity of this perspective. Moreover, the fact that, in the ACNU concentration-survival curves, the effects were greater for the spheroids than the monolayer cells supports the idea that ACNU has strong effects not only on proliferating cells but also on quiescent cells.

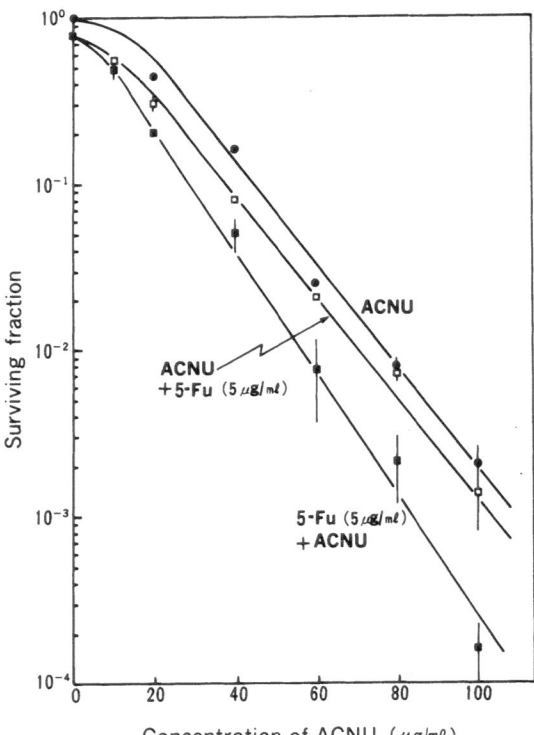

Fig. 3.61. Survival curves of RG
C-6 in spheroids for ACNU with
combined treatment by a fixed
concentration of 5-FU (5 μg/ml)

Isobologram Analysis

As discussed above, since enhanced effects were obtained for cells of both the
monolayer and spheroids using combined ACNU and 5-FU treatment, isobologram analysis [20, 90] was performed when ACNU was used 24 h after pretreatment
with 5-FU. The isobolograms illustrate the isoeffect levels of SF at 0.01 and 0.1 and
are shown in Figs. 3.62 and 3.63. At an SF of 0.01, the combined therapy produced
supra-additive effects in both the monolayer and the spheroids. It can be seen that
particularly strong enhancements were found at low 5-FU concentrations combined with high ACNU concentrations. At an isoeffect level of SF = 0.1, there were
also supra-additive effects when the 5-FU concentration was 5 μg/ml, although
those for the spheroids was small.

Figure 3.64 shows the enhancement ratio, which is the concentration of 5-FU
alone required for a certain effect (as obtained from Figs. 3.56 and 3.57) divided by
the concentration needed for the same effect (isoeffect) when ACNU and 5-FU are
administered in combination. It can be seen that a higher range of enhancement
ratios was obtained for the spheroids than for the monolayer cells. The range was an
ACNU concentration of 10–35 μg/ml and a 5-FU concentration of 2–15 μg/ml [48].
It has previously been reported that in combined chemotherapy the effects are
generally stronger on monolayer cells than on spheroids [70, 83, 96]. The effects of
combined therapy with 5-FU and ACNU in the present experiment thus were of
particular interest.

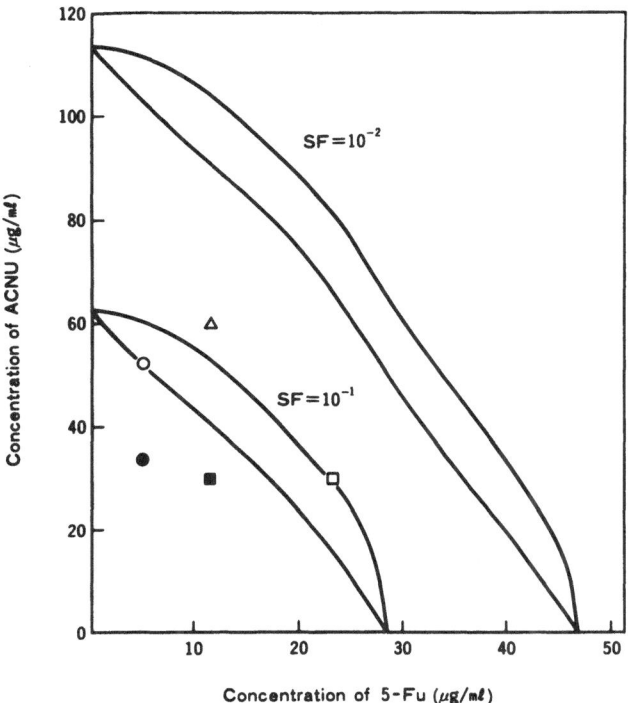

Fig. 3.62. Isobolograms of RG C-6 cells in monolayer for ACNU treatment following 24-h administration of 5-FU were constructed from Figs. 3.56, 3.57, 3.60, 3.61 for the isoeffect levels of the surviving fraction at 0.01 and 0.1, where an additive envelope was surrounded by a curve when two drugs acted independently and by a curve when two drugs interacted additively. *Symbols* in combined treatment of (o, ●) are from Fig. 3.60 for monolayer and from Fig. 3.61 for spheroid. The *symbols* △, ▲, □, ■ are from Fig. 3.56 for monolayer and from Fig. 3.57 for spheroid

Time-Survival Curves for 5-FU Treatment Followed by 2-h ACNU Posttreatment

The monolayer cells were treated with 5 μg/ml 5-FU for various lengths of time, followed immediately by 10 μg/ml ACNU treatment. Enhanced effects were already apparent within the short period of 1-2 h of 5-FU pretreatment, and these effects increased with time. After about 12 h, a constant surviving fraction was obtained (Fig. 3.65).

Using the spheroids, similar enhancement was again seen within 1–2 h of the 5-FU pretreatment. A transient plateau was found between 4 and 10 h, after which there were further decreases in the surviving fraction with prolongation of the 5-FU treatment (Fig. 3.66).

Effect of Time Intervals Between 5-FU and ACNU Treatment

In the monolayer cells, 60 μg/ml ACNU was given at intervals ranging from 1 to 24 h after 24-h treatment with 5 μg/ml 5-FU. The longer the duration between

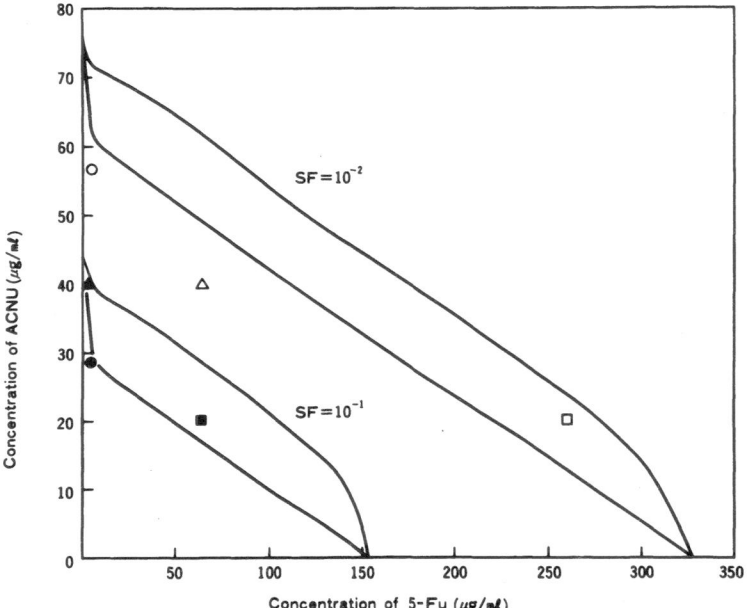

Fig. 3.63. Isobolograms of RG C-6 cells in spheroids for ACNU treatment following 24-h administration of 5-FU. For explanation, see legend to Fig. 3.62

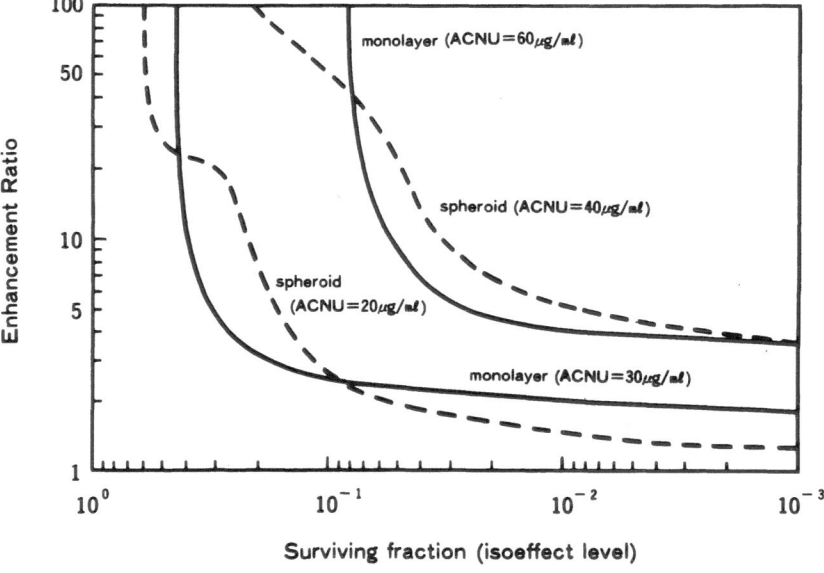

Fig. 3.64. Enhancement ratio defined in the text was plotted for RG C-6 cells in both monolayer and spheroids at various levels of the surviving fraction shown in the *abscissa*. Data were calculated from Figs. 3.56, 3.57

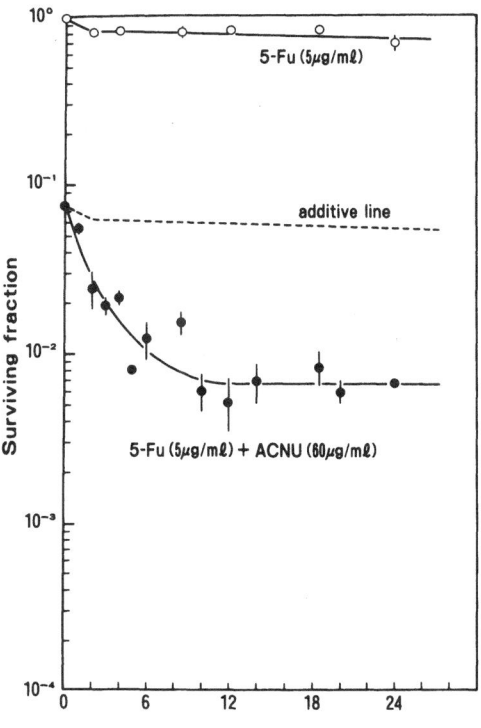

Fig. 3.65. Time-survival curve of RG C-6 cells in monolayer treated with 5-FU (5 μg/ml) followed by treatment with ACNU (60 μg/ml). The *broken line* represents the additive level calculated by the product of the surviving fraction with ACNU alone (2 h) and that with 5-FU alone

treatments, the smaller were the final effects, and after 16 h the surviving fraction had risen to above the level of the additive effects. Increases in the surviving fraction showed cyclicity with peaks at around 4 and 10 h (Fig. 3.67).

A similar study was done using the spheroids. Decreases in the lethal effects were seen with increases in the interval between treatments, but in comparison with the monolayer cells the surviving fraction increased to the additive range in a short period of time (Fig. 3.68).

Effects of ACNU on Recovery from Potentially Lethal 5-FU Damage

A study of the monolayer cells using three distinct groups: (a) those treated with 12.5 μg/ml 5-FU for 24 h and then returned to the fresh culture medium, where cells were trypsinized at various times; (b) those treated with 5-FU, immediately treated with 40 μg/ml ACNU, and then trypsinized at various times; and (c) those returned to fresh culture medium after 2-h ACNU treatment, after which the cells were trypsinized at various times. When the cells were returned to culture medium after 5-FU treatment, there were steady increases in the surviving fraction for about 6 h, after which a plateau level was reached. An increase over time was also seen in terms of the number of surviving cells per dish. This is thought to indicate recovery from potentially lethal 5-FU damage. In contrast, among those cells given ACNU treatment, there was a decrease in the surviving fraction, but even when they were

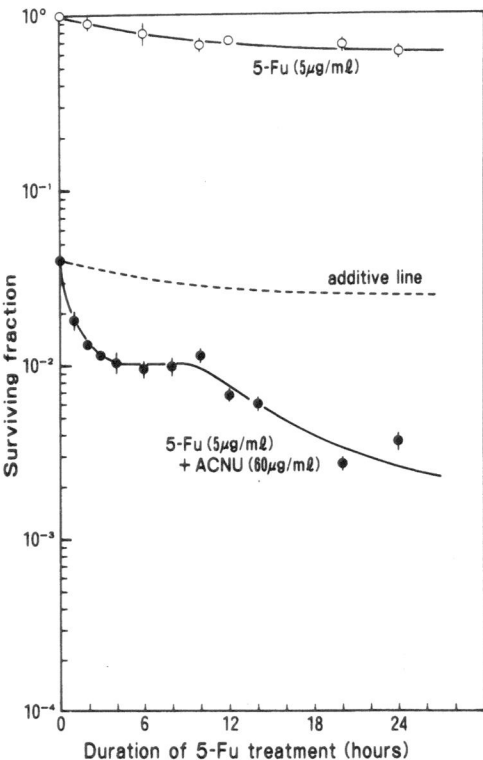

Fig. 3.66. Time-survival curve of RG C-6 cells in spheroids treated with 5-FU (5 μg/ml) followed by treatment with ACNU (60 μg/ml). The *broken line* represents the additive level calculated by the product of the surviving fraction with ACNU alone (2 h) and that with 5-FU alone

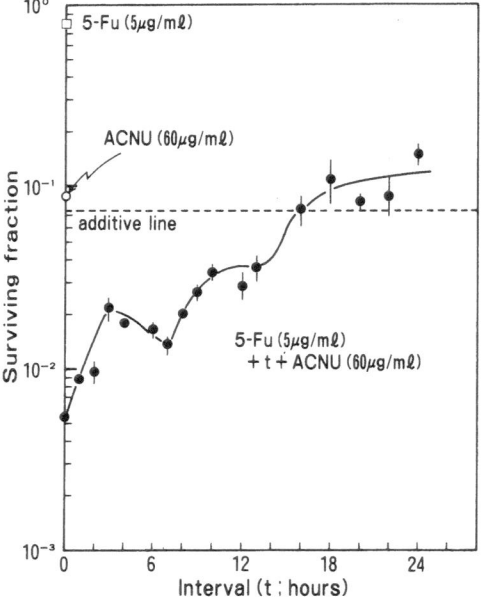

Fig. 3.67. Time-survival curve of RG C-6 cells in monolayer for 24-h treatment with 5-FU (5 μg/ml) followed by 2-h treatment with ACNU (60 μg/ml). The drug-free interval of the two treatments, 0–24 h, is shown in the *abscissa*

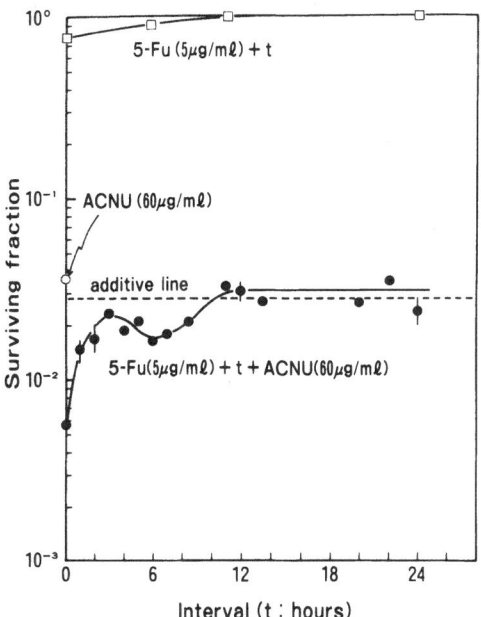

Fig. 3.68. Time-survival curve of RG C-6 cells in spheroids for 24-h treatment with 5-FU (5 μg/ml) followed by 2-h treatment with ACNU (60 μg/ml). The drug-free interval of two treatments, 0–24 h, is shown in the *abscissa*

returned to fresh culture medium after 2-h treatment by ACNU, there were no increases in the surviving fraction or the surviving cell count, suggesting that ACNU inhibits recovery from 5-FU-induced PLD (Fig. 3.69).

In the spheroids, a similar experiment was done using 50 μg/ml 5-FU and again ACNU was found to inhibit recovery from 5-FU-induced PLD (Fig. 3.70).

Variations in Cell Survival As a Function of Depth from Spheroid Surface

Experiments were done using 60 μg/ml ACNU, 50 μg/ml 5-FU, and the two drugs combined (Fig. 3.71). Sequential trypsinization was performed by transferring about 50 spheroids after drug treatment to 30 ml Erlenmeyer flasks, adding 3 ml 0.1% trypsin and 0.04% Versene solution, and shaking for 5 min at 18°–20°C. The supernatant containing single cells was then removed and treated as one fraction. These procedures were repeated nine times and single-cell suspensions for layers of various depth were prepared and plated for colony assay.

5-FU was found to have preferential effects on some 20%–30% of the cells of the first few superficial layers of the spheroids but to have much weaker effects on the deeper layers. In contrast, ACNU had greater effects on the deeper layers than on the superficial layers. This suggests that ACNU has its effects not only on proliferating cells but also on quiescent cells. These findings are in accord with reports on preferential cell killing by BCNU for noncycling Q cells [34, 39] and on a preferential cell killing in the deeper layers of spheroids by several nitrosoureas [53].

When ACNU treatment was done after 5-FU treatment, effects which were almost homogenous were obtained in both superficial and deep layers. Comparison of the effects of both drugs with the level calculated from the expected additive level showed that the effect was more than additive for the deeper layers of the spheroids.

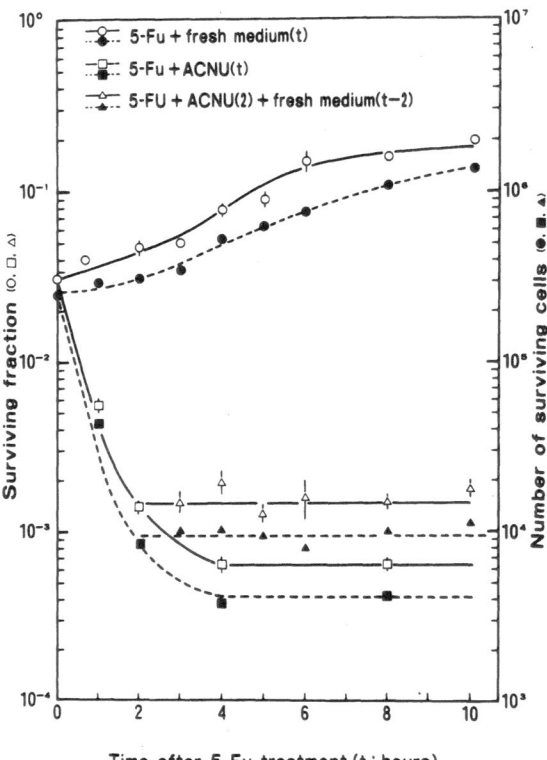

Fig. 3.69. Recovery from potentially lethal 5-FU damage (PLD recovery) and the effect of ACNU on the PLD recovery. RG C-6 cells in monolayer were treated with 5-FU for 24 h followed by treatment with fresh medium or fresh medium containing ACNU (for 2 h followed by fresh medium, or for the entire remaining period). *Solid lines* show the surviving fraction and *broken lines* show the number of surviving cells per dish

Discussion of Combination of 5-FU and ACNU

Surgery and radiotherapy have long been the principal therapeutic techniques for malignant glioma, but both techniques have the disadvantage of being most suitable for localized tumors. As supplementary therapies, chemotherapy and immunotherapy have been employed and therapeutic results have consequently improved [105]. The role of chemotherapy has, however, continued to become increasingly important. Since the 1970 report of Wilson et al. [116] on the effective BCNU treatment of malignant glioma, reports have appeared on the effectiveness of various nitrosoureas, such as BCNU, CCNU, and MeCCNU [26, 75, 109]. In Japan as well, ACNU (which was developed in 1974) [2] has come into widespread use and favorable clinical results have been reported [37, 62, 101, 105]. To obtain increased drug effects and because of the known tumor cell heterogeneity of drug sensitivity, combined drug therapy using two, three, or more drugs with different mechanisms of action has been actively pursued [105] in place of therapy with a single drug. In

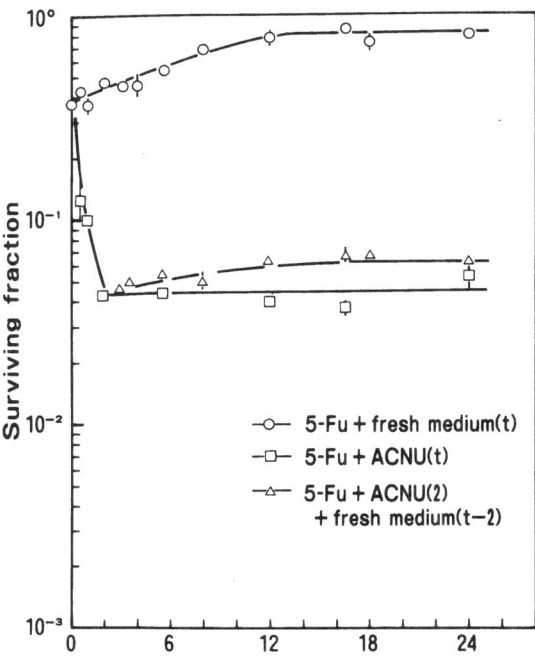

Fig. 3.70. Recovery from potentially lethal 5-FU damage (PLD recovery) of RG C-6 cells in the spheroids and the effect of ACNU on the PLD recovery

Time after 5-Fu treatment (t ; hours)

1972, Fewer et al. [25] reported good results using combined therapy with BCNU and vincristine against malignant gliomas and further improvement in clinical results using combined therapy has since been reported [32, 55–57].

With regard to combined therapy for malignant glioma using nitrosoureas and 5-FU, in 1978 Levin et al. [57] reported favorable outcomes in 24 of 29 cases of recurrent malignant glioma using BCNU and 5-FU. In Japan, improvements in therapeutic results using ACNU and 5-FU have also been reported [47, 59, 100]. In addition basic studies using nitrosoureas and 5-FU have been performed [17, 85, 97, 110]. Gerosa et al. [29] found an increased survival time as a result of BCNU and 5-FU therapy after intracerebral transplantation of 9L cells. For these reasons, it is thought that combined therapy using nitrosoureas and 5-FU is an effective means of treating malignant glioma cases. Firm conclusions about the most appropriate methods for combined therapy, however, have not yet been reached.

In the experiments reported above, it is particularly noteworthy that in the combined ACNU and 5-FU therapy, greater effects were obtained in the spheroids than in the exponentially growing monolayer cells. In combined drug techniques, the effects on the tumor tissue are of course the most important, but the damage caused to normal tissue must also be considered. In other words, the appropriateness of the combined technique should be determined from the perspective of how much more effective the therapy is against tumor tissue than against normal tissue. Since, from the perspective of cell kinetics, there are many similarities between exponentially growing monolayer cells and normal tissues, such as bone marrow

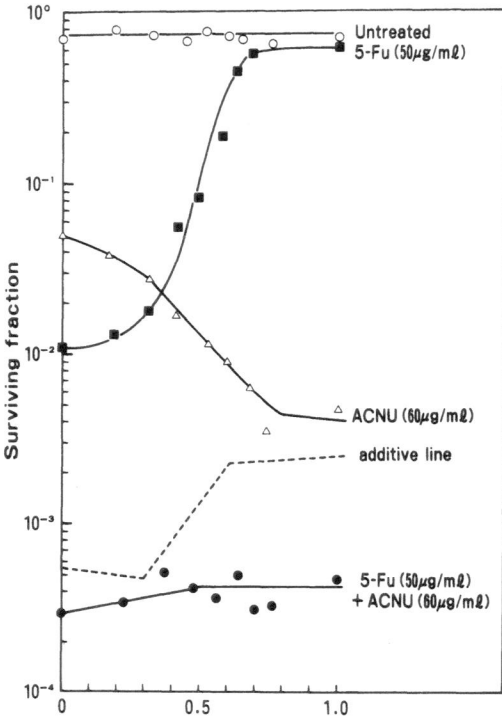

Fig. 3.71. Cell survival of RG C-6 cells as a function of cell fraction (depth into spheroid) from the spheroid surface in untreated controls, 24-h treatment with 5-FU (50 μg/ml), 2-h treatment with ACNU (60 μg/ml), and combined treatment with 5-FU and ACNU

and intestinal tissues (i.e., rapidly proliferating tissues which are often acutely damaged in therapy), it is essential that a combined therapeutic technique be found in which the effects on spheroids exceed those on exponentially growing monolayer cells [80]. In light of the experimental findings reported above, in which a greater combined effect was found in the spheroids over the monolayer cells at a concentration range where either ACNU alone or 5-FU alone showed smaller effects on cells, we believe that this combined therapeutic technique should have significant clinical implications.

Conclusion

From the mid-1970s combined radio- and chemotherapy has been widely used for the treatment of brain tumors, particularly malignant glioma, and therapeutic results have thus improved. However, together with the greater effectiveness of such therapy with regard to the tumor tissue itself, there have also been greater deleterious effects on normal tissues. Such side effects, particularly myelosuppression, remain the greatest single obstacle to the successful treatment of brain tumors. As a consequence, it is desirable that new therapeutic techniques be developed which have enhanced effects on brain tumor tissue and, moreover, act selectively on the tumor tissue. Currently, various new techniques are under development along these lines, including altered time-dose fractionation in radiotherapy, radiotherapy using radiations of high linear-energy-transfer, clinical applications of monoclonal antibodies, and new drugs for chemotherapy.

In summary, we found that in combined therapy using radiotherapy and ACNU, radiotherapy and 5-FU, or ACNU and 5-FU, greater effects can be obtained for cells in spheroids than in exponentially growing monolayers. These findings are of particular interest since they indicate the possibility that the effects will occur selectively on tumor tissue rather than on normal tissue. Based upon these experimental results, we have devised a therapeutic regimen using the combined therapies of radiotherapy, ACNU, and 5-FU and have thus far obtained favorable results. Follow-up studies are in progress.

References

1. Acker H (1984) Microenvironmental conditions in multicellular spheroids grown under liquid-overlay tissue culture conditions. Recent results in cancer research, spheroids in cancer research. Springer, Berlin—Heidelberg—New York—Tokyo, pp 116–133
2. Arakawa M, Shimizu F, Okada N (1974) Effect of 1-(4-amino-2-methyl-5-pyrimidinyl) methyl-3-(chloroethyl)-3-nitrosourea hydrochloride on leukemia L-1210. Jpn J Cancer Res 65: 191
3. Arima S, Kimura M, Shimizu H (1978) The density in blood and organ of N_1-(2-tetrahydrofuryl)-5-fluorouracil (FT-207) administered in rectum. Jpn J Cancer Clin 24: 613–617 (in Japanese)
4. Asamura M, Kanamaru R, Sato H, Saito T (1977) Mechanism of ACNU treatment. Saishin-Igaku 32: 1417–1419 (in Japanese)
5. Asamura M, Saito T (1978) Cell synchronization and chemotherapy of cancer. Jpn J Cancer Chemother 5: 737–746 (in Japanese)
6. Barranco SC, Novak JK, Humphrey RM (1973) Response of mammalian cells following treatment with bleomycin and 1, 3-bis(2-chloroethyl)-1-nitrosourea during plateau phase. Cancer Res 33: 691–694
7. Benda P, Leightbody J, Sato G, Levin L, Sweet WH (1968) Differentiated rat glial cell strain in tissue culture. Science 161: 370–371
8. Benda P, Someda K, Messer J, Sweet WH (1971) Morphological and immunological studies of rat glial tumors and clonal strains propagated in culture. J Neurosurg 34: 310–323
9. Berry RJ (1966) Effect of metabolic inhibition on X-ray dose response curve for the survival of mammalian cells in vitro, and on early recovery between fractionated X-ray doses. Br J Radiol 39: 458–463
10. Bhuyan BK, Blowers CL, Neil GL, Bono VH, Day KJ (1977) Partial synchronization of L 1210 cells by 5-fluorouracil and its use in drug combinations. Cancer Res 37: 3204–3208
11. Bhuyan BK, Fraser TJ, Day KJ (1977) Cell proliferation kinetics and drug sensitivity of exponential and stationary populations of cultured L 1210 cells. Cancer Res 37: 1057–1963
12. Bhuyan BK, Scheidt LG, Fraser TJ (1972) Cell-cycle phase specificity of antitumor agents. Cancer Res 32: 398–407
13. Brown JM (1979) Evidence for acutely hypoxic cells in mouse tumors, and a possible mechanism of reoxygenation. Br J Radiol 52: 650–656
14. Bruce WR, Meeker BE (1967) Comparison of the sensitivity of haematopoietic colony-forming cells in different proliferative status to 5-fluorouracil. J Nat Cancer Inst 38: 401–405

15. Byfield JE, Calabro-Jones P, Klisak I, Kulhanian F (1982) Pharmacologic requirements for obtaining sensitivity of human tumor cells in vitro to combined 5-fluorouracil or futoraful and X-ray. Int J Radiat Oncol Biol Phys 8: 1923–1933
16. Chaplin DJ, Olive PL, Durand RE (1987) Intermittent blood flow in a murine tumor: Radiobiological effects. Cancer Res 47: 597–601
17. Corbett TH, Griswold DP, Roberts BJ, Peckham JC, Schabel FM Jr (1977) Evaluation of single agents and combinations of chemotherapeutic agents in mouse colon carcinomas. Cancer 40: 2660–2680
18. Courtenay VD (1976) A soft agar colony assay for Lewis lung tumor and B16 melanoma taken directly from the mouse. Br J Cancer 34: 39–45
19. Deen DF, Hoshino T, Williams ME, Muraoka I, Knebel KE, Baker M (1980) Development of a 9L rat brain tumor cell multicellular spheroid system and its response to 1,3-bis(2-chloroethyl)-1-nitrosourea and radiation. J Nat Cancer Inst 64: 1373–1382
20. Deen DF, Williams ME (1979) Isobologram analysis of X-ray-BCNU interactions in vitro. Radiat Res 79: 483–491
21. Durand RE (1976) Cell cycle kinetics in an in vitro tumor model. Cell Tissue Kinet 9: 403–412
22. Durand RE, Biaglow JE (1977) Radiosensitization of hypoxic cells of an in vitro tumor model by respiratory inhibitors. Radiat Res 69: 359–366
23. Elkind MM, Sutton H (1960) Radiation response of mammalian cells grown in culture. I. Repair of X-ray damage in surviving chinese hamster cells. Radiat Res 13: 556–593
24. Elkind MM, Whitmors GF (1967) The radiobiology of cultured mammalian cells. Gordon and Breach, New York, pp 7–84
25. Fewer D, Wilson CB, Boldrey EB (1972) The chemotherapy of brain tumors, clinical experience with carmustine (BCNU) and vincristine. JAMA 222: 549–552
26. Fewer D, Wilson CB, Boldrey EB, Enot KJ (1972) A phase II study of 1-(2-chloroethyl)-3-cyclohexyl-1-nitrosourea (CCNU). Cancer Chemother Res 56: 421–427
27. Fletcher GH (1980) Textbook of radiotherapy, 3rd edn. Lea and Febiger, Philadelphia, pp 138–144
28. Fujita H, Ogawa K, Fukabe T, Kimura K (1972) Metabolism of N_1-(2'-tetrahydrofuryl)-5-fluorouracil (FT-207). Jpn J Cancer Clin 18: 917–922 (in Japanese)
29. Gerosa MA, Dougherty DV, Wilson CB, Rosenblum MR (1983) Improved treatment of a brain tumor model: II. Sequential therapy with BCNU and 5-fluorouracil. J Neurosurg 58: 368–373
30. Gerweck LE, Kornblith PL, Burlett P, Wang J, Sweight S (1977) Radiation sensitivity of cultured human glioblastoma. Radiol 125: 231–234
31. Gray LH (1957) Oxygenation in radiotherapy: I. Radiological consideration. Br J Radiol 30: 403–406
32. Gutin PH, Wilson CB, Kumar ARV, Boldrey EB, Levin VA, Powell M, Enot KJ (1975) Phase II study of procarbazine, CCNU and vincristine combination chemotherapy in the treatment of malignant brain tumors. Cancer 35: 1398–1404
33. Hahn GM (1973) Response of solid tumor cells exposed to chemotherapeutic agents in vivo: Cell survival after 2- and 24-hour exposure. J Nat Cancer Inst 50: 529–533
34. Hahn GM, Gordon LF, Kurkjian SD (1974) Response of cycling and noncycling cells to 1,3-bis(2-chloroethyl)-1-nitrosourea and bleomycin. Cancer Res 34: 2373–2379
35. Hall T (1958) Acute and chronic toxicity studies with 5-fluorouracil in man. Proc Am Ass Cancer Res 2: 305
36. Heal JM, Fox P, Schein PS (1979) A structure-activity study of seven new water soluble nitrosourea. Biochem Pharmacol 28: 1301–1306
37. Hori M, Nakagawa H, Hasegawa H (1978) Chemotherapy of malignant glioma with the new nitrosourea derivative (ACNU). Jpn J Cancer Chemother 5: 773–778 (in Japanese)
38. Hoshino T (1973) Cell kinetics of brain tumors. Brain and Nerve 1: 453–459 (in Japanese)

39. Hoshino T, Deen DF, Williams ME, Sano Y (1981) Differential response of elutriated 9L cells to treatment with 1, 3-bis-(2-chloroethyl)-1-nitrosourea. Cancer Res 41: 4404–4407

40. Inch WR, McCredie JA, Sutherland RM (1970) Growth of nodular carcinomas in rodents compared with multicell spheroids in tissue culture. Growth 34: 271–282

41. Jones AC, Stratford LJ, Wilson PA, Peckham MJ (1982) In vitro cytotoxic drug sensitivity testing of human tumor xenografts grown as multicellular tumor spheroids. Br J Cancer 46: 870–879

42. Kanazawa H, Miyamoto T (1983) Effect of ACNU, a water-soluble nitrosourea derivative, on survival and cell progression of cultured HeLa S_3 cells. Jpn J Cancer Chemother 10: 2007–2015 (in Japanese)

43. Kanamaru R, Asamura M, Sato H, Hayashi Y, Saito T, Saito S (1978) Studies on the effect of ACNU (1-(4-amino-2-methylpyrimidine-5-yl)methyl-3-(2-chloroethyl)-3-nitrosourea hydrochloride) for cultured HeLa S_3 cells. Kokenshi (Tohoku University) 30: 162–170 (in Japanese)

44. Kaneko S, Allen NJ, Clendenon NR, Kartha M (1983) Treatment schedule of combined radiation and ACNU in combination in experimental brain tumors. Neurol Med Chir (Tokyo) 23: 849–855 (in Japanese)

45. Kapp DS, Wagner FC, Lawrence R (1982) Glioblastoma multiforme: Treatment by large dose fraction irradiation and metronidazole. Int J Radiat Oncol Biol Phys 8: 351–355

46. Kaufman N, Bicher HI, Hetzel FW, Brown M (1981) A system for determining the pharmacology of indirect radiation sensitizer drugs on multicellular spheroids. Cancer Clin Trials 4: 199–204

47. Kawano H, Kubota T, Hayashi M (1986) Evaluation of ACNU and 5-Fu in the treatment of gliomas. Neurol Med Chir (Tokyo) 26: 140–146 (in Japanese)

48. Kitahara M, Katakura R, Mori T, Suzuki J, Sasaki T (1986) Combined effect of ACNU and 5-Fu on rat glioma cells in spheroids and monolayer. Int J Cancer 38: 215–222

49. Kitahara M, Katakura R, Mori T, Sazuki J, Sasaki T (1984) Combined effect of ACNU and 5-fluorouracil on spheroids of rat glioma cells. Neurol Med Chir (Tokyo) 24: 745–757 (in Japanese)

50. Kitahara M, Kuwahara K, Katakura R, Mori T, Suzuki J, Sasaki T (1983) Effect of combined therapy of ACNU and 5-Fu on multicellular spheroids—study of mechanisms and optimal administration. Proceedings of Japan Cancer Association, 42nd Annual Meeting, October 25 (Nagoya), p 228 (in Japanese)

51. Kogelnik HD, Karcher KH, Szepesi T Schratter AV (1982) High-dose irradiation and misonidazole in the treatment of malignant gliomas—A preliminary report. In: Kärcher KH, Kogelnik HD, Reinartz G (eds) Progress in radio-oncology II. Raven, New York, pp 189–195

52. Kovacs CJ, Hopkins HA, Evans MJ, Looney WB (1976) Changes in cellularity induced by radiation in a solid tumor. Int J Radiat Biol 30: 101–113

53. Kwok TT, Twentyman PR (1985) The relationship between tumour geometry and the response of tumour cells to cytotoxic drugs—An in vitro study using EMT6 multicellular spheroids. Int J Cancer 35: 675–682

54. Leenhouts HP, Chakwick KH (1980) An analysis of the interaction between two nitrosourea compounds and X-irradiation in rat brain tumor cells. Int J Radiat Biol 37: 169

55. Levin VA, Crafts DC, Wilson CB, Schultz RM, Boldrey EB, Enot KJ, Pischer TL, Seager ML, Elashoff RM (1976) BCNU and procarbazine treatment for malignant brain tumors. Cancer Treat Rep 60: 243–249

56. Levin VA, Edwards MS, Wright D, Seager ML, Pischer TL, Wilson CB (1980) Modified procarbazine, CCNU and vincristine (PCV 3) combination chemotherapy in the treatment of malignant brain tumors. Cancer Treat Rep 64: 231–241

57. Levin VA, Hoffman WF, Pischer TL, Seager ML, Boldrey EB, Wilson CB (1978)

BCNU-5-fluorouracil combination therapy for the recurrent malignant brain tumors. Cancer Treat Rep 62: 2071–2076

58. Madoc-Jones H, Bruce WR (1967) Sensitivity of L cells in exponential and stationary phase to 5-fluorouracil. Nature 215: 302–303

59. Matsumoto K, Tabuchi K, Furuta T (1983) Combined chemotherapy of ACNU and 5-Fu on malignant glioma. Neurol Med Chir (Tokyo) 23: 625–632 (in Japanese)

60. Mineura K, Mori T, Katakura R, Sasaki T (1981) Therapeutic effects of 1-(4-amino-2-methyl-5-pyrimidinyl)methyl-3-(2-chloroethyl)-3-nitrosourea hydrochloride (ACNU) and radiation on the rat glioma. Neurol Surg (Tokyo) 9: 257–265 (in Japanese)

61. Mori T, Mineura K, Katakura R (1979) A consideration on pharmacokinetics of a new water-soluble anti-tumor nitrosourea, ACNU, in patients with malignant brain tumor. Brain and Nerve 31: 601–606 (in Japanese)

62. Mori T, Mineura K, Katakura R (1979) Chemotherapy of malignant brain tumor by a water-soluble anti-tumor nitrosourea, ACNU. Neurol Med Chir (Tokyo) 19: 1157–1171 (in Japanese)

63. Moulder JE, Rocknell S (1984) Hypoxic fraction of solid tumors: Experimental technique, method of analysis, and a survey of existing data. Int J Radiat Oncol Biol Phys 10: 695–712

64. Muller-Klieser, Sutherland EM (1982) Oxygen tensions in multicell spheroid of two cell lines. Br J Cancer 45: 256–264

65. Nakamura K, Asami M, Kawada K (1979) Chromatographic studies on chemical desolation of carcinostatic nitrosourea. J Chromatogr 168: 221

66. Nakamura K, Asami M, Kawada K, Sasahara K (1977) Quantitative determination of ACNU (1-(4-amino-2-methyl-5-pyrimidinyl)methyl-3-(2-chloroethyl)-3-nitrosourea hydrochloride, a new water-soluble antitumor nitrosourea, in biological fluids and tissue of patients by high-performance liquid chromatography: I. Analytical method and pharamatokinetics. Ann Rep Sankyo Res Lab 29: 66 (in Japanese)

67. Nakamura T, Sasada M, Tashima M (1978) Mechanism of action of 1-(4-amino-2-methyl-pyrimidin-5-yl)methyl-3-(2-chloroethyl)-3-nitrosourea (ACNU) in leukemia cells. Jpn J Cancer Chemother 5: 971–1000 (in Japanese)

68. Nakajima Y, Miyamoto T, Tanabe M, Watanabe I (1979) Enhancement of mammalian cell killing by 5-fluorouracil in combination with X-ray. Cancer Res 39: 3763–3767

69. Nederman T, Carlsson J, Malqvist M (1981) Penetration of substances into tumor tissue—A methodological study on cellular spheroids. In Vitro. 17: 290–298

70. Nederman T (1984) Effects of vincristine and 5-fluorouracil on human glioma and thyroid cancer cell monolayers and spheroids. Cancer Res 44: 254–258

71. Ogawa T, Yoneda T, Sakuta M (1984) Activation of FT-207 to 5-Fu in cultured cells of human maxillary cancer (OKK). Proceedings of Japan Cancer Association, 43rd Annual Meeting, October 3 (Fukuoka), p 289 (in Japanese)

72. Paterson R (1963) The treatment of malignant disease by radiotherapy. Williams and Wilkins, Baltimore, pp 12–15

73. Phillips H (1973) Dye exclusion tests for cell viability. In: Kruse PF Jr, Patterson MK Jr (eds). Tissue culture, methods and applications. Academic, New York, pp 406–408

74. Phillips RA, Tolmach LJ (1966) Repair of potentially lethal damage in X-irradiated HeLa cells. Radiat Res 29: 413–432

75. Rosenblum ML, Reynolds AF, Smith KA, Rumack BH, Walker MD (1973) Chloro-ethyl-cyclohexyl-nitrosourea (CCNU) in the treatment of malignant brain tumors. J Neurosurg 39: 306–314

76. Sakamoto K (1976) Reoxygenation of tumor. Jpn J Cancer Clin 22: 116–119 (in Japanese)

77. Sakamoto K (1974) Radiological significance and limitation of hyperbaric oxygen radiotherapy. Jpn J Cancer Clin 20: 56–58 (in Japanese)

78. Sakamoto K (1978) Radiobiology of cancer. Chugai-Igakusha, Tokyo, pp 115–118 (in Japanese)

79. Sasaki T (1981) Implication of tumor cell kinetics in radiotherapy and radiobiology.

Jpn J Cancer Clin 27: 1507–1515 (in Japanese)

80. Sasaki T (1983) Therapeutic ratio in combined radiochemotherapy—Radiobiological consideration. Jpn J Cancer Clin 29: 1584–1593 (in Japanese)
81. Sasaki T, Sakka M (1981) Implication of thymidine labelling index in the growth kinetics of human solid tumors. Jpn J Cancer Res 72: 181–188
82. Sasaki T, Sato Y, Sakka M (1980) Cell population kinetics of human solid tumors: A statistical analysis in various histological types. Jpn J Cancer Res 71: 520–529
83. Sasaki T, Yamamoto M, Kuwahara K (1984) Lethal effect of bleomycin and peplomycin on HeLa cells in multicell tumor spheroids. Cancer Res 44: 1374–1379
84. Sasaki T (1984) Utilization of cultured solid tumor model (spheroid) on tumor-biological research. Radiobiol Res 19: 195–208 (in Japanese)
85. Schabel FM Jr, Laster WR Jr, Trader MW, Corbett TH, Griswold DP Jr (1981) Combination chemotherapy with nitrosourea plus other anticancer drugs against animal tumors. In: Prostayko AW, Grooke ST, Baker LH, Carter SK, Schein PS (eds) Nitrosourea—current status and new development. Academic, New York, pp 9–26
86. Sheldon PW, Foster JL, Fowler JF (1974) Radiosensitization of C_3H mouse mammary tumours by a 2-nitroimidazole drugs. Br J Cancer 30: 560–565
87. Shitara N, Kohno T, Nagamune A, Takakura K, Sano K (1978) Pulse-cytophotometric studies on experimental brain tumor under the effect of chemotherapeutic agents, microwave irradiation and hyperthermia. Neurol Med Chir (Tokyo) 18: 199–207 (in Japanese)
88. Skipper HE, Schabel FM Jr, Mellet LB, Montgomery JA, Welkoft LJ, Lloid HH, Brockman RW (1970) Implication of biochemical, cytokinetic, pharmacologic and toxicologic relationships in the design of optimal therapeutic schedules. Cancer Chemother 54: 431–450
89. Steel GG (1977) Growth kinetics of tumors. Clarendon, Oxford, pp 23, 24
90. Steel GG (1979) The conceptual basis for the combined uses of radiotherapy and chemotherapy. Radiat Res, Proceedings of 6th International Congress Radiat Res, Tokyo, pp 804–809
91. Steel GG, Pekham MJ (1979) Exploitable mechanism in combined radiotherapy-chemotherapy: the concept of additivity. Int J Radiat Oncol Biol Phy 5: 85–91
92. Sugiyama S, Mori T, Suzuki J, Sasaki T (1984) Lethal effect of X-ray and ACNU on cultured rat glioma cells in multicellular spheroids. Neurol Med Chir (Tokyo) 24: 758–766 (in Japanese)
93. Sugiyama S, Mori T, Suzuki J, Sasaki T (1985) Effects of combined treatment of X-ray and ACNU on rat glioma cells in monolayer and multicellular spheroids. Neurol Med Chir (Tokyo) 25: 707–714 (in Japanese)
94. Sutherland RM, McCredie JA, Inch WR (1971) Growth of multicell spheroids in tissue culture as a model of nodular carcinomas. J Nat Cancer Inst 46: 113–120
95. Sutherland RM, Durand RE (1976) Radiation response of multicell spheroids. An in vitro tumor model. Curr Top Radiat Res Q 11: 87–139
96. Sutherland RM, Eddy HA, Bareham B, Reich K, Banantwerp D (1979) Resistance to adriamycin in multicellular spheroids. Int J Radiat Oncol Biol Phys 5: 1225–1230
97. Sutton JE, Roos IAG, Hillcoat BL (1982) Combined actions of 5-fluorouracil and 1-(2-chloroethyl)-3-(4-methylcyclohexyl)-1-nitrosourea on human colonic carcinoma cells in vitro. Cancer Res 42: 5172–5175
98. Suzuki M, Hori K, Abe I, Saito S, Sato H (1981) A new approach to cancer chemotherapy: Selective enchancement of tumor blood flow with angiotensine II. J Nat Cancer Inst 67: 663–669
99. Suzuki M, Mori T, Watanabe T, Katakura R, Suzuki J, Wada T (1983) Combined radio-chemo-immunotherapy (RAFP therapy) for medulloblastoma. Neurol Surg (Tokyo) 11: 1271–1276 (in Japanese)
100. Takakura K, Shitara N, Kohno T, Yamamoto H, Sano K (1979) Cell cycle of brain tumor cells and its combined therapy. Jpn J Cancer Chemother 6: 31–40
101. Takakura K, Abe H, Tanaka R, Kitamura K, Miwa T, Takeuchi K, Yamamoto S,

Kageyama N, Handa H, Mogami H, Nishimoto A, Uozumi T, Matsutani M, Nomura K (1986) Effects of ACNU and radiotherapy on malignant glioma. J Neurosurg 64: 53–57

102. Tamura M, Inoue H, Yamasaki H, Kawafuchi J, Niibe H (1983) Evaluation of high dose radiotherapy (500 rads twice weekly) in cerebral glioblastoma. Neurol Med Chir (Tokyo) 23: 192–197 (in Japanese)

103. Tannock IF (1972) Oxygen diffusion and the distribution of cellular radiosensitivity in tumors. Br J Radiol 45: 515–524

104. Terashima T, Taolmach LJ (1961) Changes in X-ray sensitivity of HeLa cells during the division cycle. Nature (London) 190: 1210–1211

105. The committee of brain tumor registry in Japan (1984) Brain Tumor Registry in Japan, vol 5, Tokyo

106. Thomlinson RH, Gray LH (1955) The histological structure of some human lung cancers and the possible implications for radiotherapy. Br J Cancer 9: 539–549

107. Tobey RA, Crissman HA (1975) Comparative effects of three nitrosourea derivatives on mammalian cell cycle progression. Cancer Res 35: 460–470

108. Toide H, Unemi N, Kawaguchi Y, Taira K (1977) Studies of the mechanism of action of FT-207. Chemother 25: 385–391 (in Japanese)

109. Tranum BL, Haut A, Rivkin E, Quagliana JM, Shaw M, Tucker WG, Smith FE, Samson M, Gattlieb J (1975) A phase II study of methyl CCNU in the treatment of solid tumors and lymphomas: A southwest oncology group study. Cancer 35: 1148–1153

110. Valeriote FA, Bruce WR, Meeder BE (1968) Synergistic action of cyclophosphamide on a transplanted murine lymphoma. J Nat Cancer Inst 40: 935–944

111. Vaupel PW, Frink S, Bicher HI (1981) Heterogenous oxygen partial pressure and pH distribution in C3H mouse mammary adenocarcinoma. Cancer Res 41: 2008–2013

112. Wallen CA, Michaelson S, Wheel KT (1980) Evidence for an unconventional radiosensitivity of rat 9L subcutaneous tumors. Radiat Res 84: 529–541

113. Wharam MD, Phillips TL, Kane L, Utley JF (1973) Response of murine solid tumor to in vivo combined chemotherapy and irradiation. Radiol 109: 451–455

114. Wheeler GP, Bowdon BJ, Adamson DJ, Vali MH (1972) Comparison of the effects of several inhibitors of the synthesis of nucleic acids upon the viability and progression through the cell cycle of cultured H. Ep. No. 2 cells. Cancer Res 32: 2661–2669

115. Wheeler KT, Levin VA, Deen DF (1978) The concept of drug dose for in vitro studies with chemotherapeutic agents. Radiat Res 76: 441–458

116. Wilson CB, Boldrey EB, Enot KJ (1970) BCNU [1,3-bis-2-(chloroethyl)-1-nitrosourea] in the treatment of brain tumors. Cancer Chemother Rep 54: 273–281

117. Yuhas JM, Li AP, Martines AO, Landman AJ (1977) A simplified method for production and growth of multicellular spheroids. Cancer Res 37: 3639–3643

Chapter 4

The Pharmacokinetics of ACNU in Patients with Malignant Brain Tumor

T. MORI

Introduction

ACNU [1-(4-amino-2-methyl pyrimidine-5-yl)-methyl-3-(2-chloroethyl)-3-nitroso-urea hydrochloride] is a water-solube nitrosourea anticancer agent which has been developed in Japan [1, 16]. It contains nitroso (-NO), alkyl (R-CH$_2$-), and carbamoyl (R-N-CO) ligands in common with lipid-soluble nitrosoureas (NU), such as 1-(2-chloroethyl)-3-cyclohexyl-1-nitrosourea (CCNU) [5, 6, 9, 15, 20], 1,3-bis(2-chloroethyl)-1-nitrosourea (BCNU) [2, 14, 19, 22], and 1-(2-chloroethyl)-3-(4-methylcyclohexyl)-1-nitrosourea (Me-CCNU) [17, 18, 23] (Table 4.1).

Lipid-soluble NU has been shown to pass through the blood-brain barrier [11, 21] and to enter the cerebrospinal fluid (CSF). As a consequence, it has been effective in the treatment of brain tumors. If chemotherapeutic agents are to be used in brain tumor cases, it is essential to know whether or not this drug will also pass through the blood-brain barrier and what its pharmokinetics will be [4, 10, 11, 13].

In the present chapter, we report the results of clinical studies on the pharmokinetics of ACNU and its movement into the CSF.

Materials and Methods

Study was made of 14 brain tumor patients to whom ACNU was given (nine malignant gliomas, one metastatic brain tumor, one recurrent craniopharyngioma, and three meningiomas). ACNU was administered i.v. in 1–3 min at 100–150 mg/body (1.72–2.50 mg/kg). The CSF was sampled before resection of the tumor and postoperatively by means of ventricular drainage tubes. In one case only (case 10), CSF was sampled using a flushing device during ventriculoperitoneal shunt. Following i.v. administration, CSF samples of about 1 ml were obtained after 5, 15, 30, 90, and 120 min, at which times 1- to 2-ml samples of venous blood were also obtained and immediately frozen.

The blood and CSF concentrations of ACNU were measured using high-power liquid chromatography (HPLC) [12]: After 1,2-dichloroethane extraction in a darkened and frozen state, the ACNU was isolated by paired ion chromatography using a reverse-phase column (u-Bondapak C18) and quantified using the peak height method (UV 254 nm, AUFS 0.005). The limits of quantification were about 40 ng/ml.

Table 4.1. Chemical structure of nitrosourea agents

Drug	Chemical name (generic name)	Structure (molecular weight)	Solubility (Pi)	Dosage administration
CCNU	1-(2-Chloroethyl)-3-cyclohexyl-1-nitrosourea (lomustine)	cyclohexyl–NHCON(NO)CH$_2$CH$_2$Cl	Lipid soluble (2.5)	100–150 mg/m^2 p.o., 6–8 weeks
BCNU	1,3-Bis(2-chloroethyl)-1-nitrosourea (carmustine)	ClCH$_2$CH$_2$NHCON(NO)CH$_2$CH$_2$Cl (214.06)	Lipid soluble (1.39)	200 mg/m^2 drip i.v., 4–6 weeks
MeCCNU	1-(2-Chloroethyl)-3-(4-methylcyclohexyl)-1-nitrosourea (semustine)	4-methylcyclohexyl–NHCON(NO)CH$_2$CH$_2$Cl (248)	Lipid soluble (3.01)	200–225 mg/m^2 p.o., 6 weeks
ACNU	1-(4-Amino-2-methylpyrimidin-5-yl)methyl-3-(2-chloroethyl)-3-nitrosourea hydrochloride (nimustine)	(4-amino-2-methylpyrimidin-5-yl)CH$_2$NHCON(NO)CH$_2$CH$_2$Cl · HCl (309.2)	Water soluble	2–3 mg/kg i.v.,

The mean values (model-1) of the sequential changes in CSF and/or blood concentrations of ACNU for the 14 patients were investigated. In 8 of the 14 cases, measurements were made of the concentrations in both CSF and blood.

Results

ACNU Movement into CSF

Movement of ACNU into the CSF was noted 5 min after i.v. administration of the drug, and a high concentration of 0.59 ± 0.13 μg/ml was obtained after 30 min (Table 4.2; Figs. 4.1, 4.2). Thereafter, a rapid decrease was evident. There were, however, cases in which a high concentration was still found after 60 min: In one meningioma (case 12) and one malignant glioma (case 13), high concentrations of 1.26 and 0.98 μg/ml, respectively, were found.

Six of the nine cases in which CSF concentrations were measured were malignant glioma cases and their mean level 30 min after administration was 0.4 μg/ml. Although strong conclusions cannot be drawn from a sample of three cases, two of the three meningioma cases had concentrations of more than 0.88 μg/ml—well above that for the glioma cases. No other distinguishing features were detected between those cases with high concentrations and cases with low concentrations.

Model-1 analysis was done on an IBM 370-125 computer using a one-compartment model (BMDP 3R Non-linear Regression Program [3]; Fig. 4.2).

Simulation using Eq. (4.1), which expresses the relationship between the CSF concentration of ACNU and time, allowed for calculation of a transfer constant K_t and an elimination constant K_{el}:

$$C_p = [K_t/(K_t - K_{el})] \times A_0(e^{-K_{el} \cdot t} - e^{-K_t \cdot t}) \tag{4.1}$$

These values were found to be $K_t = 1.85$ h and $K_{el} = 1.42$ h and the half-life in the CSF (in the cerebral ventricles) was $t_{1/2} = 0.49$ h. The maximum concentration in the ventricles was approximately 1 μg/ml, which was estimated to occur 37 min after administration. Transfer of the drug to other tissues was found to be considerably delayed. There was a good correlation between K_{el} and the blood concentration, suggesting that there was also transfer of the drug from the CSF to the blood.

ACNU Concentration in Blood

The blood concentration of ACNU 5 min after administration was 3.86 ± 0.64 μg/ml, but it fell rapidly thereafter (Table 4.2; Figs. 4.1, 4.3). After 1 h, it had become 1.01 ± 0.12 μg/ml and it was subsequently maintained at about that level.

For the pharmacokinetic analysis, a two-compartment open model (the pharmaceutical program of Awazu-Hanano, Tokyo University [7] Fig. 4.3 was used.

In the model, the central compartment is the blood and the organs that show identical changes to those of the blood; V_1 is the volume distribution; the tissue compartment includes all other tissues; and V_2 is the volume distribution of the tissue compartment. Using velocity constants, $K_{12} \times K_{21}$, for the speed of transfer between these two compartments and an elimination constant, K_{el}, for the speed of elimination from the central compartment, the drug concentration in the central

Table 4.2. Concentration of ACNU transferred from blood to CSF in brain tumor cases

Case no.	Sex	Age (yrs)	Diagnosis	Body weight (kg)	Dose (iv) mg/body	mg/kg	Blood (µg/ml) 5	15	30	60	90 min	CSF (µg/ml) 5	15	30	60	90 min
1	F	29	Astrocytoma IV	42	100	2.38	—	—	1.52	—	—	0.14	0.45	0.64	—	—
2	F	40	" IV	55	100	1.82	—	—	—	—	—	n.d.	0.07	0.12	0.19	0.25
3	F	28	" III	45	100	2.22	—	—	—	1.47	—	0.07	0.23	0.42	0.41	0.22
4	F	45	Meningioma	45	100	2.22	—	—	—	1.52	—	n.d.	0.36	0.50	0.32	—
5	F	29	Astrocytoma IV	50	100	2.00	—	1.70	2.56	1.53	—	0.43	0.89	0.87	0.66	0.35
6	M	42	" III	65	125	1.92	2.26	1.87	1.28	0.89	0.67	—	—	—	—	—
7	F	24	" IV	40	100	2.50	4.93	—	2.60	1.14	0.78	—	—	—	—	—
8	F	46	Metstatic T.	58	100	1.72	5.65	3.10	2.35	1.11	0.89	—	—	—	—	—
9	M	51	Astrocytoma III	65	150	2.31	5.15	3.56	2.70	1.37	0.95	—	—	—	—	—
10	F	36	Craniopharyngioma (rec.)	47	100	2.13	5.58 (3 min)	3.54	1.46	0.84	0.76	n.d.	0.27	—	0.62	—
11	F	48	Meningioma	50	100	2.00	4.87 (7 min)	4.28 (18 min)	0.60	0.30	0.26	—	—	—	—	—
12	F	48	"	58	100	1.72	2.15	1.80	2.03	0.57	0.47	0.23 (150 min)	0.77	1.26	0.43	—
13	M	33	Astrocytoma III	60	150	2.50	—	—	1.24	0.71	n.d.	0.05	—	0.28	0.98	0.34
14	M	39	" IV	77	150	1.95	2.99	2.22	1.28	0.63	0.33	n.d.	0.05	0.66	0.54	0.13
Model-1			Mean ± SE (n)		113 ± 6	2.1 ± 0.08	3.86 ± 0.64 (6)	2.54 ± 0.31 (7)	1.78 ± 0.29 (11)	1.01 ± 0.12 (12)	0.57 ± 0.10 (9)	0.11 ± 0.05 (8)	0.36 ± 0.11 (8)	0.59 ± 0.13 (8)	0.52 ± 0.08 (8)	0.26 ± 0.04 (5)

rec. recurrence, n.d. < 0.04 µg/ml
Roman numerals refer to grade of astrocytoma
Model-1 is the mean value ± standard error of 14 cases

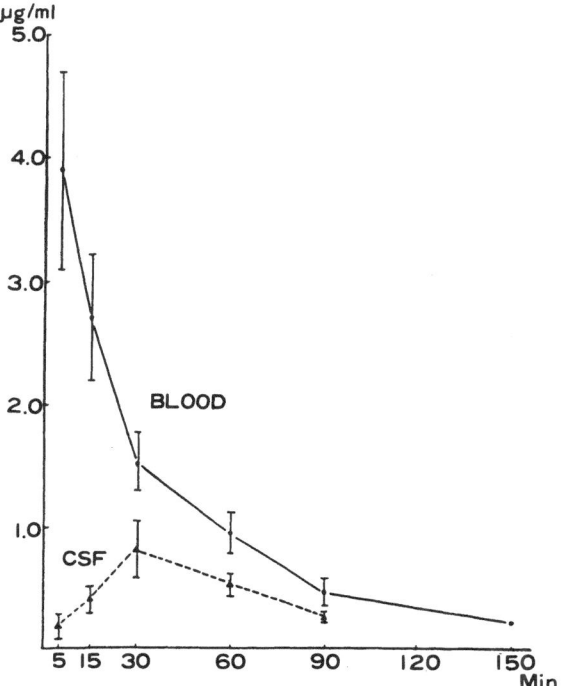

Fig. 4.1. Blood and CSF concentration of ACNU (model-1)

compartment can be calculated with Eq. (4.2):

$$C_p = Ae^{-\alpha t} + Be^{-\beta t} \qquad (4.2)$$

Variables A, B, α, and β, which satisfy the above equation, are calculated from the blood concentrations at various times (hours), and from the parameters obtained it is possible to obtain K_{12}, K_{21}, K_{el}, V_1, V_2, the half-life (t/2) and $[AUC]_0$ (Table 4.3). Both the α and β phases were calculated in cases 6, 8, 9, 10, 11, and model-1. The fact that these results could not be obtained in all cases is due to the extremely rapid diffusion of ACNU, large fluctuations in the data for samples obtained during surgery, especially immediately following drug injection, and differences in the handling of the samples.

From the results obtained, the following conclusions can be drawn concerning the changes in ACNU concentration following i.v. administration: (a) The diffusion of the drug is extremely fast, with the half-life of the phase (αt/2) being 1.3 min (0.021 h). (b) The elimination velocity was relatively fast, with the half-life of the phase (βt/2) being 35 min (0.58 h). (c) Except for those cases in which model-1 was applied, the comparison of the velocity constants showed $K_{12} > K_{el} > K_{21}$ for all patients. (d) The volume distributions showed $V_2 > V_1$, indicating a high rate of transfer into tissues.

Discussion

We have previously carried out experimental studies on ACNU, one of the drugs widely used alone or in combination for the treatment of malignant brain tumors.

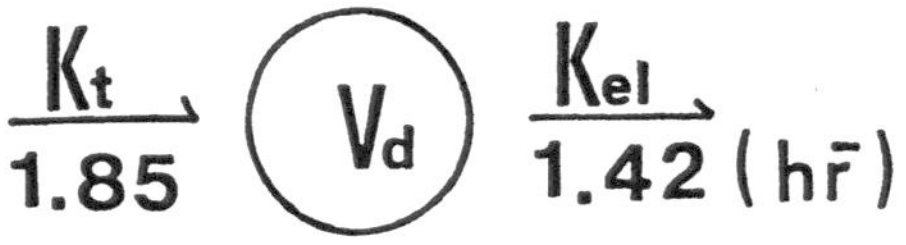

$$\frac{K_t}{1.85} \rightarrow \boxed{V_d} \xrightarrow{K_{el}} \frac{}{1.42}\ (h\bar{r})$$

Fig. 4.2. One-compartment model for the distribution of ACNU in CSF. *Kt* transition rate constant, *Kel* elimination rate constant

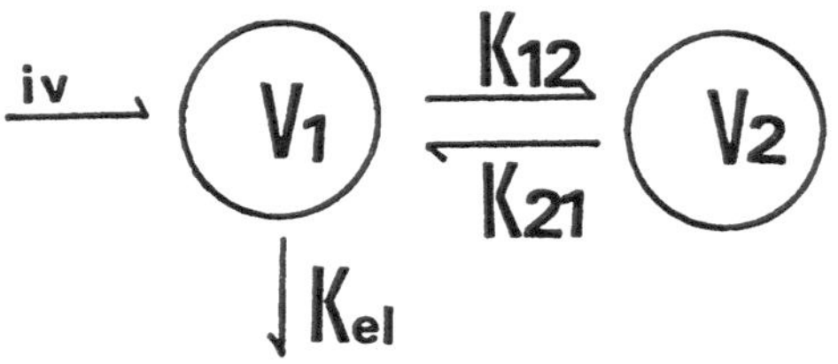

$$iv \rightarrow \boxed{V_1} \underset{K_{21}}{\overset{K_{12}}{\rightleftharpoons}} \boxed{V_2} \quad \downarrow K_{el}$$

Fig. 4.3. Two-compartment open model for the distribution of ACNU. V_1 distribution volume of central compartment, V_2 distribution volume of tissue compartment, K_{12}, K_{21} transition rate constant between the two compartments

It has been demonstrated that notable therapeutic effects can be obtained by using ACNU together with 5-fluorouracil (5-FU) and radiation therapy. The next step for bringing ACNU into clinical use involves the study of its in vivo pharmacokinetics, as reported here.

We have found that in brain tumor patients, the distribution time of ACNU is extremely rapid and the half-life of its elimination time is relatively fast (35 min). Considerable movement of the drug into the CSF has also been shown. The reason why ACNU shows good movement into CSF despite the fact that it is a water-soluble NU compound is thought to be due to the following factors. Although the water solubility of ACNU is caused by the chloride salt of the pyrimidine ligand, the alkalicity of this aminopyrimidine is weak and its pKa is 5.96 (20°C using the UV method). Under physiological conditions (pH 7.4), more than 96% of the drug exists as neutral molecules which cannot be isolated [12]. In other words, even if administered as an alkaline salt, most of the drug is thought to become neutralized. The lipophilicity of this neutral molecule (in the H_2O-octanol system frequently used for structure-activity correlations) is log p = 0.92, indicating relatively good lipid solubility [12]. The log p of ACNU is, however, low relative to that of other NU drugs of this series—CCNU (2.83), BCNU (1.53), and Me-CCNU (3.30) [8].

The intracerebral movement of drugs is said to be greater, the lower the molecular weight and lipophilicity of the compound. In an experimental study on rat tumors and NU compounds, Levin and Kabra [10] reported that the drug with the lowest lipophilicity but capable of penetrating the blood-brain barrier and with the greatest therapeutic effect had a log p of 0.37. These findings also indicate that ACNU has a lipophilicity which allows for passage through the blood-brain barrier and suggest that selective uptake by brain tumor tissue can be expected. In our clinical cases as well, penetration of ACNU to the CSF was found. However, in a comparison of the areas under the curves for blood and CSF concentrations $[AUC]_0$ ($\mu g \cdot h/ml$) in model-1, the absolute values varied between 0.90 and 2.21 (thus making direct comparisons impossible); it can be said that there was considerable movement of ACNU into the ventricles.

Table 4.3. Pharmacokinetics of ACNU calculated by two-compartment open model

Case no.	A (μg/ml)	B (μg/ml)	α (h$^-$)	β (h$^-$)	α [t $\frac{1}{2}$(h)]	β [t $\frac{1}{2}$(h)]
Model-1	12.2	3.4	32.5	1.2	0.021	0.58
(2.1 mg)	$\pm$ 1.7	$\pm$ 0.1	$\pm$ 3.1	$\pm$ 0.1		
6	9.1	1.8	24.2	2.3	0.029	0.30
	$\pm$ 0.2	$\pm$ 0.1	$\pm$ 0.9	$\pm$ 0.1		
8	10.3	1.8	23.8	2.3	0.029	0.30
	$\pm$ 0.2	$\pm$ 0.1	$\pm$ 0.8	$\pm$ 0.1		
9	21.4	2.5	27.6	1.7	0.025	0.41
	$\pm$ 0.6	$\pm$ 0.2	$\pm$ 1.1	$\pm$ 0.2		
10	57.3	8.8	27.8	1.9	0.025	0.37
	$\pm$ 3.2	$\pm$ 1.1	$\pm$ 2.3	$\pm$ 0.3		
11	53.0	8.6	26.4	1.9	0.026	0.37
	$\pm$ 2.8	$\pm$ 1.0	$\pm$ 2.2	$\pm$ 0.3		

Case no.	k12 (h$^-$)	k21 (h$^-$)	kel (h$^-$)	V1$'$ (1/B.W. kg)	V2 (1/B.W. kg)	[AUC]$_0^\infty$
Model-1	20.8	7.9	4.9	0.14	0.35	2.21
(2.1 mg)	$\pm$ 2.5	$\pm$ 0.4	$\pm$ 0.5	$\pm$ 0.02	$\pm$ 0.06	
6	11.1	5.9	9.6	2.3	4.3	1.16
	$\pm$ 1.2	$\pm$ 1.0	$\pm$ 0.7	$\pm$ 0.1	$\pm$ 1.2	
8	10.6	5.4	10.2	2.1	4.0	1.22
	$\pm$ 0.4	$\pm$ 0.4	$\pm$ 0.3	$\pm$ 0.1	$\pm$ 0.3	
9	14.0	4.4	10.9	2.1	6.7	2.25
	$\pm$ 0.7	$\pm$ 0.4	$\pm$ 0.5	$\pm$ 0.1	$\pm$ 0.7	
10	14.4	5.4	10.0	1.5	4.0	6.69
	$\pm$ 1.4	$\pm$ 0.8	$\pm$ 0.8	$\pm$ 0.1	$\pm$ 0.7	
11	13.6	5.3	9.5	1.6	4.1	6.54
	$\pm$ 1.3	$\pm$ 0.8	$\pm$ 0.7	$\pm$ 0.1	$\pm$ 0.7	

In the present study, we considered the CSF to be an independent compartment, but future research should focus on the development of analytic programs which can determine the balance between blood and CSF, blood and brain, and CSF and brain. It is also necessary to study the movement of ACNU into the brain tumor tissue itself.

Conclusion

In order to study the movement of ACNU through the blood-brain barrier, we measured the movement of the drug into the CSF and studied its pharmacokinetics following i.v. injection. It was found that ACNU moves easily and rapidly into the CSF, suggesting that therapeutic effects in malignant brain tumors can be expected.

References

1. Arakawa M, Shimizu F, Okada N (1974) Effect of 1-(4-amino-2-methyl pyrimidine-5-yl)methyl-3-(2-chloroethyl)-3-nitrosourea hydrochloride on leukemia L-1210. Jpn J Cancer Res 65: 191

2. Bloom HJG (1975) Combined modality therapy for intracranial tumor. Cancer 35: 111–120

3. Dixon WJ (1975) BMD Biochemical computer program. University of California Press, Los Angeles

4. Fenstermacher JD, Jonson JA (1966) Filtration and reflection coefficients of the rabitt blood-brain barrier. J Physiol (Lond.) 211: 341–346

5. Fewer D, Wilson CB, Boldrey EB, Enot JK (1972) Phase II study of CCNU (NSC 79037) in the treatment of brain tumors. Cancer Chemother Rep 56: 421–427

6. Garret MJ, Hughes HJ, Ryall RDH (1974) CCNU in brain tumors. Clin Radiol 25: 183–184

7. Hanano M, Awatsu S (1970) The 2nd symposium of drug metabolism and toxicity, Kyoto

8. Hansh C, Smith N, Engle R, Wood H (1972) Quantitative structure-activity relationships of antineoplastic drugs: nitrosoureas and triazenoimidazoles. Cancer Chemother Rep 56: 443–456

9. Hoogstraten B, Gottlieb JA, Caoili E, Tucher WG, Talley RW, Haut A (1973) CCNU (NSU 79037) in the treatment of Cancer-Phase II study. Cancer 32: 38–43

10. Levin VA, Kabra P (1974) Effectiveness of the nitrosourea as a function of their lipid solubility in the chemotherapy of experimental rat brain tumors. Cancer Chemother Rep 58: 787–792

11. Mellet LB (1977) Physicochemical considerations and pharmacokinetic behavior in delivery of drugs to the central nervous system. Cancer Treat Rep 61: 527–531

12. Nakamura K, Asami M, Kawada K, Sasahara K (1977) Quantitative determination of ACNU (1-(4-amino-2-methyl-5-pyrimidinyl)methyl-1-(2-chloroethyl)-1-nitrosourea hydrochloride), a new water-soluble anti-tumor nitrosourea, in biological fluids and tissues of patients by high-performance liquid chromatography: I. Analytical method and pharmacokinetics. Ann Rep Sankyo Res Lab 29: 66–74

13. Rall DP, Zubrod CG (1962) Mechanisms of drug absorption and excretion: passage of drugs in and out of the central nervous system. Ann Rev Pharmacol 2: 109–128

14. Rall DP, Ben M, McCarthy DM (1963) 1.3-bis- β-chloroethyl-1-nitrosourea (BCNU): Toxicity and intial cranial trial. Proc Am Ass Cancer Res 4: 55

15. Rosenblum ML, Reynold AF Jr, Smith KA, et al. (1973) chloroethyl-cyclo-hexyl-nitrosourea (CCNU) in the treatment of malignant brain tumors. J Neurosurg 39: 306–316

16. Shimizu F, Arakawa M (1975) Effects of 3-[(4-amino-2-methyl-5-pyrimidinyl)methyl]-1-(2-chloroethyl)-1-nitrosourea hydrochloride on lymphoid leukemia L-1210. Jpn J Cancer Res 66: 149–154

17. Sponzo RW, DeVita VT, Oliverio VT (1973) Physiological disposition of CCNU and MeCCNU in man. Cancer 3: 1154–1159

18. Taylor SG, Nelson L, Baxter D, Rosembaum C (1975) Treatment of grade III and IV astrocytoma with dimethyl triazenoimidazole carboxamide (DTIC, NSC-45388) alone and in combination with CCNU (NSC-79037) or methyl CCNU (MeCCNU, NSC-95441). Cancer 36: 1269–1276

19. Walker MD, Hurwitz BS (1970) BCNU (1.3-Bis (2-chloroethyl)-1-nitrosourea: NSC-409962) in the treatment of malignant brain tumor—a preliminary report. Cancer Chemother Rep 54: 264–271

20. Walker MD. Rosenblum ML, Smith KA, Reynolds AF Jr (1971) The treatment of brain tumor with 1-(2-chloroethyl)-3-cyclohexyl-1-nitrosourea (CCNU). Proc Am Ass Cancer Res 12: 51

21. Walker MD, Hilton J (1976) Nitrosourea pharmacodynamics in relation to the central nervous system. Cancer Treat Rep 60: 725–728

22. Wilson CB, Bordrey EB, Enot KJ (1970) 1.3-Bis (2-chloroethyl)-nitrosourea (NSC-409962) in the treatment of brain tumors. Cancer Chemother Rep 54: 273–281

23. Young RC, Walker MD, Canellos GP, Schein PS, Chabner BA, DeVita VT (1973) Initial clinical trial with MeCCNU. Cancer 31: 2264–2269

Chapter 5

The Effects of Induced Hypertension on the Uptake of ACNU in Experimental Brain Tumor

Y. Tsurumi

Introduction

There have been improvements in chemotherapy for malignant brain tumors in recent years, but there still remain many problems and limitations in such therapy when considered from the perspective of therapeutic effectiveness. Not only must the sensitivity of tumor tissues to various anticancer drugs be tested, but also studies must be made of the in vivo pharmacokinetics of such drugs, including their uptake by tumor cells. In other words, no matter how large the administered dose of a drug is, if the effective volume entering the tumor tissue is insufficient, then satisfactory therapeutic results cannot be expected. From this perspective, the development of new techniques for the administration of such drugs that would result in increased uptake achieved selectively by the brain tumor tissue without an increase in systemic side effects would be desirable.

In the light of recent findings concerning deficits in autoregulation in brain tumor tissue [2], the present study was undertaken to investigate the effect hypertension has on the uptake of anticancer drugs by brain tumor cells.

Materials and Methods

Brain Tumor Model

Male Wistar King Aptekman rats [4] weighing 200 g were used. Under the administration of diethylether anesthesia, a 1-mm-diameter burr hole was made over the left parietal area and KEG-1 cells (rat glioma cells induced by N-nitrosomethylurea) $(1 \times 10^5$ cells/10 μl) were transplanted into the brain using a semistereotactic technique. The rats were used in the experiment 10 days after transplantation. Successful transplants were seen in virtually all animals, and the tumors were found to be solid, subcortical growths (Fig. 5.1).

Effects of Induced Hypertension

Under the administration of sodium pentobarbital anesthesia (30 mg/kg. i.p.), a femoral artery and vein were cannulated, the rats were immobilized with pancuronium bromide and regulated respiration was instituted. The anticancer drug used

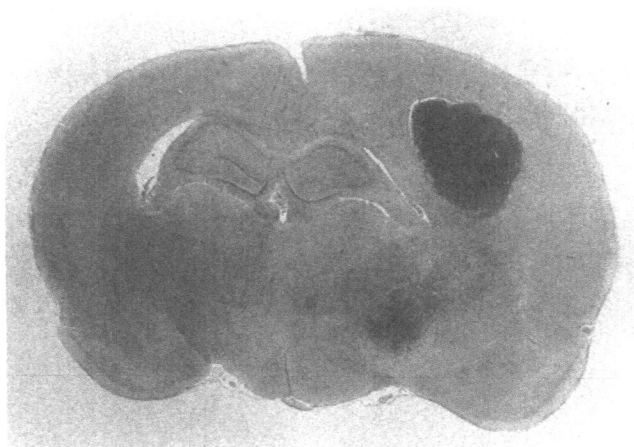

Fig. 5.1. Control section of the rat brain 10 days after transplantation of KEG-1 cells

in this study was the ^{14}C-labeled, ethylene radical of 1-(4-amino-2-methyl-5-pyri-midyl)-methyl-3-(2-chloroethyl)-3-nitrosourea hydrochloride (ACNU), i.e., ^{14}C-ACNU, with a specific activity of 26.1 μCi/mg. In order to prevent a loss of its activity, 383 μg of the drug was dissolved in 0.6 ml physiological saline immediately prior to administration and was given i.v. over a period of 1 min.

Angiotensin II was administered continuously through the femoral vein and the mean blood pressure was raised 35–40 mmHg and maintained at that level. The rats were decapitated 2, 5, 10, 20, or 30 min after ^{14}C-ACNU had been administered, and brain tissue was sampled from both the region of the tumor and the contra-lateral region of normal brain tissue.

After burning the tissue in a sample oxidizer (Aloka ASC-113), the ^{14}C concentration was measured using a liquid scintillation counter (Aloka, LSC-903) and comparisons were made between the animals which had undergone hypertension and those that had not. During the experiments, blood gases and rectal temperature were monitored and maintained as follows: PaO_2, 100 ± 20 mmHg; $PaCO_2$, 40 ± 4 mmHg; pH, 7.35 ± 0.05; and rectal temperature; $36.5° \pm 0.5°$C. Blood pressure was also monitored continuously.

ACNU Content

Comparisons were made of the ^{14}C-ACNU content between animals undergoing continuous induced hypertension until killing and those undergoing only 5 min of hypertension following ^{14}C-ACNU administration and then decapitation after 20 or 30 min.

Survival Time

Study was also made of the survival times of animals given ACNU with induced hypertension and those given ACNU without hypertension. For this experiment, rats were given i.v. doses of ACNU (5 mg/kg) under sodium pentobarbital anesthe-sia on the 5th day following KEG-1 transplantation. The hypertension was induced with angiotensin II and was of 5-min duration. Blood pressure and body temperature were monitored, but in order to facilitate the study of survival times regulated respiration using tracheotomy was not carried out.

Results

Effects of Induced Hypertension

The ^{14}C-content of the brain tumor tissue 5 min after administration of ^{14}C-ACNU in a control (normotension) group of six animals was 0.32% $\pm$ 0.03% dose/g tissue (mean $\pm$ SE). After 10 min in seven rats, the content was 0.53% $\pm$ 0.10% dose/g tissue.

In contrast, after 5 and 10 min in hypertension groups of five and seven rats, respectively, the contents were 1.20% $\pm$ 0.09% and 1.12% $\pm$ 0.07% dose/g tissue. Thus, fourfold and twofold increases were seen in the ACNU uptake after 5 and 10 min, respectively, both of which were statistically significant at the $P < 0.01$ level using Student's t-test. Significant differences in the ^{14}C content were not found between the groups 2, 20, or 30 min after drug administration (Fig. 5.2).

Although there was a tendency for the animals which underwent hypertension to have slightly higher ^{14}C-ACNU accumulation in the contralateral, normal brain tissue, there were no statistically significant differences between these animals and those in the normotension group (Fig. 5.3).

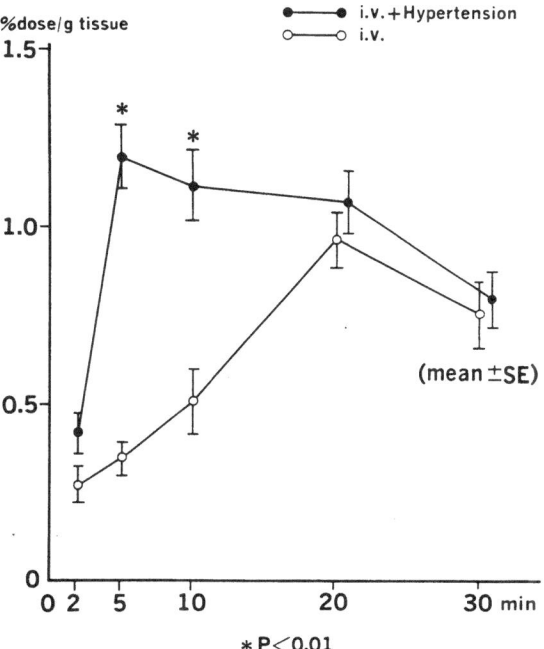

Fig. 5.2. Uptake of ^{14}C-ACNU by the experimental brain tumor with and without induced hypertension

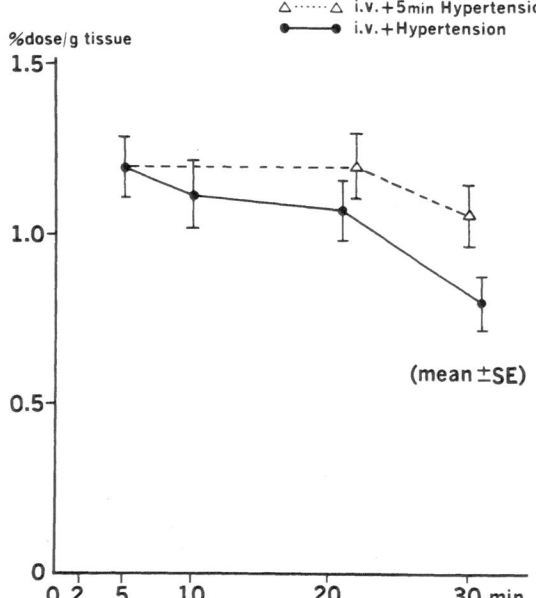

Fig. 5.3. Uptake of ^{14}C-ACNU by the experimental brain tumor and the duration of induced hypertension

ACNU Content

The animals undergoing only 5 min of hypertension showed a tendency toward a higher ACNU content than those undergoing 20 or 30 min of hypertension (Fig. 5.4). This tendency was not, however, statistically significant.

Survival Time

The survival time of the 13 untreated control animals was 12.3 $\pm$ 0.53 days, whereas that of the 14 animals given ACNU at normotension was 14.1 $\pm$ 0.59 days and that of the seven rats given ACNU and hypertension was 18.1 $\pm$ 0.60 days. Comparison of the hypertension group with the normotension groups showed a statistically significant difference ($P < 0.005$; Fig. 5.5).

Discussion

Despite the fact that ACNU is an alkylating agent drug and is lipid soluble, it also has lipophilic properties. It is an anticancer agent which can be administered intravenously and has found wide usage in cancer therapy in Japan. Previously, we have reported several experimental and clinical studies on its therapeutic effectiveness [5, 7, 8].

Alkylating agents such as ACNU are thought to have nonspecific effects on the cell cycle of cancer cells [10]. Administration of a single large dose is said to produce fewer side effects and to suppress the rate at which recurrence of the brain tumor will occur more effectively than when multiple small doses are administered [11]. There

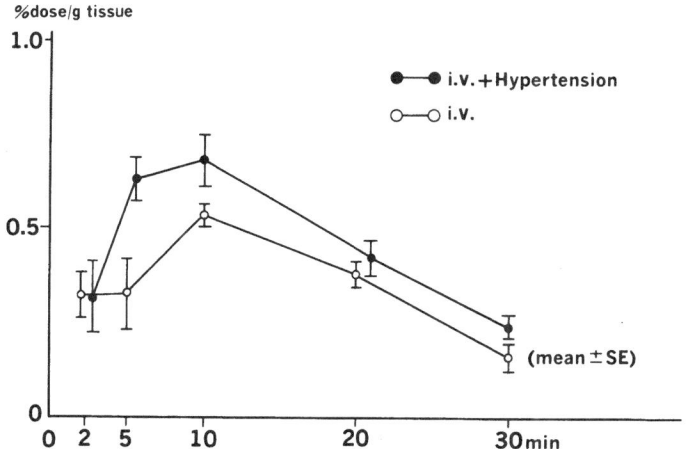

Fig. 5.4. Uptake of ^{14}C-ACNU by the contralateral normal cortex

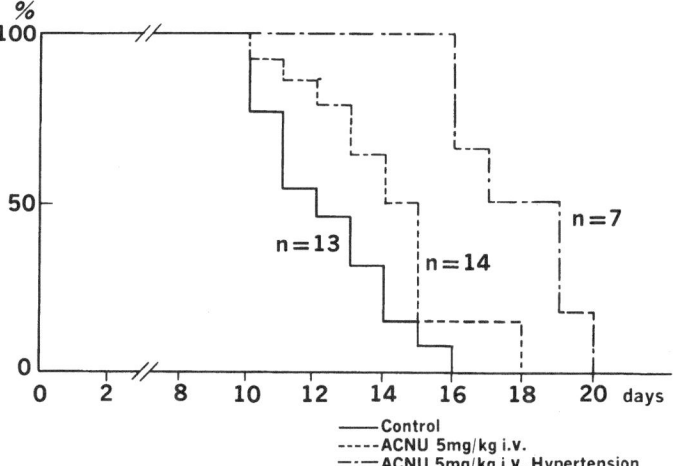

Fig. 5.5. Survival times in the untreated control, ACNU-treated and ACNU-treated induced hypertension groups

are of course limits to the size of the total drug dose and consideration of the dose-dependent side effects, particularly myelosuppression due to ACNU, has led to an accepted clinical dose of 1–2 mg/kg i.v. However, according to studies in which the ACNU concentration in brain tumor tissue was measured from tissue samples obtained at surgery, it is necessary to administer "one shot" of ACNU of 3–4 mg/kg i.v. in order to achieve clinically the effective drug concentration which has been found capable of suppressing tumor cell proliferation in vitro [3]. In other words, in order to deliver a dose of ACNU to tumor tissue which can be expected to produce therapeutic effects in brain tumor patients, it is necessary to devise methods to go beyond the currently accepted maximum dose of ACNU. This dose would have to be 1.5–4.0 times greater.

It has been pointed out that one of the characteristics of tumor tissue is a loss of autoregulation of blood flow [2]. In experiments where angiotensin II is used to induce hypertension, the autoregulatory capability of the blood vessels maintains blood flow at a constant level in the brain and other organs, provided that the mean blood pressure does not exceed 150 mmHg. There is, however, a 5.7-fold increase in blood pressure in tumor tissue which has been transplanted to subcutaneous regions [12, 13]. In the light of such findings, we considered that the uptake of ACNU by brain tumor tissue might be increased by means of induced hypertension and we consequently undertook the experiments described above.

It was found that a two- to fourfold increase in the ACNU concentration in tumor tissue could be brought about by such hypertension, whereas in the contralateral normal brain tissue statistically significant increases were not found. These findings demonstrate that using the same dosage it may be possible to increase the amount of ACNU delivered to tumor tissue without bringing about systemic side effects or deleterious effects on normal brain tissue. Furthermore, since the active site on the ethylene-^{14}C-ACNU used in this experiment contained the radioactive label, the increases in ^{14}C accumulation which were obtained are thought likely to correlate well with the anticancer effectiveness of the drug.

One of the characteristics of the nitrosourea anticancer drugs is their relatively short biological half-life within the systemic circulation [6]; that of ACNU is particularly short at only 12 min [14]. For this reason, if the administered ACNU is not delivered rapidly to the tumor tissue, sufficient therapeutic effects cannot be expected.

In the present study, at normotension a peak concentration in the tumor tissue was found 20 min after i.v. administration, whereas the peak was between 5 and 10 min after administration when hypertension was induced. In light of the known biological half-life of ACNU, this result concerning the peak concentration indicates that its anticancer effects should exceed those expected solely from the increase in ^{14}C uptake when hypertension is employed.

In addition, it was also found that by means of induced hypertension of only 5-min duration, a higher concentration of ACNU was delivered to the tumor tissue than when prolonged hypertension was employed. It may be the case that due to the halt in induced hypertension, the blood flow in the tumor tissue, which had lost its autoregulation functions, decreased and as a consequence there was prolongation of the "wash out" of the ACNU already taken up by the tumor tissue. However, although it is thought that the uptake of lipid-soluble drugs such as ACNU is determined by the blood flow and the distribution rate [9], there have been reports indicating that the blood flow is lower in experimentally induced brain tumors than in contralateral normal tissue [1]. Moreover, the fact that we found a higher concentration of ACNU in the tumor tissue than contralaterally in the groups treated at normotension suggests that the uptake of ACNU by tumor tissue is not regulated solely by the volume of blood flow.

It is evident that a future topic for research on the mechanisms of ACNU taken up into brain tumor tissue must include questions concerning the blood-brain barrier, which is said to be absent in brain tumor tissue. In any case, the extremely short 5-min increase in blood pressure of this method of ACNU administration is, from a clinical viewpoint, extremely convenient and we have found this technique to be effective in producing significant increases in survival time in a brain tumor model using the rat.

We believe that the induced hypertension technique, which has been demonstrated to be effective both in terms of pharmacokinetics and in terms of survival time in our experiments, is an invaluable method which should find widespread usage in the treatment of malignant brain tumors.

Conclusion

In light of previous experimental data on the widely used anticancer drug ACNU, it is thought desirable to administer a single large dose of the drug. Consideration of the associated side effects, however, makes it virtually impossible to administer clinically a single large dose which would be of a sufficient size to lead to the desired therapeutic effects. In the present study, we investigated the effects of induced hypertension on the uptake of ACNU by brain tumor tissue autoregulation functions, which are lost in tumor tissue.

Using a rat brain tumor model, it was found that the uptake of ^{14}C-ACNU following 5 min of induced hypertension was four fold greater than that of a group of animals administered ACNU at normotension. In normal brain tissue on the contralateral side, significant increases in ACNU uptake were not found, indicating that the induced hypertension technique leads to a selective increase in the delivery of ACNU to the brain tumor tissue. As a result of 5 min of induced hypertension following administration of the ACNU, a significant increase in the survival time of the rats was also found. We conclude that this induced hypertension technique should be tried in the chemotherapy of various brain tumors.

References

1. Blasberg RG, Kobayashi T, Horowitz M, Rice JM, Groothuis D, Molnar P, Fenstermacher JD (1983) Regional blood flow in ethylnitrosourea-induced brain tumors. Ann Neurol 14: 189–201
2. Endo H, Larsen B, Lassen NA (1977) Regional cerebral blood flow alterations remote from the site of intracranial tumors. J Neurosurg 46: 271–281
3. Hara M, Takeuchi K (1979) Pharmacokinetic analysis of ACNU in brain tumors. Brain and Nerve 31: 1279–1289 (in Japanese)
4. Kaneko S, Abe H, Aida T, Tsuru M, Kodama T, Kobayashi H (1980) Experimental study of immunochemotherapy of brain tumors—experimental brain tumor model and immunochemotherapy by a combination of PSK and ACNU. Neurol Med Chir (Tokyo) 20: 997–1005 (in Japanese)
5. Kitahara M, Katakura R, Mori T, Suzuki J, Sasaki T (1984) Combined effect of ACNU and 5-fluorouracil on spheroids of rat glioma cells. Neurol Med Chir (Tokyo) 24: 747–757 (in Japanese)
6. Levin VA, Hoffman W, Weinkam RJ (1978) Pharmacokinetics of BCNU in man: a preliminary study of 20 patients. Cancer Treat Rep 62: 1305–1312
7. Mineura K, Mori T, Katakura R, Suzuki J, Sasaki T (1981) Therapeutic effects of 1-(4-amino-2-methyl-5-pyrimidinyl)methyl-3-(2-chloroethyl)-3-nitrosourea hydrochloride (ACNU) and radiation on the rat glioma. Neurol Surg (Tokyo) 9: 257–265 (in Japanese)
8. Mori T, Mineura K, Katakura R (1979) Chemotherapy of malignant brain tumors by a water-soluble anti-tumor nitrosourea, ACNU. Neurol Med Chir (Tokyo) 19: 1157–1171 (in Japanese)
9. Rall DP, Zubrod CG (1962) Mechanism of drug absorption and excretion: passage of drugs in and out of the central nervous system. Ann Rev Pharmacol 2: 109–128

10. Schabel FM (1974) New experimental drug combination with potential clinical utility. Biochem Pharmacol (Suppl 2) 23: 163–176
11. Schabel FM (1975) Synergism and antagonism among antitumor agents. In: Pharmacological basis of cancer chemotherapy. Williams and Wilkins, Baltimore, pp 595–623
12. Suzuki M, Hori K, Abe I, Saito S, Sato H (1981) A new approach to cancer chemotherapy: Selective enhancement of tumor blood flow with angiotensin II. J Nat Cancer Inst 67: 663–669
13. Suzuki M, Hori K, Abe I, Saito S, Sato H (1984) Functional characterization of the microcirculation in tumors. Cancer Metastasis Rev 3: 115–126
14. Tanaka M, Nishigaki T, Nakajima E, Totsuka S, Nakamura K (1980) Distribution, excretion, and metabolism of 3-[(4-amino-2-methyl-5-pyrimidinyl)methyl]-1 (2-chloroethyl)-1-nitrosourea (ACNU) in rats and mice after iv administration. Cancer Treat Rep 64: 575–580

Chapter 6

A Study of Intratumoral Oxygen Pressure in Brain Tumors

T. KAYAMA

Introduction

Even today with the development of various immunochemotherapies, radiation therapy remains the principal treatment for malignant brain tumors [27, 35]. It is well known, however, that prevention of recurrence or complete cure in such cases is often not attainable, even with extensive radiation therapy. One cause for this is said to be the presence of hypoxic cells within the tumor tissue. Following the early (1955) advocacy of the concept of hypoxic cells by Thomlinson and Gray [29], the cells have been observed experimentally in monolayers [10, 13, 36] and spheroids [6, 23], but in all such cases experimental work has been confined to the in vitro situation, rather than the actual measurement of oxygen pressure (PO_2) within tumor tissue. In experimental tumors as well, the transplanted tissue tends to be small and it becomes technically difficult to measure PO_2 [7]. Futhermore, there have been no reports of PO_2 measurements of tumor tissue in a clinical setting [9, 26].

In the present study, we used a 700-μm-diameter tube sensor to make sequential measurements simultaneously of the PO_2 of tumor tissue surrounding normal brain tissue and arterial blood during surgery on brain tumors. We report our findings on the various correlations among these measurements.

Research Methods

Prior to the intracranial surgery, an intravascular PO_2 sensor (Kontron Co., Ltd., Module 636, Basel, Switzerland) was inserted into the femoral artery and sequential measurements of the arterial oxygen pressure (PaO_2) were made. After craniotomy, the region of the brain tumor and its surrounding tissue was exposed, and one or two identical sensors were inserted into the tumor. A plate-type sensor (Kontron Co., Ltd., Module 632 Basel, Switzerland) was placed on the tissue surrounding the tumor and sequential measurements were made of both the tumor tissue oxygen pressure (TuO_2) and that of the surrounding normal brain tissue (BrO_2).

Ethrane anesthesia was used and maintained at a constant concentration during the measurements. Systolic blood pressure was kept at approximately 120 mmHg. During this period, the $O_2 : N_2O$ rate was maintained at 1 : 3 and observations were made on the changes in PaO_2, TuO_2, and BrO_2 (Fig. 6.1).

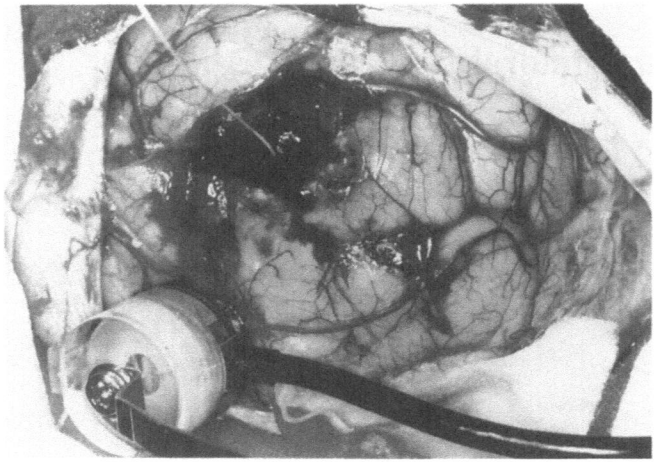

Fig. 6.1. Method of measurement of intratumoral O_2 pressure and tissue O_2 pressure of the brain tissue surrounding the tumor. A needle-type O_2 sensor is inserted into the tumor tissue and a plate-type O_2 sensor is placed on the surface of the brain during surgery for total removal

Clinical Materials

The clinical materials consisted of 16 cases of untreated brain tumor. The histopathological types consisted of three cases of glioblastoma multiforme, three grade III and four grade II astrocytomas, and two oligodendrogliomas. The remaining four cases were metastatic brain tumors originating in the lungs: two were adenocarcinomas, one was a squamous cell carcinoma, and one was an undifferentiated cancer. The locations of the tumors were as follows: ten in the frontal lobe, one in the temporal lobe, one in the Sylvian fissure, and four in the posterior fossa.

The ages of the patients ranged from 2 to 71 years, with a mean of 41 years. With regard to the vascularity of the tumors as seen in cerebral angiograms, the tumor shadow was not visualized in seven cases, faintly visualized in five cases, and markedly visualized in four cases. Computed tomography (CT) enhancement effects were faint in a portion or all of the tumor in nine cases and distinct in seven cases (Table 6.1).

Results

Tumor PO_2

When the $O_2 : N_2O$ ratio was kept at 1 : 3, the PaO_2 varied between 80 and 140 mmHg (the mean and standard error being 109.2 $\pm$ 5.8 mmHg). In contrast, the TuO_2 of the 16 cases ranged between 5 and 38 mmHg (15.3 $\pm$ 23 mmHg). Four of the 16 cases had TuO_2 levels of 20–30 mmHg, five had levels of 10–20 mmHg, and six cases had TuO_2 levels below 10 mmHg (Fig. 6.2).

Table 6.1. Summary of cases

Case no.	Initials	Age (yrs)	Sex	Site	Pathological classification[a]	Vascularity[b]	Enhancement[c]
1	N. S.	52	M	Fr	Glioblastoma	−	+
2	H. T.	10	M	Fr	Glioblastoma	+	+
3	M. S.	13	F	Fr	Glioblastoma	+ +	+ +
4	T. S.	36	F	Fr	Astrocytoma gr. III	−	+
5	S. K.	28	F	FP	Astrocytoma gr. III	+	+
6	T. I.	51	M	Fr	Astrocytoma gr. III	−	+ +
7	T. S.	19	M	Fr	Astrocytoma gr. II	+ +	+ +
8	C. S.	2	F	C	Astrocytoma gr. II	−	+ +
9	T. N.	64	M	C	Astrocytoma gr. II	−	+
10	E. O.	12	M	C	Astrocytoma gr. II	−	+
11	T. K.	60	M	Fr	Oligodendroglioma	+	+
12	R. T.	50	F	T	Oligodendroglioma	−	+
13	M. E.	65	F	Fr	Adenocarcinoma	+	+
14	K. H.	63	M	C	Adenocarcinoma	+ +	+ +
15	S. S.	57	M	Fr	Squamous carcinoma	+ +·	+ +
16	S. K.	71	M	Fr	Undifferentiated carcinoma	+	+ +

Fr frontal, *FP* frontoparietal, *C* cerebellum, *T* temporal
[a] According to WHO criteria
[b] − no vascularization, + slight vascularization, + + strong vascularization
[c] + partial and/or slight diffuse enhancement, + + strong diffuse enhancement

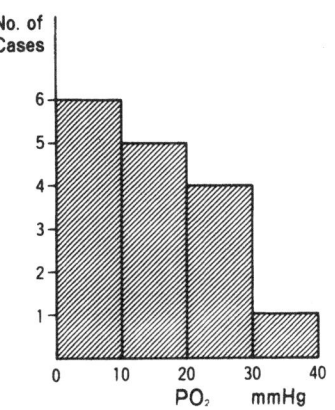

No. of Cases

PO$_2$ mmHg

Fig. 6.2. Frequency distribution of PO$_2$ in all cases of brain tumor. The intratumoral O$_2$ pressure was 15.3 ± 2.3 (mean ± SE) mmHg when the PaO$_2$ value was similar to that in the physiological state—109.2 ± 5.8 mmHg ($n = 16$)

When the TuO$_2$ levels were studied separately for the glioma and metastatic brain tumor cases, no statistically significant difference between the two groups was found. Nevertheless, there were slightly higher TuO$_2$ levels for the four metastatic brain tumor cases (16.5 ± 2.0 mmHg) than for the 12 glioma cases (14.9 ± 3.2 mmHg; Figs. 6.3, 6.4).

A clear correlation between the TuO$_2$ level and the vascularity seen in angiograms

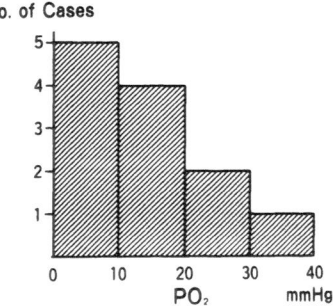

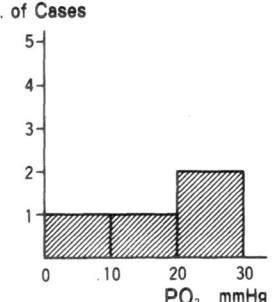

Fig. 6.3. Frequency distribution of PO_2 in glioma tissue. The intratumoral O_2 was 14.9 ± 3.2 mmHg when the PaO_2 value was similar to that in the physiological state—114.8 ± 3.5 mmHg ($n = 12$)

Fig. 6.4. Frequency distribution of PO_2 in metastatic brain tumor. The intratumoral O_2 pressure was 16.5 ± 2.0 mmHg when the PaO_2 value was similar to that in the physiological state—108.8 ± 7.0 mmHg ($n = 4$)

or enhancement effects in CT scans was not found in the present study. For example, in case 7, which showed both distinct vascularity and marked enhancement effects, the TuO_2 level was low at 12 mmHg, whereas in case 1, where the vascularity was faint and the enhancement effects weak, the TuO_2 level was high at 38 mmHg (Table 6.2).

PO₂ Levels in Surrounding Normal Brain Tissue

Measurements of BrO_2 were possible in 11 of the 16 cases. With on $O_2 : N_2O$ ratio of 1 : 3, the PaO_2 level was 112.7 ± 5.2 mmHg and BrO_2 was 59.8 ± 6.5 mmHg. These values were much higher than the 15.3 ± 2.3 mmHg of TuO_2. Nine of the eleven cases had high levels of between 40 and 70 mmHg (Fig. 6.5). A statistically significant difference between the TuO_2 and BrO_2 levels was found using Student's t-test ($P < 0.025$; Fig. 6.6).

Discussion

Research on hypoxic tissue within malignant tumors began with histopathological studies [29] and was further motivated by the in vitro identification of the susceptibility of hypoxic cells to various levels of irradiation [10, 13]. It was then found that the influence of oxygen on the therapeutic effects of irradiation, particularly X-ray irradiation, is large [3, 5]. These research results were then applied clinically and have been used in the treatment of lung cancer, brain tumors, tongue cancers, skin cancers, esophageal cancers, etc., using hyperbaric oxygenation therapy [2, 7, 16, 18] and hypoxic cell radiosensitizers, together with high-electron-affinity imidazole inducers [4, 11, 19, 25, 31]. Most studies on such therapy, however, have reported that the clinical results were not as good as had been anticipated. As a consequence, the presence of hyperoxic cells within malignant tumor tissue has been looked upon with scepticism by some researchers [e.g., 30].

Table 6.2. Results of study

Case no.	PaO_2 (mmHg)	TuO_2 (mmHg)	BrO_2 (mmHg)
1	110	38	54
2	99	12	47
3	102	28	—
4	130	8	—
5	136	8	114
6	124	6	56
7	114	12	87
8	110	18	—
9	110	5	50
10	102	6	—
11	128	16	—
12	112	22	54
13	95	22	60
14	120	24	42
15	140	8	54
16	80	12	40

PaO_2 arterial O_2 pressure, TuO_2 intratumoral pressure, BrO_2 pressure of normal brain tissue surrounding tissue

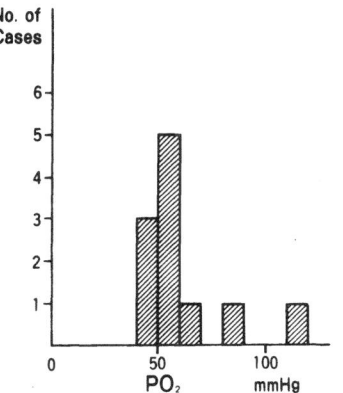

Fig. 6.5. Frequency distribution of PO_2 on the cortex surrounding the brain tumor. The cortical PO_2 pressure was 59.8 ± 6.5 mmHg when the PaO_2 value was similar to that in the physiological state—112.7 ± 5.2 mmHg ($n = 11$)

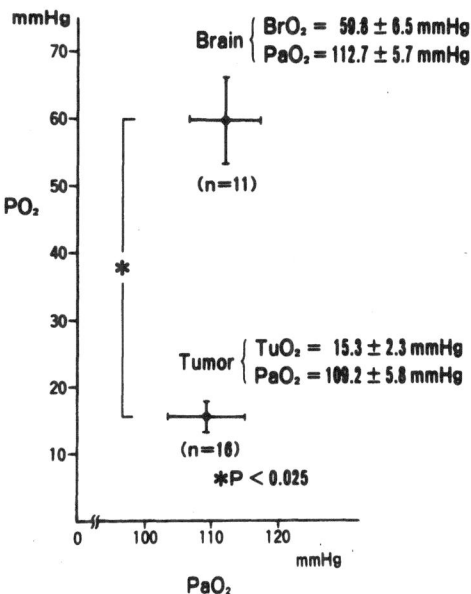

Fig. 6.6. Comparison of PO_2 intratumoral tissue and cortex surrounding the tumor; the difference was significant

The first reported attempt to measure the tissue pressure O_2 of a malignant tumor in vivo was that of Gullino and Grantham [14] in 1961. They compared the venous oxygen pressure of isolated tumor tissue (i.e., transplanted tumor tissue) and the feeding arterial oxygen pressure. Such research, however, was performed solely on isolated tumors and it was not until 1974 that Ardenne and Reitraver [1], Vaupel and Thews [32], and Vaupel [34] reported on the measurement of the O_2 pressure in mammary gland tissue transplanted to the peritoneal cavity of the mouse, using a gold needle as the PO_2 sensor. They reported that more than 50% of the tumors showed reduced susceptibility to radiation.

In such studies, problems familiar in much experimental oncology concerning differences in the environment of the tumor, its vascular structure, and surrounding tissues have remained. Moreover, there have been no reports of measurements of PO_2 in human malignant tumors and there has been no research which strongly supports the idea of hypoxic tissue present within human malignant tumors [9]. Although there have been several reports [12, 20, 21] on the oxygen extraction fraction and $CMRO_2$ in cancer tissues, there have been no observations on tissue PO_2.

In the present study, we made PO_2 measurements during surgery in 16 cases of untreated malignant brain tumor. The PO_2 sensor used was that developed by Clark [8], in which PO_2 is determined from the electrostatic potential between a cathode and an anode within a 700-μm-diameter tube inserted into the tumor. The temperature at the time of measurement is known to affect the results, but temperature influences can be largely avoided if the electrode is inserted deeply into the tumor. The time lag until measurement using this method is 90 s, and so sequential measurements can be made and the correlation with arterial PO_2 (PaO_2) studied simultaneously.

The $O_2 : N_2O$ ratio which we used for TuO_2 measurements was 1 : 3—a ratio at which PaO_2 was maintained at approximately 110 mmHg. This value was slightly above the PaO_2 obtained at atmospheric pressure when room air was used, nevertheless the TuO_2 obtained in this manner for the 16 cases had a low value of 15.3 ± 2.3 mmHg. Statistically, this TuO_2 value was significantly lower than the 59.8 ± 6.5 mmHg value for BrO_2, the latter being similar to the PaO_2 values. These results clearly indicate that there is a region of hypoxic tissue within the brain tumor tissue. Moreover, if it is considered that, after oxygen enters brain tissue from the blood it disperses due to PO_2 differences in the tissue [24], it can be inferred that hypoxic tissue with a value still lower than the region showing 15.3 ± 2.3 mmHg exists. From these facts, we believe that the present experiments demonstrate the presence of a hypoxic region within human malignant brain tumors, as first surmised by Gray in 1955.

Following reports by Deschner and Gray [10] and Gray [13] concerning the radiosensitivity of hypoxic cells, it has been established that there is a significant decrease in tumor radiosensitivity at PO_2 levels below 30 mmHg. In other words, it can be said that in radiotherapy of brain tumors, complete cure or prevention of recurrence is difficult due to the presence of tumor cells in a hypoxic state, such as in the present study (15.3 ± 2.3 mmHg). It is also apparent that since the surrounding normal brain tissue has a much higher PO_2 level (59.8 ± 6.5 mmHg), it will be unaffected by oxygen effects on the radiosensitivity during radiotherapy. These findings indicate that the presence of hypoxic tissue cannot be ignored when treating brain tumors and, furthermore, that methods for increasing the radiosensitivity of hypoxic tissue in tumors using hyperbaric techniques or imidazole inducing agents should be further developed.

In the present study, significant correlations were not found between the PO_2 of the tumor tissue in our 16 cases and the degree of vascularity as seen in angiograms or CT scans. Among the reasons for this lack of correlation may be the formation of an arteriovenous shunt by the vessels proliferating within the tumor, a histopathologically well-defined phenomenon [15, 17, 22, 28, 33]. It can, therefore, be assumed that even if there is abundant vasculature within the tumor, there will be little development of capillaries, and blood oxygen will not enter the tumor tissue, resulting in a hypoxic region. Even when angiograms show little vascularity, it is thought that a relatively high PO_2 value will be found in cases where an effective vascular network has developed.

Conclusion

Simultaneous measurements were made of the oxygen pressure within brain tumor tissue, in the surrounding normal brain tissue, and in the arterial blood in 16 patients undergoing excision of brain tumors.

When the $O_2 : N_2O$ ratio was maintained at $1 : 3$, it was possible to keep the arterial PO_2 at around 110 mmHg. Similar PaO_2 values were obtained when the patients were breathing room air at atmospheric pressure. Under such conditions, the TuO_2 was 15.3 ± 2.3 mmHg (mean $\pm$ SE), which statistically was significantly lower than the 59.8 ± 6.5 mmHg value obtained in the normal tissue surrounding the brain tumor.

Statistically significant differences between the TuO_2 values in metastatic brain tumors and glioma were not found.

Correlations between TuO_2 and the degree of CT enhancement effects or the vascularity of the tumor as seen in angiograms were also not found.

References

1. Ardenne M, Reitnauer PG (1974) Measuring the PO_2 time behaviour in tumors as a valuable tool in cancer therapy. Oncol 29: 364–375
2. Atkins HL, Seaman WB, Jacox HW, Matteo RS (1965) Experience with hyperbaric oxygenation in clinical radiotherapy. Am J Roentgenol Rad Therapy Nuclear Med 93: 651–663
3. Barendsen GW, Koot CJ, Van Kersen GR, Bewley DK, Field SW, Parnell CJ (1966) The effect of oxygen on impairment of the proliferative capacity of human cells in culture by ionizing radiations of different LET. Int J Radiat Biol 10: 317–327
4. Belli JA, Hellman S (1976) Hypoxic cell sensitizers. N Eng Med 294: 1399–1400
5. Broerse JJ, Barendsen GW, Van Kersen GR (1967) Survival of cultured human cells after irradiation with fast neutrons of different energies in hypoxic and oxygenated conditions. Int J Radiat Biol 13: 559–572
6. Byfield JE, Barone RM, Calabro-Jones P, Lim P, Murane J, Ward JF (1980) Human tumor spheroid model for evaluating agents active against hypoxic cells. In: Brady LW (ed) Radiation sensitizers. Masson, New York, pp 465–471
7. Chang CH (1977) Hyperbaric oxygen and radiation therapy in the management of

glioblastoma. Nat Cancer Inst Monogr 46: 163–169
 8. Clark LC Jr (1956) Monitor and control of blood and tissue oxygen tension. Trans Am Soc Artif Internal Organs 2: 41–48
 9. Denekamp J (1983) D_0 hypoxic cells matter ? In: Steel GG, Adams GE, Reckham MJ (eds) The biological basis of radiotherapy. Elsevier, Amsterdam. pp 139–155
10. Deschner E, Gray LH (1959) Influence of oxygen tension on X-ray-induced chromosomal damage in Ehrlich ascites tumor cells irradiated in vitro and in vivo. Radiation Res 11: 115–146
11. Dische S (1979) Misonidazole—A drug for trial in radiotherapy and oncology. Int J Radiat Oncol Biol Phys 5: 851–860
12. Frackowick RSJ, Lenzi GL, Jones T, et al. (1980) Quantative measurement of regional cerebral blood flow and oxygen metabolism in man using ^{15}O and positron emission tomography: theory, procedure and normal values. J Comput Assist Tomogr 4: 727–736
13. Gray LH (1957) Oxygenation in radiotherapy: I. Radiological considerations. Br J Radiol 30: 403–406
14. Gullino PM, Grantham FH (1961) Studies on exchange of fluids between host and tumor: I. A method for growing 'tissue-isolated' tumors in laboratory animals. J Nat Cancer Inst 27: 679–693
15. Guillno PM, Grantham FH, Courtrey AH (1967) Utilization of oxygen by transplanted tumors in vivo. Cancer Res 27: 1020–1030
16. Henk JM (1981) Does hyperbaric oxygen have a future in radiation therapy? Int J Radiat Oncol Biol Phys 7: 1125–1128
17. Hirano A, Matsui T (1975) Vascular structure in brain tumors. Human Pathol 6: 611–521
18. Kapp JP, Routh A, Cotton D (1982) Hyperbaric oxygen as a radiation sensitizer in the treatment of brain tumors. Surg Neurol 17: 233–235
19. Kapp DS, Wagner F, Lawrence R (1982) Glioblastoma multiforme: Treatment by large dose fraction irradiation and metronidazole. Int J Radiat Oncol Biol Phys 8: 351–355
20. Lammertsma AA, Jones T (1983) Correction for the presence of intravascular oxygen-15 in the steady state technique for measuring regional oxygen extraction ratio in the brain: I. Description of the method. J Cereb Blood Flow Metabol 3: 416–424
21. Lammertsma AA, Wise RJS, Heathar JS (1983) Correction for presence of intravascular oxygen-15 in the steady state technique for measuring regional oxygen extraction ratio in the brain: II. Results in normal subjects and brain tumor and stroke patients. J Cereb Blood Flow Metabol 3: 425–431
22. Long DM (1970) Ultrastructure and the blood-brain barrier in human malignant brain tumors. J Neurosurg 32: 127–144
23. Pourreau-Schneider N, Malaise EP (1981) Relationship between surviving fractions using the colony method, the LD_{50} and the growth delay after irradiation of human melanoma cells grown as multicellular spheroids. Radiat Res 85: 321–334
24. Siesjo BK (1978) Hypoxia. In: Siesjo BK (ed) Brain energy metabolism. Wiley, Chichester, pp 398–452
25. Stalder B, Karcher H, Kogelnik HD, Szepesi T (1984) Misonidazole and irradiation in the treatment of high grade astrocytomas; Future report of the Vienna study group. Int J Rad Oncol Biol Phys 10: 1713–1717
26. Stewart FA, Rojas A, Denekamp J (1983) Radioprotection of two mouse tumors by WR-2721 in single and fractionated treatment. Int J Radiat Oncol Biol Phys 9: 507–513
27. Takakura K, Abe H, Tanaka R, Kitamura K, Miwa T, Takeuchi K, Yamamoto S, Kageyama N, Handa H, Mogami H, Nishimoto A, Uozumi T, Matsutani M, Nomura K (1986) Effects of ACNU and radiotherapy on malignant glioma. J Neurosurg 64: 53–57
28. Tanaka Y (1973) Microcirculation of the tumor and radiosensitivity—significance in clinical application. Jpn Cancer Clin 19: 922–928 (in Japanese)
29. Thomlinson RH, Gray LH (1955) The histological structure of some human lung cancers and the possible implications for radiotherapy. Br J Cancer 9: 539–549
30. Tsuchidoya T (1982) Approach to radiotherapy from pathological findings: II. Radio-

sensitivities of mixed cancer and brain tumor. Clin Rad 27: 1481–1482 (in Japanese)
31. Urtasun R, Band P, Chapman JD, Feldstein ML, Mielke B, Fryer C (1976) Radiation and high-dose metronidazole in supratentorial glioblastomas. N Engl J Med 294: 1364–1367
32. Vaupel P, Thews G (1974) PO_2 distribution in tumor tissue of DS-carcinoma. Oncol 30: 475–484
33. Vaupel P (1977) Hypoxia in neoplastic tissue. Microvascular research. 13: 399–408
34. Vaupel P (1977) Heterogenous responses to combination of hyperthermia and radiation. Radiology 123: 463–474
35. Walker DM (1975) Adjuvant to surgery and radiation therapy. Seminars in Oncol 2: 69–72
36. Wright EA, Howard FP (1957) The importance of oxygen on the radiosensitivity of mammalian tissue. Acta Radiol 48: 26–32

Part III
Clinical Studies

Chapter 7

An Outline of RAFP Therapy

T. Mori

Introduction

The principles of surgical therapy for primary malignant brain tumors, especially malignant gliomas, were established by Cushing in the 1930s, but today more than half a century later, the survival rate following surgery in such cases has been extended by no more than a few months. The treatment of malignant gliomas thus remains one of the most difficult, unsolved problems in neurosurgery today.

By the 1940s, however, radiation therapy had been introduced and in the 1960s effective chemo- and immuno- therapies were developed. By the 1970s, research into the tumor cell kinetics of malignant tumors [8, 9] had advanced considerably, the nitrosourea agents were synthesized, fundamental concepts of pharmacokinetics were introduced [10], and there were many new developments in treatment based upon a fundamental understanding of drug therapy [45, 54].

During this same period, computed tomography (CT) was coming into wide us, microsurgical techniques were being developed, and there were improvements in postoperative care. Together, these have led to a gradual but noteworthy improvement in therapeutic results. Most recently, the circulation and metabolism of brain tumor tissues have been greatly clarified by means of various imaging techniques, including magnetic resonance imaging (MRI), emission CT, Xenon (Xe), and N-isopropyl-p-[^{123}I] iodoamphetamine (IMP). These techniques may play a major role in the development of new therapeutic methods.

As was discussed in the previous chapter on findings reported in the neurosurgical literature, the best clinical results are obtained when surgical removal, radiation therapy, and chemotherapy are all employed. In particular, the developments in adjuvant therapy using radiochemotherapy have been remarkable. In order to obtain the most effective results from such therapies, however, various problems such as the optimal combination method, optimal doses, and the side effects of radiation therapy and chemotherapy must be studied with regard to tumor cell kinetics, pharmacokinetics, toxicity, and drug resistance.

From basic experimental data [19–21, 31, 37, 50, 51] and an analysis of our own clinical results [30, 36], we have developed a combined radiochemotherapy, which we refer to as RAFP therapy, for the treatment of malignant gliomas. Thus far, we have obtained favorable results [22, 23, 52]. This chapter presents the fundamental theory and clinical combination of RAFP therapy.

Fundamentals of RAFP Therapy

RAFP therapy is a combination of radiation therapy, chemotherapy using 1-(4-amino-2-methyl pyrimidine-5-yl)-methyl-3-(2-chloroethyl)-3-nitrosourea hydrochloride (ACNU) and N_1-(2-tetrahydrofuryl)5-fluorouracil (FT-207), and immunotherapy using polysaccharide Kureha (PSK) designed to exploit the different mechanisms of these therapies in order to enhance cytotoxicity synergistically. In the following sections, we describe the therapies and drugs which are a part of RAFP therapy and discuss their mechanisms of action, the effects of combined usage, and the reasons for their usage.

Radiation Therapy

Radiation therapy is essential for the treatment of brain tumors and is indisputably responsible for the prolongation of the survival time which has been obtained over the past few decades. A wide variety of developments in radiation therapy designed to improve therapeutic results have been introduced. One notable example is the treatment based on tumor cell kinetics.

According to cell kinetics studies on glioblastoma by Hoshino et al. [11, 12], 60%–70% of the brain tumor cells they examined were nonproliferating pool cells (G_0 cells), and the remaining 30%–40% were proliferating pool cells. Among these, G_2-M phase cells, which show sensitivity to irradiation, accounted for only 10% of the proliferating pool cells. So, it is thought that the therapeutic effect of irradiation is extremely poor.

These findings suggest that the effectiveness of radiation therapy could be improved by means of synchronization of tumor cells to the G_2-M phase using drugs such as ACNU and Vincristin. Shidara [46], therefore, devised a treatment for brain tumors called cellular synchronization radiation therapy. RAFP therapy is a combined treatment in which the additional effects of chemotherapy and immunotherapy are exploited.

As a rule, radiation therapy employs equal fractionation of irradiation to achieve a whole-brain dose of 30 Gy and a local dose of 30 Gy to give a total dose of 60 Gy. An interval of 1 week is normally allowed between the whole-brain and local irradiation to allow for tissue repair processes and the repopulation of tumor cells. During this period, it is considered that G_0 cells will enter the proliferating pool. Moreover, this interval allows for some recovery of the patient's general condition and some psychological respite. CT scans and other examinations can also be done during this interval. In cases of medulloblastoma, irradiation to the spinal cord is also performed.

The significance of chemotherapy in combination with radiation therapy has already been summarized by Phillips [41]. The main advantages are: (a) Tumor cells outside the field of irradiation can be killed; (b) radiation therapy can be used in regions not accessible to the drug; (c) the radiochemotherapy may have supraadditive effects, or the radiotherapy itself may be more effective due to the drug treatment.

We have previously found experimentally that each of the drugs (ACNU, FT-207, and PSK) used in RAFP therapy enhances the effect of the radiation therapy synergistically. Moreover, the combination of these drugs led to enhancement of their cytotoxic effects, which are discussed below.

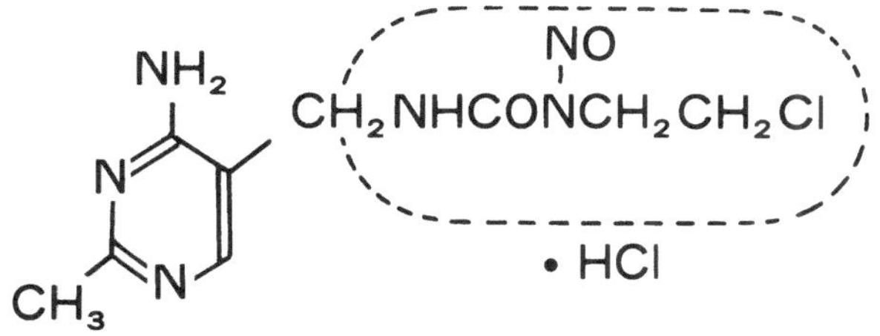

NH₂

N

N

CH₃

NO
CH₂NHCONCH₂CH₂Cl

• HCl

Fig. 7.1. Chemical structure of ACNU

ACNU (Nimustin)

ACNU is a water-soluble nitrosourea first synthesized by Nakao et al. [39] and Arakawa et al. [2] in 1974. It has a molecular weight of 309.2, the formula is $C_9H_{14}O_2N_6Cl_2$, and the structure is illustrated in Fig. 7.1. Under physiological conditions (pH 7.4), most molecules of ACNU are not ionized and about 96% do not decompose but exist as neutral molecules. At a log P of 0.92, ACNU is lipid soluble. It passes through the blood-brain barrier and is known as an anticancer agent with a high penetrance into the cerebrospinal fluid (CSF) and brain tumor tissue [13, 34].

The main mechanism of ACNU is thought to be its extremely slow alkylization of intracellular DNA, the blockage of DNA synthesis, and subsequent impairment of RNA and protein synthesis [14, 60]. Carbamoylization of DNA may also be involved [60].

With regard to the effects of ACNU on the cell cycle, Asamura and Saito [3] found that cultured mouse L cells had the greatest sensitivity to ACNU in the G_1 to early S phases and that ACNU blocked the progression of cells from the S phase to the G_2 phase, and from the G_2 phase to the M phase. Nakagawa et al. [38] found that mouse glioma MGB cells showed the greatest sensitivity to ACNU in the S phase and the least sensitivity in the M phase. Moreover, Takakura et al. [54] have reported that, using c-6 glioma cells, pretreatment of G_2-M phase cells with ACNU produced a proliferation of 10.6%, whereas 24 and 72 h after 10 µg/ml ACNU treatment, there was 30.1% and 40.5% proliferation, respectively. In vivo experiments have produced similar results.

Yamamoto and Matsutani [63] have reported strong synchronization to the middle S phase in glioma cells due to ACNU—a finding which suggests that effective antitumor results might be expected with the combined use of the cell-synchronizing capacities of ACNU combined with irradiation.

In our own experiments using rat glioma RG C-6 cell spheroids, we obtained the interesting finding that ACNU greatly reduces the size of the X-ray resistant hypoxic cell fraction. Since it is thought that hypoxic cells lie near a region of necrotic cells, these findings suggest that the therapy is more effective on quiescent hypoxic cells than on the proliferating cells [53]. For all the reasons discussed above, ACNU is used in our combined radiochemotherapy.

We will now discuss the effects of ACNU in combination with other therapies.

There have been many experimental and clinical studies on the synchronizing effects of ACNU on the tumor cell cycle to the G_2-M phase and on the effectiveness of ACNU in combination with radiation therapy [10, 25]. In both in vitro and in vivo experiments, additive or synergistic enhancement of the effects of ACNU has been found when it was combined with radiation therapy.

With regard to the timing of ACNU administration in relation to radiation therapy, we found in an experiment using monolayer cultured rat glioma (RGc-6) cells that the strongest effects were obtained when ACNU was administered 2-6 h prior to irradiation [51]. Suzuki and Tanaka [53] reported large antitumor effects when irradiation was done simultaneously with ACNU administration in an experiment on mice. Using a rat glioma model, Kaneko et al. [17] found a prolonged survival time when the drug was given 1 or 72 h before irradiation. With respect to enhancement of the effect occurring with administration of ACNU 1 h before irradiation, Leenhouts and chadwick [27] reported that the mechanism was the result of interactions at the level of cellular DNA. In the light of these findings, it is thought that there are two optimal timings for ACNU administration—0–6 h before irradiation and 72 h prior to irradiation.

Clinically, we have used the following protocol. Between 2 and 6 h prior to radiation therapy, ACNU is administered and some 24–72 h later at the beginning of the week when irradiation is possible ACNU is again given. In order to obtain the maximum effects of such combined therapy, it is desirable to increase the number of doses of ACNU, but this is difficult because of side effects such as delayed myelosuppression [44]. As a consequence, we normally administer a total of four doses of ACNU (1 mg/kg/dose) during the period of radiation therapy. Currently, favorable therapeutic results in the treatment of brain tumors are being reported by various groups employing a combination of ACNU and radiation therapy [28, 56, 59, 62].

FT-207 (Futraful)

FT-207 is a masked compound of 5-fluorouracil (5-FU) with a molecular weight of 200.17; the formula of $C_8H_9FN_2O_3$ (Fig. 7.2). It was first synthesized by a Soviet team [9] in 1966. FT-207 is decomposed into 5-FU via three different mechanisms, i.e., spontaneous decomposition, cytoplasmic decomposition, and actions of the liver macrosome enzyme, P-450. In turn, 5-FU has anticancer effects due to its blockage of DNA synthesis and disruption of RNA synthesis.

With regard to the cytotoxic effects of 5-FU, Skipper et al. [47] maintain that it is a cell cycle-specific (CCS) drug acting on the S phase, whereas Bhuyan et al. [4] argue that it is a cell cycle-nonspecific drug which has partial synchronization at nonlethal doses. Thus, it is considered that 5-FU is a drug with various modes of action, depending upon the type of cells used and the experimental system.

The reasons we chose FT-207 for use in our combined radiochemotherapy are as follows. Most importantly, FT-207 is highly lipid soluble and passes easily through the blood-brain barrier. Since its uptake by brain tumor tissue is also high [6, 7, 29, 40, 49] and there is little breakdown of 5-FU within tumor cells, the accumulation of 5-FU by such tissues can be anticipated. Secondly, since FT-207 is a masked compound, it has one-fifth to one-sixth the toxicity of 5-FU, its blood concentration is maintained for an extended period, its effects are twice those of 5-FU, and it is a time-dependent antimetabolite. Thirdly, the mechanism of action of FT-207 and its side effects differ from those of irradiation and ACNU, suggesting that supra-additive effects might be obtained in combination with those therapies. Fourthly, FT-207 can be administered either orally or rectally and can be given daily over an extended period.

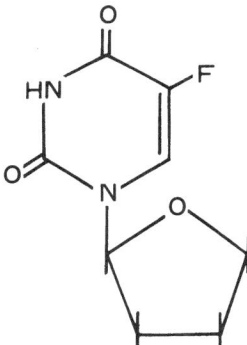

Fig. 7.2. Chemical structure of FT-207

Reasons for rectal administration of FT-207 include the fact that this route is easier than intravenous injection and fewer gastrointestinal side effects are encountered than with oral administration. Secondly, when administered orally, FT-207 enters the portal system and a large proportion of the drug is metabolized into an inactive substance. When delivered via the rectum, a large proportion is absorbed directly into the vena cava and the "fast-pass" effects on drugs due to the portal system are avoided. A high concentration of the drug can, therefore, be delivered to tissues other than the liver, especially tumor tissues. Thirdly, even with long-term usage, damage to the normal tissues of the rectum is not incurred and it is thus possible to give relatively large single daily doses and total doses which are far greater than those of other types of FT-207.

The effects of FT-207 in combination with other therapies will now be discussed.

We have performed experiments on the combined effects of radiation therapy and 5-FU in RGc-6 cells and have found that supra-additive effects are first found when irradiation is given 12 h after 5-FU administration. These effects are thought to be due to partial synchronization of the cell cycle to the G_1-S boundary due to the 5-FU treatment. In contrast, when glioma spheroids were used, maximal enhancement of cytotoxic effects were obtained when the irradiation was given 3–6 h after 5-FU administration. Moreover, our data suggest that this timing also produces the least amount of acute damage in normal tissue [26].

The combined administration of 5-FU and ACNU also produced supra-additive effects, and the cytotoxic effects were stronger when the 5-FU was given prior to ACNU [19, 20]. This finding is thought to be due to the fact that 5-FU treatment helps to accumulate proliferating cells at the G_1-S boundary. In addition, ACNU is known to have a strong cytotoxic effect on cells in the G_1 and early S phases [3]. It is also possible that ACNU blocks the recovery of cells damaged by 5-FU [21].

The above findings clearly indicate that combined therapy of FT-207 with either irradiation or ACNU can be expected to produce supra-additive effects. To maximize such effects, the timing of these combinations should be as follows. First, 5-FU should be administered, then ACNU, and, finally, irradiation should be done some 3–6 h later.

Since the report of Blokhina et al. [5], many studies on the effects of FT-207 in brain tumor cases have appeared. The majority have been effective in 33%–100% of cases, using combined irradiation and other anticancer agents [1, 13, 24, 35, 48, 55, 58].

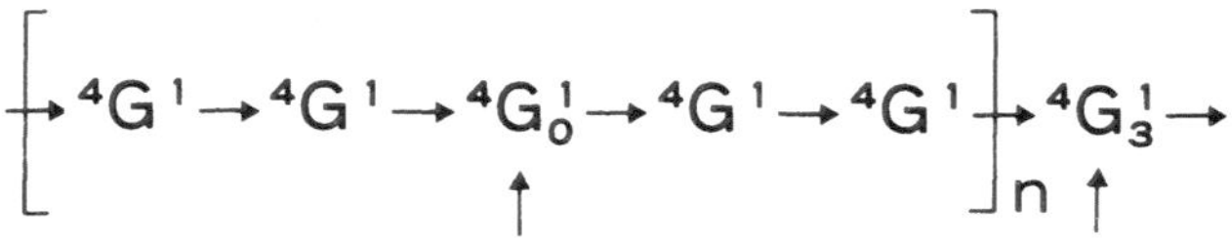

$$\left[\rightarrow {}^4G^1 \rightarrow {}^4G^1 \rightarrow {}^4G_0^1 \rightarrow {}^4G^1 \rightarrow {}^4G^1 \right. \left. \rightarrow {}^4G_3^1 \rightarrow \right]_n$$

G : β—D—Glucopyranose

Fig. 7.3. Chemical structure of Krestin (PSK)

PSK (Krestin)

PSK is a protein-bound polysaccharide extracted from cultured Kawaratake (*Coriolus versicolor Quel*), which is a basidiomycete [57]. It has a molecular weight of 9.4×10^4 and has immunopotentiating actions. It was first developed and marketed by Kureha Kogyo, Ltd., Tokyo in 1977. The presumed molecular structure of the main polysaccharide is shown in Fig. 7.3. The amino acid and monosaccharide content of PSK are given in Tables 7.1 and 7.2, respectively.

The mechanisms of action of PSK are multifaceted. It strengthens the activity of killer T cells, natural killer (NK) cells, and macrophages, increases the production of interleukin (Il-1 and Il-2), migration inhibitory factor (MIF), and tumor necrotizing factor (TNF), suppresses thromboxan A_2 (TXA_2) production, increases prostaglandin I_2 (PGI_2) production, ameliorates the side effects of antitumor drugs, prevents reduced resistance to infection during cancer therapy, increases the antitumor effects of other anticancer agents given in combination, and suppresses metastasis.

The antitumor effects of PSK are seen with oral administration and it is a unique biological response modifier (BRM) in not having side effects when used clinically [32].

Our reasons for using PSK include the fact that it is easily given orally, it facilitates many immune actions and it reduces the side effects of anticancer agents. It has also been found experimentally to enhance the antitumor effects of irradiation. In metastatic mammary mouse cells (MM46), this occurred when PSK was administered following irradiation. On sarcoma 180 transplanted to a mouse, the antitumor effects were produced by simultaneous administration and irradiation [33].

With regard to the combined use of ACNU and PSK on malignant mixed glioma in the rat, Kaneko et al. [16] reported that there was prolonged survival when PSK was administered both after and before ACNU treatment. It is thought that such effects are due to the capacity of PSK to prevent the decreases in immune functions normally caused by ACNU. Suzuki and Tanaka [53] reported that such combined therapy prolonged survival and suppressed the decreases in body weight. This latter finding is consistent with our own experimental results (Fig. 7.4).

Yamada et al. [61] reported on the effects of combined therapy using PSK and FT-207 in metastatic mouse sarcoma tissue (MCA-K3). They found greater suppression of the proliferation of the tumor cells when FT-207 was administered after PSK administration.

There have been many previous reports on the therapeutic effects of PSK on malignant tumors, and several studies have reported favorable results using combined radiochemotherapy with PSK in brain tumors [14, 18, 42, 43].

Table 7.1. Amino acid composition in the protein portion of PSK

Amino Acid	Composition (%)
Aspartic acid	13.2
Threonine	4.5
Serine	4.7
Glutamic acid	14.4
Proline	+
Glycine	7.8
Alanine	9.2
Cystine	+
Valine	9.6
Methionine	1.9
Isoleucine	5.9
Leucine	13.4
Tyrosine	2.9
Phenylalanine	6.7
Tryptophan	+
Lysine	2.8
Histidine	2.3
Arginine	0.7

+ trace

Table 7.2. Monosaccharide composition in the sugar portion of PSK

Monosaccharide	Composition (%)
Glucose	74.6
Galactose	2.7
Mannose	15.5
Xylose	4.8
Fucose	2.4

Practical Aspects of RAFP Therapy

With regard to the total dose of irradiation, a time dose fractionation (TDF) of 95–100 and 60 Gy with the Lineac or ^{60}Co is normally used (Fig. 7.5). First, whole-brain irradiation at a dose of 30 Gy is completed. As a rule, two-window opposing irradiation (2.0 Gy/dose) is given 5 days/week. After the completion of whole-brain irradiation, a week's rest is allowed and then a total of 30 Gy local irradiation is done over the following 3 weeks. If neurological symptoms are aggravated after the beginning of irradiation, mannitol and steroids are administered.

ACNU, 1 mg/kg, is dissolved in 20 ml distilled water immediately before administration either intravenously or by an intracarotid injection to the side of the tumor. As a rule, ACNU is given on Monday or Tuesday and irradiation is given 6 h after ACNU administration. During the period of whole-brain irradiation, ACNU is given once a week for 2 consecutive weeks. Then, after a period of 4 weeks, rest has been allowed to confirm that myelosuppression has not occurred, a similar schedule is used during the period of local irradiation.

ACNU therapy is either halted or delayed if the white blood cell count falls below 3000 or platelets below 80 000. Usually, the platelet count falls 3–4 weeks after ACNU administration, followed by a decrease in white blood cells. Subsequently, 4–5 weeks later, there is spontaneous recovery of both blood cell types. In cases where severe myelosuppression occurs 1–2 weeks following ACNU administration, great care is required. It is then essential to determine whether or not bone marrow functions are at the point of recovery or taking an unfavorable course. In contrast,

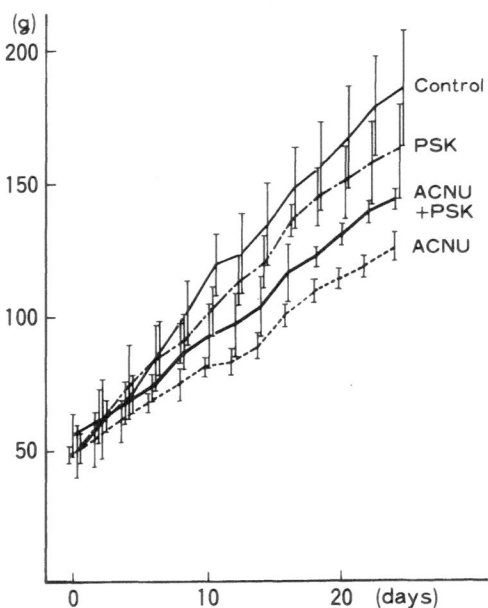

Fig. 7.4. Examination of changes in the body weight of rats treated with 10 mg/kg ACNU administered three times every 2 days and 1000 mg/kg PSK administered every day for a week. PSK inhibited the reduction of the body weight

headache and symptoms of the gastrointestinal tract, such as nausea and vomiting, within 24 h of ACNU administration are usually transitory and can be improved by conservative treatment.

We used to give 1000 mg/day of FT-207 as a suppository prior to sleep. However, since the appearance of recent experimental results, we have begun to administer it in the early morning and irradiate 3–6 h later. For extremely corpulent patients, we give two 750-mg suppositories, one in the morning and one in the evening. Patients who have difficulties with the suppository receive FT-207 orally. In such cases, it is given prior to the beginning of radiation therapy and continuously for the entire period of radiation therapy. When symptoms of the gastrointestinal tract, such as a loss of appetite, appear, FT-207 administration should be temporarily suspended or delayed.

PSK (Krestin) is given three times daily in 1-g doses; administration is done 30 min after meals per os. PSK is given continually throughout the period of therapy, and side effects are not usually encountered. During RAFP therapy, serological examinations are done once weekly and biochemical examinations once every 2 weeks. Various tests of the immune system and CT scans are done prior to therapy and after the completion of whole-brain and local irradiation. When necessary, additional tests are carried out.

We have outlined the fundamental theory and practice of RAFP therapy. Although the mechanisms of action of the therapies involved are known to a large extent, great care is still needed with regard to the doses, timing, side effects, etc. of each aspect of this method. It is worth emphasizing that the full effectiveness of RAFP therapy cannot be obtained simply by combining these techniques haphazardly. On the contrary, the duration of each part of the therapy and its proper

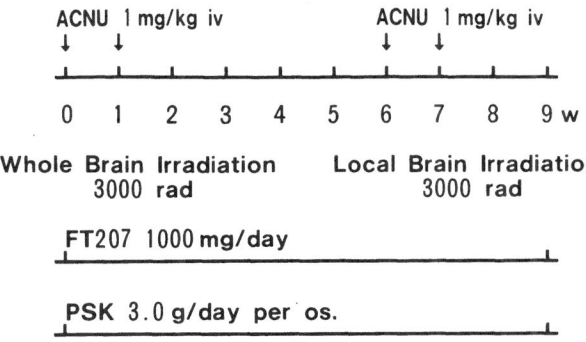

Fig. 7.5. Protocol of RAFP therapy

sequential order with respect to other parts are of extreme importance. We believe that in future studies of therapeutic techniques for brain tumors the RAFP therapy outlined above will be provide an instructive example of a therapy for which a good theoretical understanding based upon basic research has been obtained and then applied clinically.

References

1. Aoki Y (1981) Radiotherapy combined with Tegafur (FT-207) for brain tumors. Jpn J Cancer Chemother 8: 624–632 (in Japanese)
2. Arakawa M, Shimizu F, Okada N (1974) Effect of 1-(4-amino-2-methylpyrimidin-5-yl)methyl-3-(2-chloroethyl)-3-nitrosourea hydrochloride on leukemia L-1210. Jpn J Cancer Res 65: 191
3. Asamura M, Saito T (1977) Cell synchronization and chemotherapy of cancer. Jpn J Cancer Chemother 5: 737–746 (in Japanese)
4. Bhuyan BK, Scheidt LG, Fraser TJ (1972) Cell-cycle phase specificity of antitumor agent. Cancer Res 32: 398–407
5. Blokhina NG, Vozny EK, Garin AM, (1972) Results of treatment of malignant tumors with Futrafur. Cancer 30: 390–392
6. Fujita H, Ogawa K, Sawabe T, Kimura M (1972) Metabolism of N_1-(2'-tetrahydrofuryl)-5-fluorouracil (FT-207). Jpn J Cancer Clin 18: 917–922 (in Japanese)
7. Fujita H, Ogawa K, Akimoto H, Tahira K, Fukunaga I, Takakura K, Kohono T, Kimura M (1976) Distribution of FT-207 and its active substance into the brain and cerebrospinal fluid. Jpn J Cancer Chemother 3: 551–555 (in Japanese)
8. Fujiwara K, Taomoto K, Tamaki N, Matsumoto S, Chihara T (1973) Uptake of FT-207 by the brain tumor and its clinical trials. Jpn J Cancer Chemother 5: 361–368 (in Japanese)
9. Hiller SA, Zhuk RA, Lidak MY (1967) Analogous of pyrimidine nucleosides 1. N-(α-furanydyl)-derivatives of natural pyrimidine bases and their antimetabolite. Dokl Akad Nauk (USSR) 176: 332–335
10. Hori M, Nakagawa H, Hasegawa H, Hayakawa T, Mogami H, Nakata Y (1978) Chemotherapy of brain tumor combined with radiotherapy. Neurol Med Chir (Tokyo) 18: 649–654 (in Japanese)
11. Hoshino T, Barker M, Wilson CB, Boldrey EB, Fewer D (1972) Cell kinetics of human gliomas. J Neurosurg 37: 15–26
12. Hoshino T (1973) Cell kinetics of brain tumor. Neurol Surg 1: 453–459 (in Japanese)
13. Hoshino T (1980) Chemotherapy of malignant brain tumors: Biology and pharmacoki-

netics. Neurol Surg 8: 1007–1016 (in Japanese)

14. Imagawa K, Tochio H, Toda M, Hayashi S, Asai A, Nomura R (1972) Clinical studies on PSK combined therapy with surgery and adjuvant chemotherapy for brain tumor. Shinyaku Rinsho 26: 2109–2113 (in Japanese)

15. Kanamaru R, Asamura M, Sato H, Saito S, Wakui A, Saito T (1980) Studies on mechanism of action of ACNU, 1-(4-amino-2-methylpyrimidine-5-yl)-methyl-3-(2-chloroethyl)-3-nitrosourea hydrochloride: Effects on cultured Hela S_3 cells. Tohoku J Exp Med 132: 431–441

16. Kaneko S, Abe H, Aida T, Tsuru M, Kodama T, Kobayashi H (1980) Fundamental study of immunochemotherapy of brain tumors—Experimental brain tumor model and immunochemotherapy by a combination of PSK and ACNU. Neurol Med Chir (Tokyo) 20: 997–1005 (in Japanese)

17. Kaneko S, Allen NJ, Clendenon NR, Kartha M (1983) Treatment schedule for combined therapy using radiation and ACNU in experimental brain tumors. Neurol Med Chir (Tokyo) 23: 849–855 (in Japanese)

18. Kida Y, Shibuya N, Okada C, Umenura A, Kobayashi T, Kageyama N, Kamei H (1977) Immunological therapy for brain tumors by protein polysaccharide (PSK). Jpn J Cancer Chemother 4: 863–867 (in Japanese)

19. Kitahara M, Katakura R, Mori T, Suzuki J, Sasaki T (1984) Combined effect of ACNU and 5-fluorouracil on spheroids of rat glioma cells. Neurol Med Chir (Tokyo) 24: 747–757 (in Japanese)

20. Kitahara M, Katakura R, Mori T, Suzuki J, Sasaki T (1986) Combined effect of ACNU and 5-Fu on rat glioma cells in spheroids and monolayer cultures. Int J Cancer 38: 215–222

21. Kitahara M, Katakura R, Suzuki J, Sasaki T (1987) Experimental combination chemotherapy of ACNU and 5-Fu against cultured glioma model (spheroid) and subcutaneous rat glioma. Int J Cancer 40: 557–563

22. Kitahara M, Katakura R, Mashiyama S, Niizuma H, Yoshimoto T, Suzuki J, Mori T, Wada T (1987) Results of oligodendroglioma combined with radiochemotherapy. Neurol Surg 15: 397–403 (in Japanese)

23. Kitahara M, Katakura R, Shingai J, Niizuma H, Yashimoto T, Suzuki J, Mori T, Wada T (1987) Clinical results of supratentorial low-grade astrocytoma combined with radiochemotherapy. Neurol Surg 15: 597–604 (in Japanese)

24. Kohno T, Shitara N, Takakura K, Fujita H (1976) Role of FT-207 in the treatment of metastatic brain tumors. Jpn J Cancer Chemother 3: 729–734 (in Japanese)

25. Kohno T, Matsutani M, Hoshino T, Takakura K (1985) Effects of anticancer drugs on multicellular spheroids of 9L rat brain tumor. Brain and Nerve 37: 991–997 (in Japanese)

26. Kuwahara K, Katakura R, Sasaki T, Suzuki J (1987) Effect of combined treatment of X-rays and 5-Fu on rat glioma cells in multicellular spheroids. Neurol Med Chir (Tokyo) 27: (in press) (in Japanese)

27. Leenhouts HP, Chadwick KH (1980) An analysis of the interaction between two nitrosourea compounds and X-irradiation in rat brain tumor cells. Int J Radiat Biol 37: 169–181

28. Matsumoto K, Tabuchi K, Furuta T (1983) Combination chemotherapy of brain tumors with ACNU and 5-Fu. Neurol Med Chir (Tokyo) 23: 625–632 (in Japanese)

29. Matsuura H, Nakazawa S (1983) FT-207 and 5-Fu concentration in brain tumor tissues, plasma and CSF after administration of FT-207 suppository. Jpn J Cancer Chemother 11: 912–916 (in Japanese)

30. Mineura K, Mori T, Katakura R, Suzuki J (1979) Follow-up study of glioblastoma—A review of 179 cases. Neurol Med Chir (Tokyo) 19: 229–237 (in Japanese)

31. Mineura K, Mori T, Katakura R, Sasaki T (1981) Therapeutic effects of 1-(4-amino-2-methyl-5-pyrimidinyl)methyl-3-(2-chloroethyl)-3-nitrosourea hydrochloride (ACNU) and radiation on the rat glioma. Neurol Surg 9: 257–265 (in Japanese)

32. Mitomi T, Ogoshi K (1987) PSK and clinical application. The Saishin-Igaku 42: 314–318 (in Japanese)

33. Miyaji C, Ogawa Y, Imajo Y, Kimura S (1982) Combination therapy of radiation and immunomodulators in the treatment of MM46 tumor transplanted C3H/He mice. J Jpn Soc Cancer Ther 17: 1035–1042 (in Japanese)
34. Muraoka K (1983) ACNU delivery to malignant brain tumor tissue and serum—route of administration and effect of phenobarbital. Brain and Nerve 35: 1199–1206 (in Japanese)
35. Mori T, Fukawa O, Sato T, Hori S, Wada T (1977) Regression of recurrent malignant glioma by combined chemoradiotherapy utilizing Carboquone, FT-207 and Telecobalt—Report of a case. Neurol Surg 5: 865–869 (in Japanese)
36. Mori T, Mineura K, Katakura R (1979) Chemotherapy of malignant brain tumor by a water-soluble anti-tumor nitrosourea, ACNU. Neurol Med Chir (Tokyo) 19: 1157–1171 (in Japanese)
37. Mori T, Mineura K, Katakura R (1979) A consideration on pharmacokinetics of a new water-soluble anti-tumor nitrosourea, ACNU, in patients with malignant brain tumor. Brain and Nerve 31: 601–606 (in Japanese)
38. Nakagawa H, Hori M, Hasegawa H, Mogami H, Hayakawa T, Nakata Y (1979) The anti-tumor effet of ACNU and X-irradiation on mouse glioma. Brain and Nerve 31: 927–936 (in Japanese)
39. Nakao H, Fukushima M, Shimizu F (1974) Antileukemic agents: III. Synthesis and antitumor activity of N-(2-chloroethyl)-N-nitrosourea derivatives. Yakugaku Zasshi 94: 1032–1037 (in Japanese)
40. Nogaki H, Taomoto K, Tamaki N, Matsumoto S (1983) 5-FU concentration in brain tumors after co-administration of FT and uracil. Jpn J Cancer Chemother 10: 1007–1012 (in Japanese)
41. Phillips TL (1979) Current status, opportunities and problems in clinical combined chemoradiotherapy. Radiat Res, Proc of IVth international congress of radiation research, Tokyo, pp 822–829
42. Saito Y, Takami M, Muraoka K, Hokama Y (1981) Postoperative immuno-chemotherapy of brain tumors which ACNU and PSK. Jpn J Cancer Chemother 8: 1066–1075 (in Japanese)
43. Saito Y, Hori T, Takami M, Muraoka K, Hokama Y, Numata H (1984) Long-term survival of brain tumor patients treated postoperatively with ACNU and PSK , and immunological follow-up. Jpn J Cancer Chemother 11: 2185–2192 (in Japanese)
44. Saito T, Yokoyama M, Himori T, Ujiie S, Sugawara N, Sugiyama Z, Kitada K (1977) Phase I and preliminary phase II study of 1-(4-amino-2-methyl-5-pyrimidinyl)methyl-3-(2-chloroethyl)-3-nitrosourea hydrochloride (ACNU) administered by intermittent dose schedule. Jpn J Cancer Chemother 5: 991–1004 (in Japanese)
45. Sano K (1976) Chemotherapy on brain tumors. Neurol Med Chir (Tokyo) 16: 379–386 (in Japanese)
46. Shitara N (1978) Experimental and clinical study of cellular synchronization-radiation therapy for malignant brain tumors. Adv Neurol Sci 22: 119–131 (in Japanese)
47. Skipper HE, Schabel EM Jr, Mellet LB, Montgomery JA, Wekoff LJ, Lloid HH, Brockman RW (1970) Implications of biochemical cytokinetic pharmacologic and toxicologic relationships in the design of optimal therapeutic schedules. Cancer Chemother Rep 54: 431–450
48. Sueyoshi K, Uozumi A, Majima H (1979) Clinical experience with nitrosourea and FT-207. Suppository combination therapy against glioma. Jpn J Cancer Chemother 6: 1083–1088 (in Japanese)
49. Sueyoshi K, Majima H (1983) Cerebrospinal fluid distribution of systemically administered fluorinated pyrimidines. Jpn J Cancer Chemother 10: 818–823 (in Japanese)
50. Sugiyama S, Mori T, Suzuki J, Sasaki T (1984) Lethal effect of X-ray and ACNU on cultured rat glioma cells in multicellular spheroids. Neurol Med Chir (Tokyo) 24: 758–766 (in Japanese)
51. Sugiyama S, Mori T, Suzuki J, Sasaki T (1985) Effect of combined treatment, X-rays and ACNU on rat glioma cells in monolayer and multicellular spheroids. Neurol Med Chir

(Tokyo) 25: 707–714 (in Japanese)
52. Suzuki M, Mori T, Watanabe T, Katakura R, Suzuki J, Wada T (1983) Combined radio-chemo-immunotherapy (RAFP therapy) for medulloblastoma. Surg Neurol 11: 1271–1276 (in Japanese)
53. Suzuki Y, Tanaka R (1980) Anti-tumor effect of ACNU on experimental mouse brain tumors. Neurol Med Chir (Tokyo) 20: 405–413 (in Japanese)
54. Takakura K (1979) Chemotherapy on brain tumors. Neurol Med Chir (Tokyo) 19: 933–940
55. Takakura K, Sano K, Hojo S, Hirano A (1982) Metastatic tumors of the central nervous system. Igaku-Shoin, Tokyo
56. Tanaka R, Murakami N, Suzuki Y, Takeda N, Arai H, Konno K, Tanimura K (1984) Radiotherapy using bleomycin, ACNU and vincristine for malignant brain tumors. Neurol Med Chir (Tokyo) 24: 557–563 (in Japanese)
57. Tsukagoshi S, Hashimoto Y, Fujii G, (1984) Krestin (PSK). Cancer Treatment Reviews 11: 131–155
58. Tsuchida T, Watanabe E, Nakayama H, Sasaki R, Nakamura M, Sasaki M, Fujiwara T, Nemoto S, Fujiwara K, Yagihashi M, Hayakawa I, Nomura K (1980) FAR therapy in brain tumors—FT-207—vitamin A—radiation therapy, Neurol Med Chir (Tokyo) 20: 453–461 (in Japanese)
59. Ushio Y, Abe H, Suzuki J, Tanaka R, Kitamura K, Miwa T, Matsutani M, Takeuchi K, Takakura K, Nomura K, Yamamoto S, Kageyama N, Handa H, Mogami H, Matsumoto S, Nishimoto A, Uozumi T, Hori T, Mori T, Mori K, Matsukado Y (1985) Evaluation of ACNU alone and combined with Tegafur as addition to radiotherapy for the treatment of malignant gliomas—A cooperative clinical trial. Brain and Nerve 37: 999–1006 (in Japanese)
60. Wakui A (1982) Cancer chemotherapy with special reference to pharmacokinetics of nitrosoureas. Jpn J Cancer Chemother 9: 1327–1338 (in Japanese)
61. Yamada Y, Kitazato K, Unemi N (1979) Combination treatment with Futraful and Krestin. Jpn J Cancer Chemother 6: 127–131 (in Japanese)
62. Yamamoto H, Nakamura O, Kohno T, Shitara N, Takakura K, Sano K, Maehara T, Akanuma A, Sato F (1984) Synchronization chemotherapy for malignant gliomas. Neurol Surg 12: 795–805 (in Japanese)
63. Yamamoto H, Matsutani M (1981) Cell kinetic studies on synchronized glioma cells in vitro with special reference to the mode of action of chemotherapeutic agents. Brain and Nerve 33: 781–793 (in Japanese)

Chapter 8

Results of RAFP Therapy on CT Scan

J. Shingai

Introduction

Many studies on the effectiveness of therapy in glioma cases have been reported thus far [1–7, 9–12], but several problems in the analysis of such results have been apparent. In our attempt to avoid such difficulties, we evaluated the effectiveness of radiation + ACNU + FT-207 + PSK (RAFP) therapy in 72 glioma cases by means of computed tomography (CT). Here, we report our results and discuss the various problems encountered in the treatment of glioma and the evaluation of therapeutic results.

Clinical Materials and Methods

From October 1977, when CT scanning was begun at the Division of Neurosurgery of Tohoku University, until December 1985, 182 glioma cases of the following types were experienced: 75 glioblastoma, 46 anaplastic astrocytoma, 30 low-grade astrocytoma, 15 medulloblastoma, 12 oligodendrocytoma, and four ependymoma. Among the glioblastoma cases, therapy following the recurrence of the tumor was done in 11 patients, 11 patients died during treament, and there were 23 cases in whom complete excision of the lesion was done prior to additional therapy. Evaluation of the therapy by means of CT, however, was inconclusive. Similar results were obtained in eleven, six, and eighteen of the anaplastic astrocytoma cases; one, three, and one of the medulloblastoma cases; one, two, and seven of the oligodendroglioma cases; zero, two, and two of the ependyoma cases; and three, zero, and eleven of the low-grade astrocytoma cases, respectively.

The above cases were excluded from the present analysis, and there were another five cases of low-grade astrocytoma which were not treated with RAFP therapy, but since they constituted a small number of cases they also were excluded from the analysis. Among the cases in which the therapeutic results could be evaluated by means of CT scan, there were 30 glioblastoma, 21 anaplastic astrocytoma, 11 low-grade astrocytoma, ten medulloblastoma, and two oligodendroglioma cases. The two oligodendroglioma cases were excluded from the present study, however, because the number available was insufficient for meaningful analysis. Therefore, a total of 72 cases were analyzed. Evaluation of the therapeutic results was undertaken following the criteria of Mogami et al. [8]: Complete remission (CR), disappearance of the lesion which can be evaluated; partial remission (PR), more than a 50% reduction in the overall area of the lesion measured in two orthogonal dimensions and no aggravation of secondary lesions; no change (NC), less than a 50% reduction of the overall area of the lesion measured in two dimensions or an increase of less than 25%, but no aggravation of lesions secondary to the brain tumor; progressive disease (PD), more than 25% increase in the area of the measured lesion, aggravation of other lesions, and/or the appearance of new lesions. Complete remission and partial remission were regarded together as cases of remission, and the remission rate was calculated from the total number of each histological type of lesion.

Results

A low remission rate of 13.3% was seen in the glioblastoma cases. There were no cases of complete remission, five of partial remission, 14 of no change, and 12 of progressive disease. The remission rate was 38.1% (8 of 21 cases) in anaplastic astrocytoma and 54.5% (6 of 11 cases) in low-grade astrocytoma, indicating that more favorable results were obtained in the less malignant forms of glioma. Among the glioblastoma cases known to have the greatest malignancy, some 40% (12 cases) showed increases in the tumor size despite the fact that treatment was in progress. All ten of the medulloblastoma cases had favorable outcomes (eight cases of complete remission and two of partial remission; Table 8.1). Among the cases of remission, all showed improvements in neurological deficits.

Discussion

There are two notable problems which are encountered when comparisons are made among the therapeutic results in glioma cases reported by different groups. The first concerns differences in the criteria for evaluating the therapeutic results. Some researchers have placed emphasis on changes in neurological findings [4, 9] and others have evaluated the results both from neurological findings and those of radionucleotide brain scans [5], but there is an inescapable subjective factor in the evaluation of neurological symptoms.

Subsequent to the introduction of the CT scan, Levin et al. [6] have advocated a method in which the scores of three indices are added together: neurological findings, radionucleide brain scans, and CT scans. While such a method allows for evaluation from several perspectives, the summation of unrelated scores makes the interpretation difficult and reduces the objectivity.

The criteria for evaluating brain tumors advocated by Mogami et al. [8] and widely used in Japan is based solely upon the image provided by CT scans. Although there are cases in which the CT scans do not accurately reflect the actual condition, the Mogami method has the advantage of being entirely objective and quantitative. Using that method, Tanaka et al. [11] reported remission rates (the summation of complete and partial remission) of 67% in astrocytoma and 29% in anaplastic glioma, and Matsumoto et al. [7] reported remission rates of 50% in astrocytoma

Table 8.1. Response of RAFP therapy for evaluable cases

	No. of cases[a]	CR	PR	NC	PD	Remission rate (%)
Glioblastoma	30	0	4	14	12	13.3
Anaplastic astrocytoma	21	0	8	9	4	38.1
Low-grade astrocytoma	11	2	4	5	0	54.5
Medulloblastoma	10	8	2	0	0	100

[a] Number of patients available for response
CR complete remission, *PR* partial remission, *NC* no change, *PD* progressing disease

and 23% in glioblastoma. Because of differences in the histopathological diagnosis, a direct comparison with our results is not possible. Nevertheless, these findings are similar to ours with regard to the high remission rate for relatively low malignancy cancers and the low remission rate for the more malignant types.

A second problem involved in the comparison of therapeutic results concerns the classification used for histological diagnosis. In most previous studies, the evaluation of therapeutic results has been done with glioblastomas and other anaplastic gliomas classified together as malignant glioma [4, 5, 9, 10, 12]. Among those studies, one reports favorable results in as much as 72% of such cases [9]. In recent years, however, a distinction between these lesions has been made [3, 6] and Levin et al. [6] reported favorable results in 36% of gliobastomas and 31% of other anaplastic gliomas, using PCV therapy together with Procarbazine, CCNU, and Vincristine.

The results of the present study pertain solely to RAFP therapy and cannot, therefore, be directly compared with most other therapeutic methods, but it is worth noting that a relatively favorable remission rate of 38.1% was obtained in anaplastic astrocytoma and a relatively poor remission rate of 13.3% was obtained in glioblastoma. These results indicate that RAFP therapy has little effectiveness in glioblastoma.

Favorable results in medulloblastoma cases have been obtained by Craft et al. (63%) and Duffner et al. (100%) and we had remission in all ten of our cases. At least with regard to the outcome immediately following RAFP therapy, our results are similar to those found in the literature. It must be emphasized, however, that the results of combined radio-chemotherapy in malignant gliomas are notably different in glioblastoma and anaplastic astrocytoma cases; evaluation of therapeutic results should be reported while making appropriate distinctions between them. It is also evident that the criteria for evaluation still differ among various research institutes and countries, indicating the desirability of a consistent and internationally agreed set of criteria.

Conclusion

The results of RAFP therapy in 30 cases of glioblastoma, 21 cases of anaplastic astrocytoma, 11 cases of low-grade astrocytoma, and ten cases of medulloblastoma were evaluated by means of CT scans.

The remission rate was 100% for medulloblastoma, 54.5% for low-grade astrocytoma, 38.1% for anaplastic astrocytoma, and 13.3% for glioblastoma.

References

1. Craft DC, Levin VA, Edwards MS, Pischer TL, Wilson CB (1978) Chemotherapy of recurrent medulloblastoma with combined procarbazine, CCNU, and vincristine. J Neurosurg 49: 589–592
2. Duffner PK, Cohen ME, Thomas PRM, Sinks LF, Freeman AI (1979) Combination chemotherapy in recurrent medulloblastoma. Cancer 43: 41–45
3. Gutin PH, Wilson CB, Kumar ARV, Boldrey EB, Levin VA, Powell M, Enot KJ (1975) Phase II study of procarbazine, CCNU, and vincristine combination chemotherapy in the treatment of malignant brain tumors. Cancer 35: 1398–1404
4. Hildebland J, Brihaye J, Wagenknecht L, Mitchel J, Kenis Y (1973) Combination chemotherapy with 1-(2-chloroethyl-3-chlorohexyl-1-nitrosourea) (CCNU), vincristine and methotrexate in primary and metastatic brain tumors—a preliminary report. Eur J Cancer 9: 627–634
5. Levin VA, Hoffman WF, Pischer TL, Seager ML, Boldrey EB, Wilson CB (1978) BCNU-5-fluorouracil combination therapy for recurrent malignant brain tumors. Cancer Treat Rep 62: 2071–2076
6. Levin VA, Wara WM, Davis RL, Vestmys P, Resser KJ, Yatsko K, Nutik S, Gutin PH, Wilson CB (1985) Phase III comparison of BCNU, and vincristine administered after radiotherapy with hydroxyurea for malignant gliomas. J Neurosurg 63: 218–223
7. Matsumoto K, Tabuchi K, Furuta T, Fujiwara T, Nakasome S, Onishi R, Moriya Y, Nishimoto A, Doi A, Asari S, Suga T (1983) Combination chemotherapy of brain tumors with ACNU and 5-FU. Neurol Med Chir (Tokyo) 23: 625–632
8. Mogami H, Ushio Y, Sano K, Takakura K, Handa H, Yamashita J, Uekik, Tanaka R, Hatanaka H, Nomura K (1986) Criteria for evaluating treatment regimens for patients with brain tumors. Neurol Med Chir (Tokyo) 26: 191–194
9. Pouillart P, Mathe G, Thy TH, Lheritier J, Poisson M, Huguenin P, Gauthier H (1976) Treatment of malignant gliomas and brain metastases in adults with a combination of adriamycin, VM-26, and CCNU: results of a phase II trial. Cancer 38: 1909–1916
10. Seiler RW, Greiner RH, Zimmerman A, Markwalder H (1978) Radiotherapy combined with procarbazine, bleomycin and CCNU in the treatment of high-grade supratentorial astrocytomas. J Neurosurg 48: 861–865
11. Tanaka R, Murakami, N Suzuki N, Takeda N, Arai H, Konnok, Tanimura K (1984) Radiotherapy using bleomycin, ACNU, and vincristine for malignant brain tumors; efficacy for tumor regression. Neurol Med Chir (Tokyo) 24: 557–563
12. Zanger E, de Tribolet N, Wagenknecht L (1978) Combined chemotherapy with VM-26 and BCNU for recurrent malignant gliomas after operation and irradiation. Acta Neurochirur (Wien) 42: 97–101

Chapter 9

Clinical Analysis of Glioma: Anaplastic Astrocytoma and Glioblastoma

J. Shingai and M. Kanno

Introduction

There have been many reports on the effects of radiotherapy and chemotherapy and on the factors influencing the prognosis of malignant gliomas [1, 3, 5, 6, 10–12, 15, 17, 18]. The approach of most early investigations was historical [e.g., 3, 17, 18], but in recent years the number of randomized studies reporting on the effects of radiotherapy or chemotherapy has increased [1, 5, 10–12]. Among such studies, some have acknowledged the effectiveness of adjuvant chemotherapy [1, 3, 10, 15, 18], but others report negative findings in this regard [5, 12, 17]. In contrast, there has been some uniformity of opinion concerning the effectiveness of radiotherapy [2, 3, 13, 16, 18, 19]. Among such studies, however, many have reported the effects of adjuvant therapy for a group in which glioblastoma and other anaplastic gliomas were discussed together as a single disease entity [1, 3, 5, 12, 17, 18].

From among our own cases of malignant glioma, we have made a study of the effects of adjuvant therapy and factors influencing the prognosis in glioma cases, where glioblastoma and anaplastic astrocytoma have been analyzed separately.

Clinical Materials and Methods

Between January 1965 and June 1985, 101 cases of glioblastoma and 102 cases of anaplastic astrocytoma were treated at the Division of Neurosurgery of Tohoku University School of Medicine. Among the glioblastoma cases, there were six operative fatalities, three postoperative deaths while the patients were still in hospital, two patients received further therapy due to recurrence of the glioma, two patients were lost to follow-up, and there were three other fatalities due to factors unrelated to the glioma. Among the anaplastic astrocytoma cases, there were eight operative deaths, seven patients who were lost to follow-up, and five other fatalities due to other disorders. The survival rate could, therefore, be evaluated in a total of 84 glioblastoma and 82 anaplastic astrocytoma cases. Aspects of the survival rates for these 166 cases were studied as described below.

Age and Sex Distribution

Study was made of the sex and ages of the patients at the time of onset in both kinds of glioma.

Overall Survival Rate

The overall survival rates for the 84 glioblastoma and 82 anaplastic astrocytoma cases were studied separately.

Age

There were 11 glioblastoma patients less than 20 years of age, ten between the ages of 20 and 39, 11 between 40 and 49, 30 between 50 and 59, and 22 were over the age of 60. The numbers of anaplastic astrocytoma patients at these ages were, respectively, 10, 29, 20, 15, and 8. Survival rates for each decade of life were calculated.

Site of Lesion

The sites of the 84 glioblastoma cases were as follows: 22 in the frontal lobe, six in the temporal lobe, four in the parietal lobe, four in the occipital lobe, eight in the thalamus, two in the lower brain stem, one in the cerebellum, and 20 with the tumor located at two or more lobes. The sites of the 82 anaplastic astrocytoma cases were: 29 in the frontal lobe, seven in the temporal lobe, seven in the parietal lobe, two in the occipital lobe, eight in the thalamus, four in the cerebellum, one in the lower brain stem, one in the lateral ventricle, one in the centrum semiovale, and 24 were located at two or more lobes.

Survival rates were calculated for the four sites where a relatively large number of cases were found, i.e., the frontal lobe, the temporal lobe, the parietal lobe, and the thalamus.

Duration of Disease

The duration of the glioblastoma ranged from 0 to 61 months, with a mean of 6.2 months, whereas that of the anaplastic astrocytoma ranged from 1 to 108 months, with a mean of 11.9 months. For the purpose of analysis, the glioblastoma cases were classified into four categories according to the duration of the disease: less than 3 months (41 cases), between 3 and 6 months (23 cases), between 6 and 12 months (eight cases), and more than 12 months (12 cases). The anaplastic astrocytoma cases were classified into three groups: less than 3·months (44 cases), between 3 and 12 months (16 cases), and more than 12 months (21 cases). Again, survival rates for each of these subgroups were calculated.

Clinical Symptoms

Classification according to the clinical symptoms at the time of admission to hospital gave the following four categories for the glioblastoma cases: six cases with convulsions but no neurological deficits: 22 with focal signs, such as motor deficits ro aphasia: 22 with symptoms suggestive of intracranial hypertension, such as headache, nausea, or vomiting; and eight with disturbances of consciousness, such as a semicomatose or confused state. Among the anaplastic astrocytoma cases, the numbers of cases with such symptoms were 13, 34, 26, and 9, respectively. Survival rates for each category were calculated.

Performance Status

The so-called performance status of the patients on admission was grouped into five categories using the ECOG classification: grade 0, social activity possible without limitations and the patient's condition is similar to that prior to onset; grade 1, limitations on heavy physical labor, but walking and light work still possible; grade 2, walking and daily chores possible and more than one half of the day is spent actively, but even light work is impossible; grade 3, daily chores possible, but patient is bedridden for more than half of the day; grade 4, daily chores impossible, assistance required for walking, and the patient is largely bedridden.

By classifying the glioblastoma cases into three groups according to the performance status (grades 0–1, grades 2–3, and grade 4), a total of 19, 39, and 25 cases, respectively, were found. For the anaplastic astrocytoma cases, these figures were 36, 26, and 19, respectively, and the survival rates were calculated.

Degree of Surgical Excision

Among the glioblastoma patients, there were 51 which underwent total resection of the glioma, 13 with subtotal resection, 13 with partial resection or biopsy, and seven without surgical intervention. For the anaplastic astrocytoma cases, there were 37 patients with total resection, 23 with subtotal resection, 16 with partial resection or biopsy, and six without surgery. The influence of the extent of the surgery on the survival rates was studied.

Method of Adjuvant Therapy

Among the glioblastoma cases, there were eight fatalities in which, despite the fact that radiochemotherapy was in progress, the size of the tumor continued to increase and death came in the middle of adjuvant therapy. Excluding these eight cases, the relationship between the survival rate and the method of adjuvant therapy could be evaluated in a total of 76 glioblastoma cases and 82 anaplastic astrocytoma cases. The adjuvant therapy in the glioblastoma cases included 44 receiving combined radiotherapy and ACNU, FT-207, and PSK (RAFP) therapy, 13 receiving combined radiotherapy and chemotherapy (three receiving CQ and FT-207, six receiving FT-207 and PSK, two receiving BLM and two receiving BAR therapy), 15 receiving radiotherapy alone, one receiving chemotherapy (BLM) alone, and three going untreated. Among the anaplastic astrocytoma cases, 32 received RAFP therapy, 19 received radiotherapy and chemotherapy (five receiving CQ and FT-207, eight receiving FT-207 and PSK, two receiving BLM, and four receiving BAR therapy), 15 received only radiotherapy, six received only chemotherapy, and ten went untreated. Survival rates were calculated only for those therapeutic groups with a relatively large number of cases (RAFP therapy, combined radiochemotherapy, and radiotherapy alone).

The histological diagnosis was made using the WHO classification. Glioblastoma multiforme (grade IV) and gliosarcoma (grade IV) were considered together as glioblastoma; astrocytoma (grade III) was considered as anaplastic astrocytoma. All lesions were evaluated by the same neuropathologist.

Survival rates were calculated using the Kaplan-Meier method [9] and evaluation of the significance between survival rates was done using the Cox-Mantel method [4].

Results

Age and Sex Distribution

The ages of the glioblastoma patients at the time of hospitalization ranged from 3 to 74 years, with a mean of 47.4 years. The decade of life during which the most cases were found was 50–59 years. For the anaplastic astrocytoma cases, ages ranged from 2 to 75 years, with a mean of 40.5 and a peak in the 30s and 40s, suggesting a tendency for anaplastic astrocytoma patients to be somewhat younger than glioblastoma patients (Fig. 9.1).

Of the 84 glioblastoma cases, 52 were male and 32 were female (a ratio of 1.7 : 1) and there was also a slight preponderance of males among the anaplastic astrocytoma cases—47 males and 35 females (1.4 : 1).

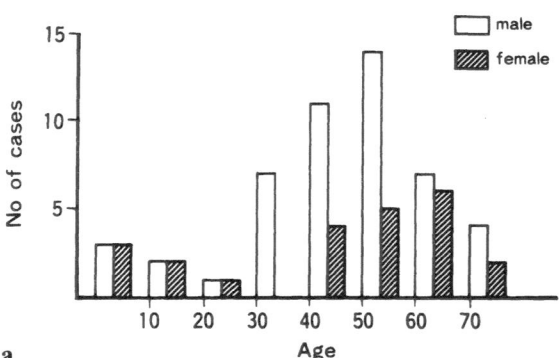

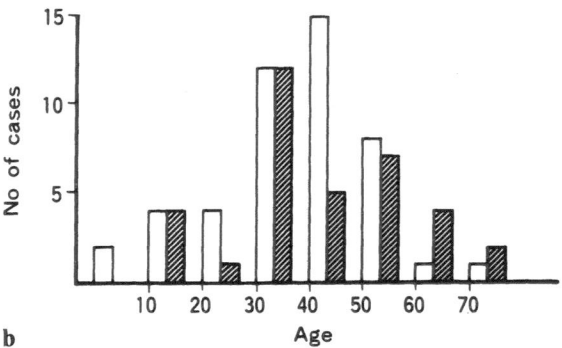

Fig. 9.1a, b. Distribution by age and sex. a Glioblastoma; b anaplastic astrocytoma

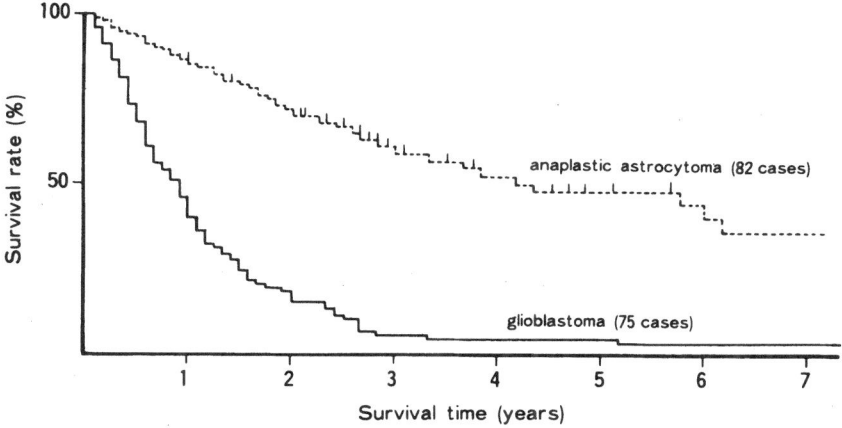

Fig. 9.2. Overall survival rates

Overall Survival Rate

The 1-, 3-, and 5-year survival rates for the anaplastic astrocytoma cases were 87%, 61%, and 48%, respectively, whereas they were 46%, 5%, and 4% for the glioblastoma cases. Clearly, a very small percentage of the glioblastoma patients survived for more than 3 years and the prognosis was generally much worse than for the anaplastic astrocytoma cases (Fig. 9.2).

Age

The prognosis for the glioblastoma cases was worst for those patients over the age of 60, where a rapid fall in the survival rate to only 9% 1 year from diagnosis was seen. The survival rates for the patients in their 20s or 30s, 40s and 50s, however, were relatively good and significantly better than the rate for patients in their 60s ($P < 0.017$, $P < 0.017$, and $P < 0.001$, respectively; Fig. 9.3a).

Among the anaplastic astrocytoma cases, the prognosis was poor for patients in their 40s, 50s, or 60s and best for patients in their 20s or 30s. Like glioblastoma, the prognosis was favorable for the youngest patients. Significant differences in the prognosis were found in a comparison of the 20- to 39-year-old group and the 40- and 50-year-old groups ($P < 0.034$; Fig. 9.3b).

It has often been reported that the prognosis in glioblastoma is poor in elderly patients—unfavorable for those over 50 years [5], but favorable for young patients [14]. Our findings are in general agreement with these previous reports but contrast with at least one report in which no relationship between age and prognosis was found among glioma cases [18]. It has also been reported that the survival rate is higher for young astrocytoma patients, as we have found in the present study.

Site of Lesion

The prognosis among the glioblastoma cases was worst for those with thalamic tumors—with a 1-year survival rate of only 13%. This rate was significantly poorer

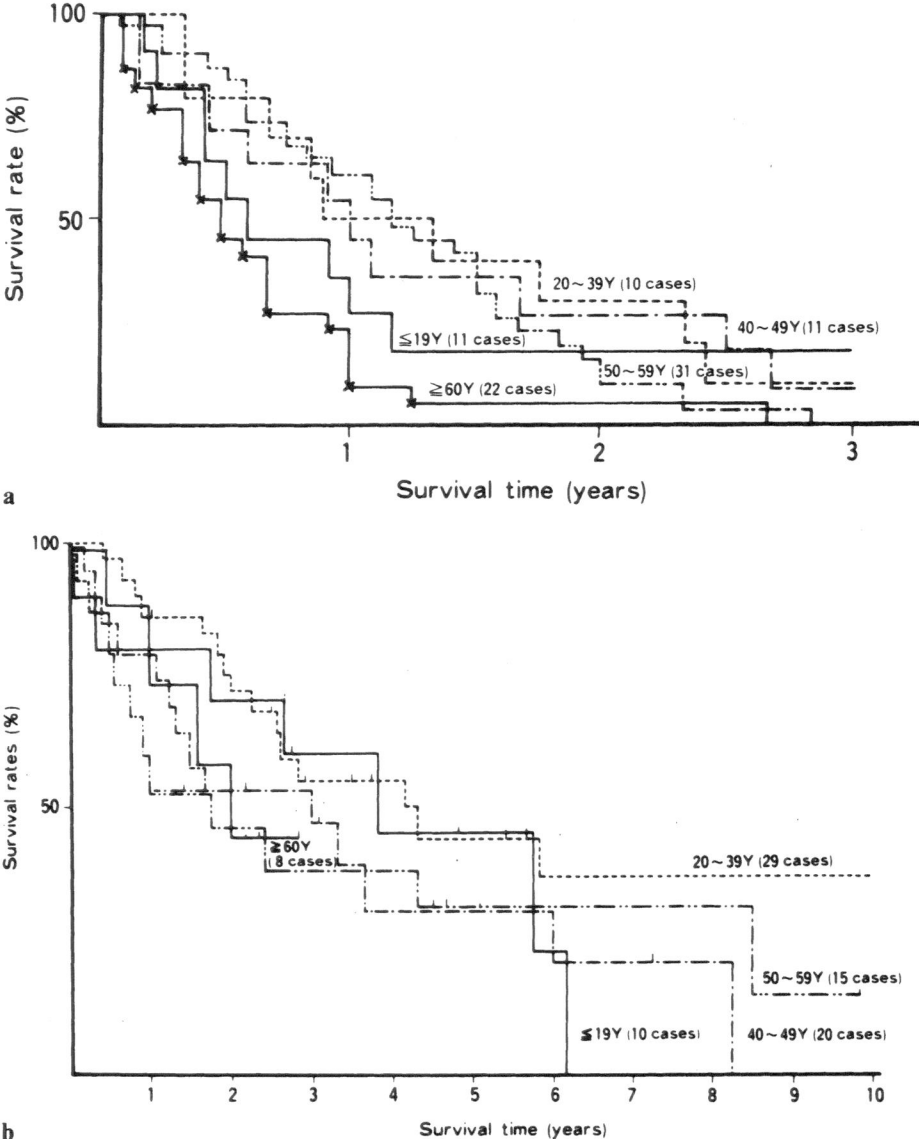

Fig. 9.3a, b. Relationship between survival rate and age. **a** Glioblastoma; **b** anaplastic astrocytoma

than that found at other sites: frontal ($P < 0.001$), temporal ($P < 0.006$), and parietal ($P < 0.03$; Fig. 9.4a).

Among the anaplastic astrocytoma patients, the survival rate was short for both the thalamic and parietal tumor cases but quite favorable for both frontal and temporal locations. A significantly higher survival rate was found in the frontal

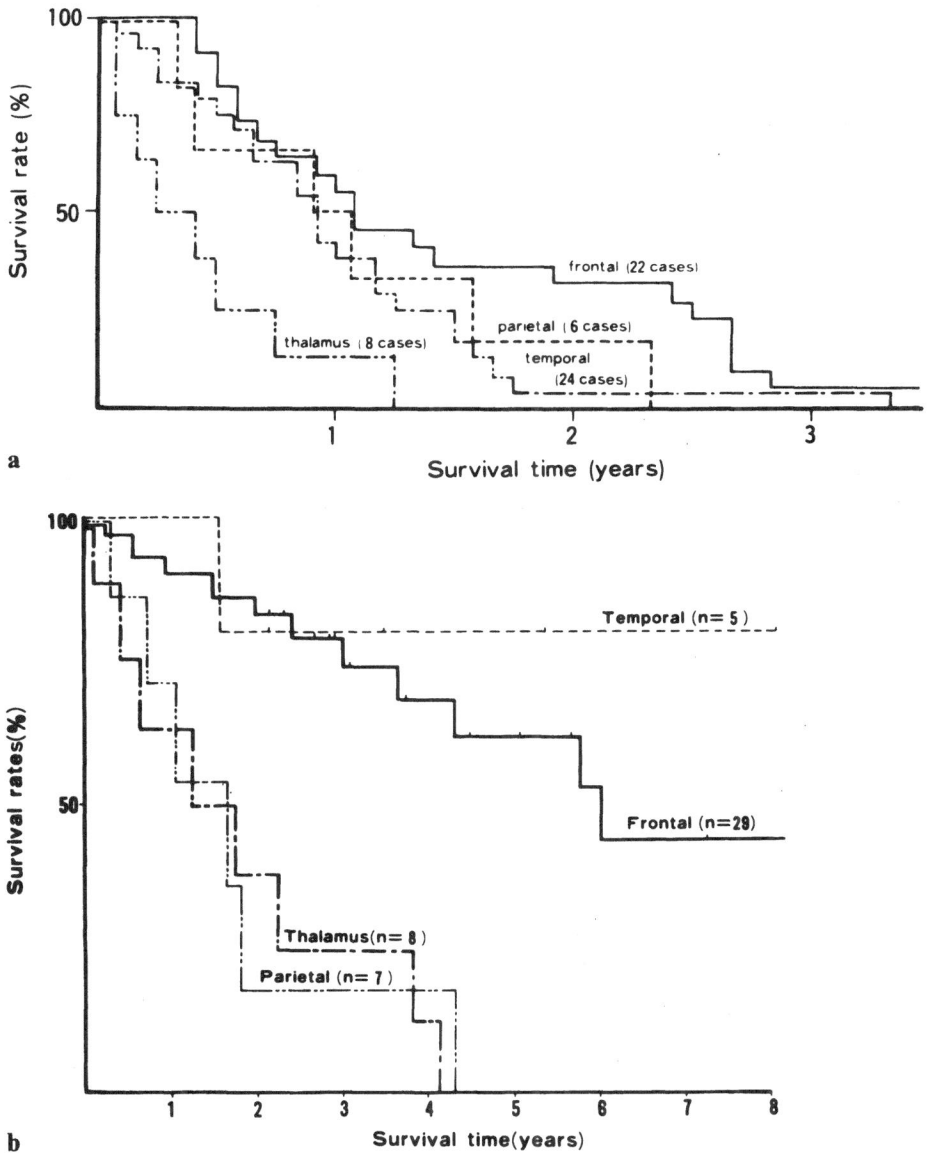

Fig. 9.4a, b. Relationship between survival rate and locations. **a** Glioblastoma; **b** anaplastic astrocytoma

lobe cases than in either the thalamic ($P < 0.001$) or parietal ($P < 0.001$) cases (Fig. 9.4b).

 Study of the relationship between the degree of extirpation and the site of the tumor showed that 12.5% of glioblastomas located in the thalamus were totally or subtotally extirpated, and some 25% of the anaplastic astrocytoma cases at that site were extirpated—well below the rate for total or subtotal extirpation at other sites

Table 9.1. Relationship between location and rate of extirpation

	Method of extirpation				No operation	Total number	Percent[a]
	Total	Subtotal	Partial	Biopsy			
Glioblastoma							
Frontal	14	7	1	0	0	22	95.5
Temporal	12	7	2	2	1	24	79.1
Parietal	4	2	0	0	0	6	100
Thalamus	1	0	1	2	4	8	12.5
Anaplastic astrocytoma							
Frontal	22	6	0	1	0	29	96.6
Temporal	3	2	0	0	0	5	100
Parietal	4	3	0	0	0	7	100
Thalamus	2	0	0	6	0	8	25.0

[a] This signifies the *Total* plus the *Subtotal* divided by the *Total number*

(Table 9.1). It is thought likely that this low rate of surgical removal of the thalamic tumors is responsible for the relatively poor prognosis. It is noteworthy, however, that the survival period was shorter in cases of parietal anaplastic astrocytomas, despite the fact that total or subtotal extirpation was done in all cases (Table 9.1). This suggests that factors other than the extent of the surgical removal play an important role in the final outcome. Walker et al. [18] reported that the prognosis in parietal lobe cases was poor in their cooperative study on anaplastic glioma, and there has also been a report of significantly better results in frontal lobe cases [5]. Our results are in agreement with those studies, but it remains uncertain why the period of survival among the parietal cases is so short.

Duration of Disease

Among the glioblastoma cases, a tendency toward prolonged survival periods was seen in those which had a duration of the disease in excess of 12 months, but this effect did not reach statistical significance because of the small number of cases (Fig. 9.5a). In the anaplastic astrocytoma group, the prognosis was worst for the cases with a duration of less than 3 months, whereas there was a significant prolongation of the period of survival time among the cases with a duration in excess of 12 months ($P < 0.024$; Fig. 9.5b).

Stage and Stein [17] reported a close relationship between the duration of the disease, degree of malignancy, and survival period in grades I–IV astrocytoma cases. Our results on the grade of the glioma, in which a distinction was made between the glioblastoma and anaplastic astrocytoma cases, showed trends similar to those reported by Stage and Stein [17] and significant differences among the grades in the anaplastic astrocytoma group.

Clinical Symptoms

In the glioblastoma group, the survival period was significantly longer in patients who had only suffered convulsions and no neurological symptoms except those seen

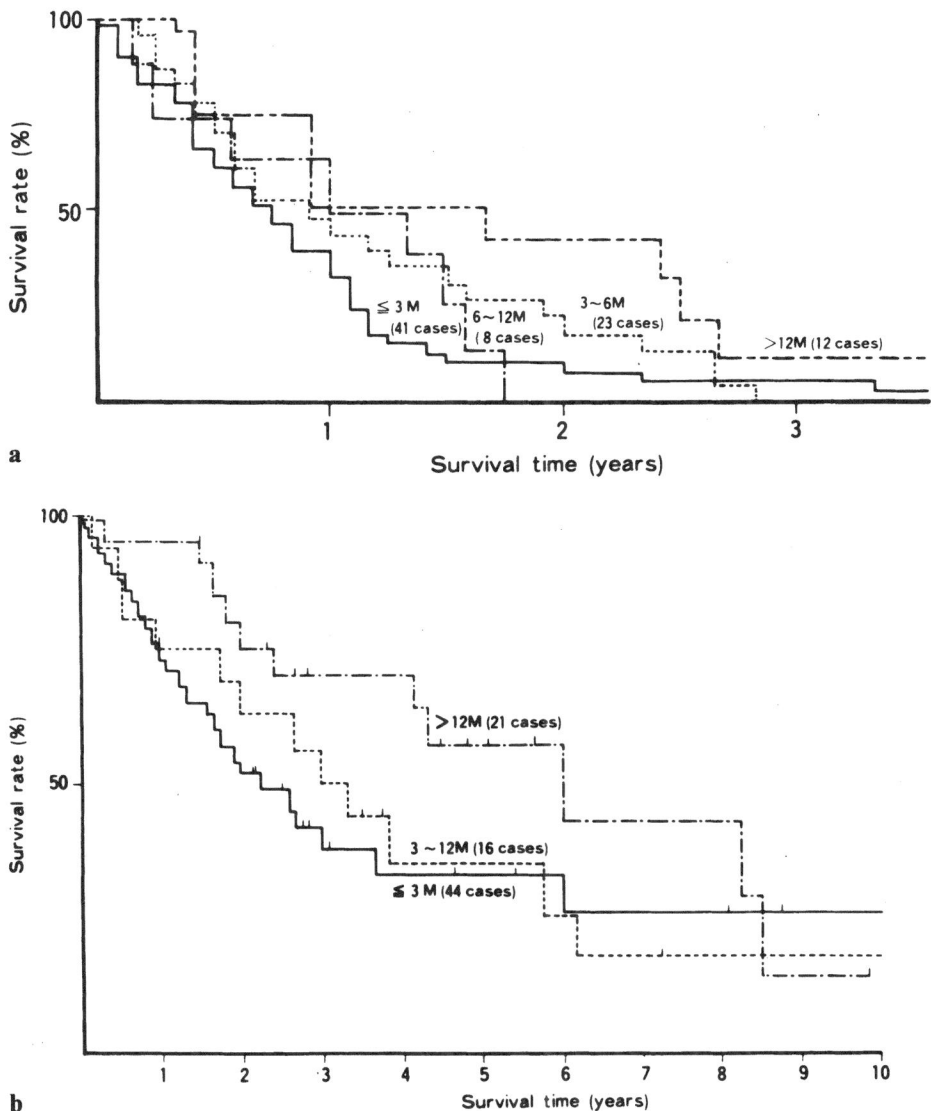

Fig. 9.5a, b. Relationship between survival rate and duration from onset to admission. **a** Glioblastoma; **b** anaplastic astrocytoma

in the group with focal signs ($P < 0.037$) or those with headache, nausea, or vomiting ($P < 0.013$). The survival period was still shorter among patients with disturbances of consciousness, but the results were not statistically significant due to the small number of cases (Fig. 9.6a).

In the anaplastic astrocytoma group, a significantly longer survival time was found in the group with no neurological symptoms, in contrast to that with either the group with focal signs ($P < 0.009$), the group with headache, nausea, and

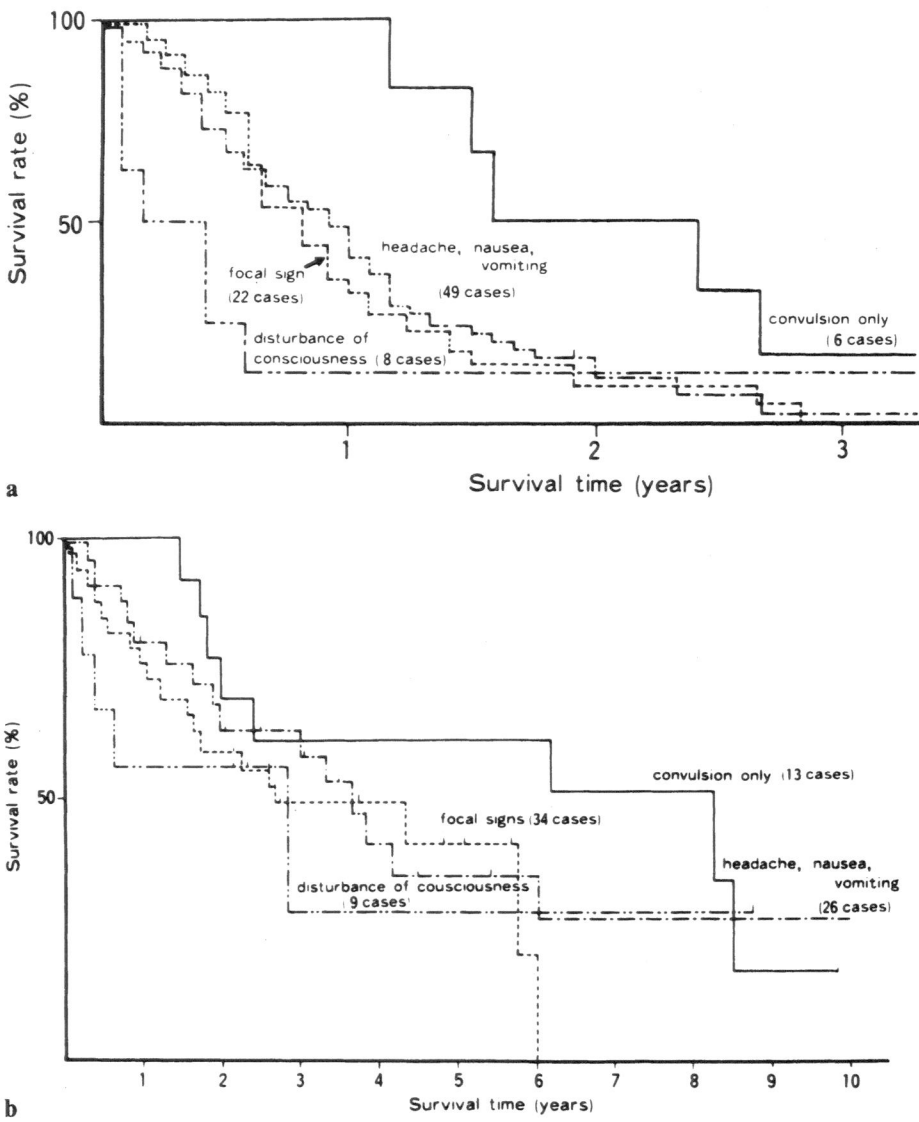

Fig. 9.6a, b. Relationship between survival rate and clinical symptoms. **a** Glioblastoma; **b** anaplastic astrocytoma

vomiting ($P < 0.009$), or the group with disturbances of consciousness ($P < 0.05$) (Fig. 9.6b).

There have been several previous reports of favorable outcomes among patients showing convulsions [14, 15]. Scott and Gilbert [15] reported that the prognosis was good in a group with convulsions, regardless of the histological malignancy and our results are similar.

Performance Status

Among the glioblastoma cases, the performance status was grouped into three categories (grades 0–1, grades 2–3, and grade 4). Generally, the better the performance status, the better the prognosis, with significant differences being found among the three groups ($P < 0.001$ between grades 0–1 and grades 2–3 and $P < 0.015$ between grades 2–3 and grade 4; Fig. 9.7a).

In the anaplastic astrocytoma group, the survival rate was highest for the grade 0–1 group and lowest for the grade 4 group ($P < 0.019$). There was a tendency for the grade 2–3 group to have a shorter survival period than the grade 0–1 group, but the difference was not statistically significant (Fig. 9.7b). Several studies have previously shown that the prognosis is better among cases with good performance status [e.g., 11, 18], as we have found in the present study.

Extent of Extirpation

The survival rate was highest among the glioblastoma cases undergoing total extirpation of the tumor, and the prognosis was poor in cases of partial extirpation or biopsy and the unoperated cases. The differences between these groups and the total extirpation group were both statistically significant at the $P < 0.001$ level. The survival rate was next greatest in the subtotal extirpation group, where again significant differences from those in the partial resection or biopsy group and the unoperated group were found (both $P < 0.016$). Although nearly all the patients died within 3 years, the median survival times were 3 months for the unoperated cases, 5 months for the partial extirpation or biopsy cases, and 14 months for the total extirpation cases. It can, therefore, be concluded that total extirpation prolongs life for at least 9–11 months (Fig. 9.8a). There was a tendency for total extirpation to prolong survival somewhat more than subtotal extirpation, but the effect was not statistically significant.

Among the anaplastic astrocytoma cases, again the most favorable outcomes were recorded in the cases undergoing total extirpation, followed by subtotal extirpation, partial extirpation or biopsy, and, finally, the unoperated cases. The differences between the total extirpation group and the other groups were statistically significant ($P < 0.018$ in comparison with the subtotal extirpation group, and $P < 0.001$ in comparison with the other groups). The median survival times were 10 months for the partial extirpation or biopsy group, 16 months for the unoperated group, 36 months for the subtotal extirpation group, and 74 months for the total extirpation group. In other words, survival was prolonged for some 5 years as a result of total extirpation (Fig. 9.8b).

In the neurosurgical literature, there is at least one report of no relationship between the surgical method and the survival rate [5], but most previous studies have found better outcomes among cases with operated tumors [e.g., 14, 16]. Stage and Stein [17] reported that the prognosis is good in patients where surgical extirpation is performed. We also found that surgical resection, particularly total resection, produces a significant prolongation of survival time.

Adjuvant Therapy

The characteristics of the glioblastoma and anaplastic astrocytoma patients in the various treatment groups are shown in Table 9.2. In glioblastoma, there were no

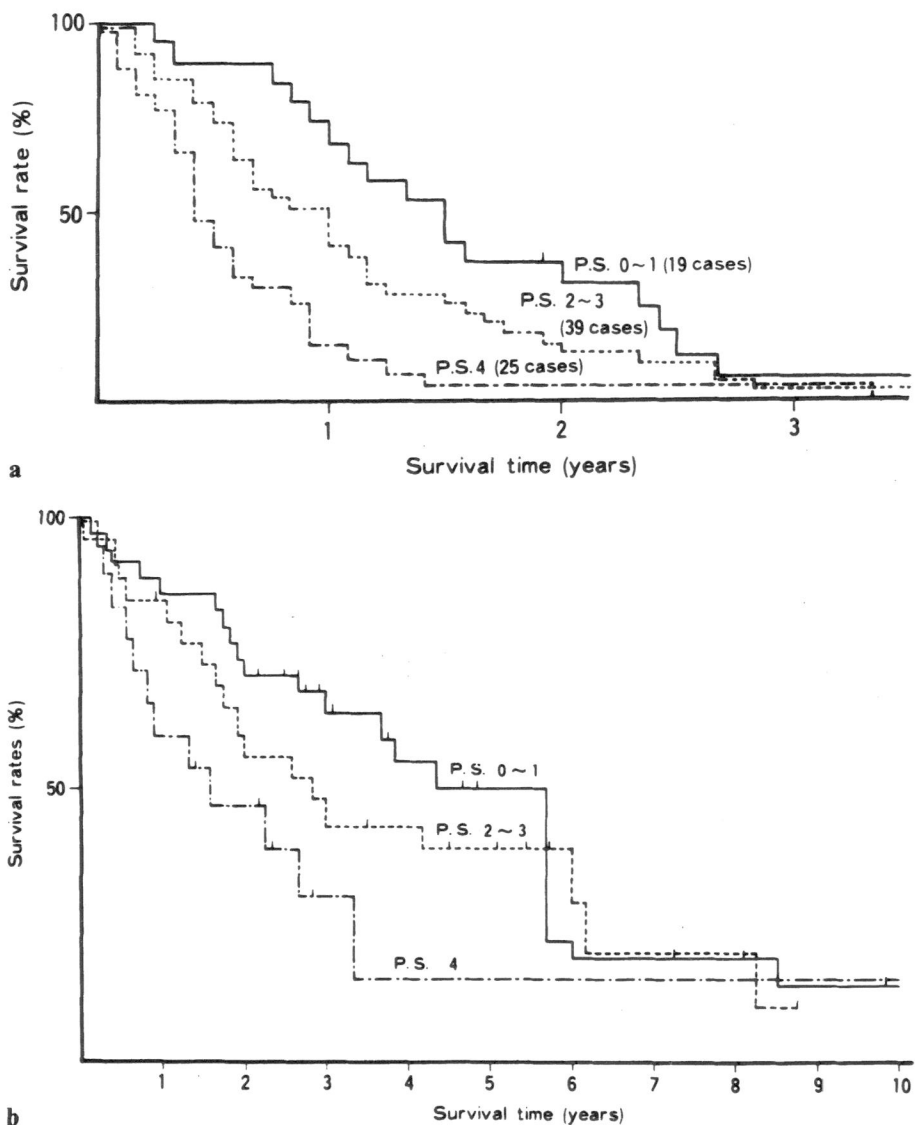

Fig. 9.7a, b. Relationship between survival rate and performance status. **a** Glioblastoma; **b** anaplastic astrocytoma

significant differences in the distribution of the patients with regard to sex, performance status, clinical symptoms, or site of the tumor (χ^2-tests), but the age of patients in the RAFP group was significantly higher than that of patients in the radiotherapy only group ($P < 0.05$, student's t-test). Among the anaplastic astrocytoma cases, no significant difference was seen with regard to age, sex, performance status, clinical symptoms, or site of the tumor, but there were significant differences in the groups undergoing various degrees of surgical treatment (χ^2-test).

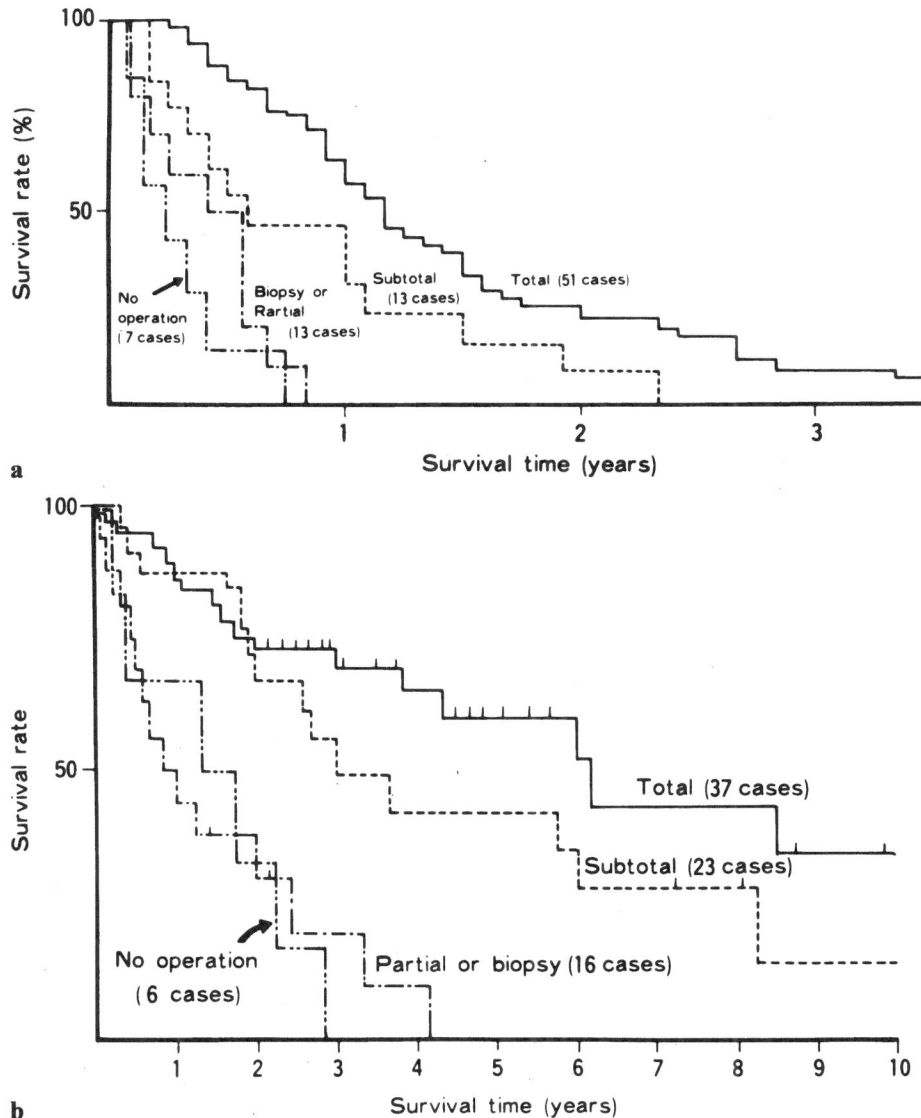

Fig. 9.8a, b. Relationship between survival rate and method of extirpation. **a** Glioblastoma; **b** anaplastic astrocytoma

Significant differences were not seen in the survival rate among the glioblastoma patients treated with RAFP therapy, combined radiochemotherapy, or radiotherapy alone (Fig. 9.9a). Similarly, for the anaplastic astrocytoma patients, significant differences were not found for the RAFP therapy, radiochemotherapy, and radiotherapy alone groups (Fig. 9.9b).

Since differences among the three groups were found with regard to the surgical methods in anaplastic astrocytoma, a similar analysis was done solely on the

Table 9.2. Characteristics of patients in the various treatment groups in evaluable cases

Parameter	Glioblastoma				Anaplastic astrocytoma			
	RAFP	RC	R	χ^2-test	RAFP	RC	R	χ^2-test
No. of cases	44	13	15		32	19	15	—
Age (years)								
Mean	51.5	43.3	39.3	—	41.5	40.2	37.4	
Range	3–74	9–62	5–64		2–75	15–58	9–69	
		(NS)	(NS)			(NS)	(NS)	
		($P < 0.05$)				(NS)		
Sex								
Male	28	10	10	NS	15	12	9	NS
Female	16	3	5		17	7	6	
Performance status								
0–1	7	3	7	NS	11	11	8	NS
2–3	18	6	6		11	5	5	
4	15	4	2		10	2	2	
Operative procedure								
Total removal	26	10	10	NS	13	10	5	$P < 0.05$
Subtotal removal	6	2	2		4	7	8	
Partial removal	3	0	1		3	1	0	
Biopsy	4	1	2		7	1	2	
None	5	0	0		5	0	0	
Symptom								
Convulsion	3	1	2	NS	1	7	4	NS
Focal sign	19	1	3		16	5	7	
Headache	22	10	9		8	7	3	
Consciousness disturbance	0	1	1		7	0	1	
Location								
Frontal	15	4	2	NS	10	9	7	NS
Temporal	10	5	5		3	1	0	
Parietal	4	0	2		2	2	0	
Thalamus	4	1	0		5	1	1	
Other	11	3	6		12	6	7	

NS not significant, *RAFP* radiation + ACNU + FT-207 + PSK, *RC* radiochemotherapy, *R* radiation therapy

patients undergoing total resection, in order to avoid questions concerning the influence of the tumor remaining prior to adjuvant therapy.

The characteristics of patients in the totally extirpated groups for both glioblastoma and anaplastic astrocytoms cases are shown in Table 9.3. Among the glioblastoma cases, significant differences in the distribution of sex, performance status, clinical symptoms, or site of lesion were not found, but a difference (significant at about the $P \fallingdotseq 0.05$ level) was found in the ages of the RAFP and radiotherapy only groups. No significant differences were found among the anaplastic astrocytoma cases.

Among the total resection cases, no significant differences were found in the survival rates of the glioblastoma cases, regardless of whether the therapy was

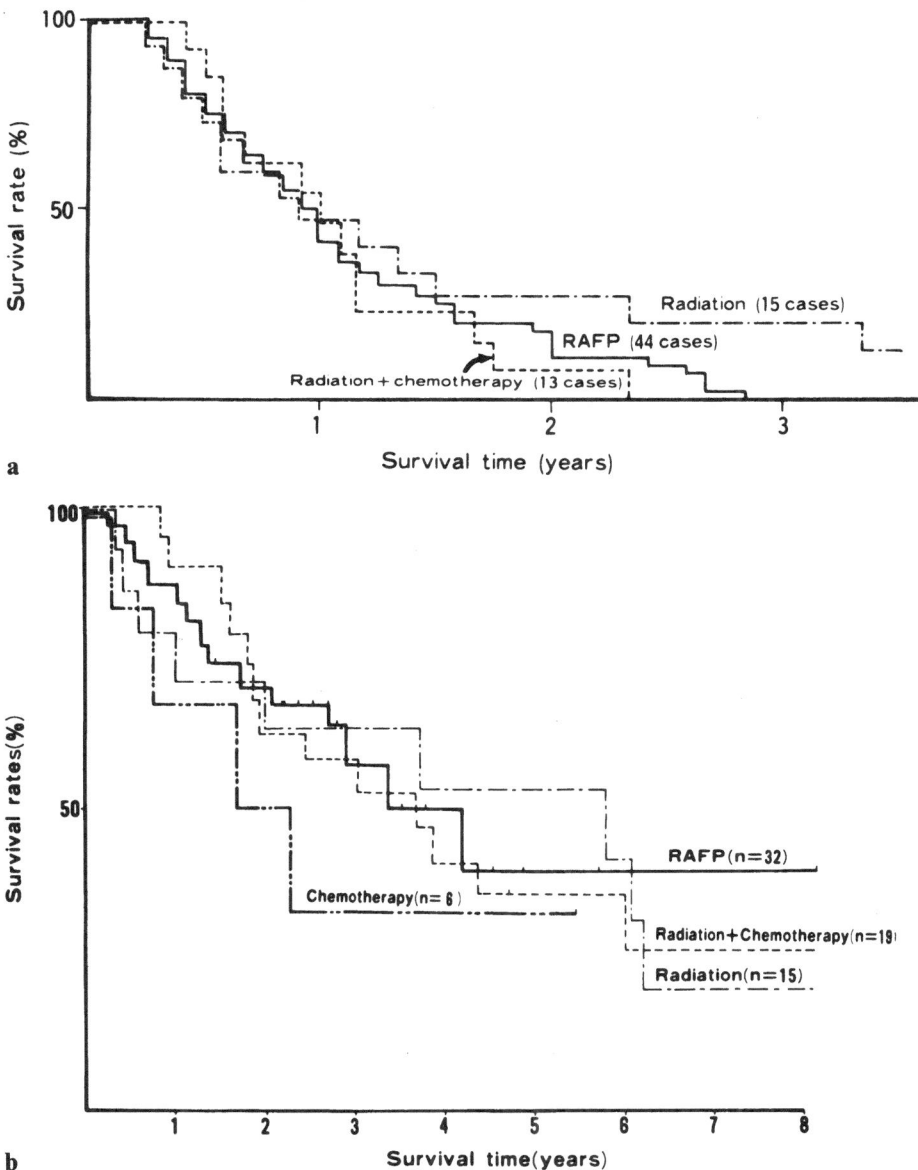

Fig. 9.9a, b. Relationship between survival rate and method of adjuvant therapy (in evaluable cases). **a** Glioblastoma; **b** anaplastic astrocytoma

RAFP, radiochemotherapy, or radiotherapy alone (Fig. 9.10a). In contrast, the 5-year survival rate for anaplastic astrocytoma total resection was 30% in the radiochemotherapy, 60% in the radiotherapy alone, and 92% in the RAFP therapy group. The survival rate of the RAFP therapy group was significantly longer than those of the radiochemotherapy group ($P < 0.005$) and the radiotherapy alone group ($P < 0.05$; Fig. 9.10b).

Table 9.3. Characteristics of patients in the various treatment groups in total extirpated cases

Parameter	Glioblastoma				Anaplastic astrocytoma			
	RAFP	RC	R	χ^2-test	RAFP	RC	R	χ^2-test
No. of cases	24	10	10		13	10	5	
Age (years)								
Mean	51.2	42.2	35.7	—	37.2	38.0	40.5	—
Range	3–69	9–62	5–64		2–75	15–54	19–69	
	⎣(NS)⎦	⎣(NS)⎦			⎣(NS)⎦	⎣(NS)⎦		
	⎣____($P < 0.05$)____⎦					⎣____(NS)____⎦		
Sex								
Male	16	8	5	NS	6	8	2	NS
Female	8	2	5		7	2	3	
Performance status								
0–1	7	2	6	NS	6	6	3	NS
2–3	13	4	2		4	3	2	
4	4	4	2		3	1	0	
Symptom								
Convulsion	2	1	1	NS	0	4	1	NS
Focal sign	6	1	1		8	4	1	
Headache, nausea	16	7	7		3	2	2	
Consciousness disturbance	0	1	1		2	0	1	
Location								
Frontal	7	4	1	NS	9	4	3	NS
Temporal	6	5	3		1	1	0	
Parietal	3	0	2		1·	1	0	
Thalamus	0	1	0		0	1	0	
Other	8	0	4		2	3	2	

NS not significant, *RAFP* radiation + ACNU + FT-207 + PSK, *RC* radiochemotherapy *R* radiation therapy

Discussion

In recent years, the therapeutic results of glioblastoma and other malignant glioma have been studied separately [10, 11]. In a randomized study, in which the results of radiotherapy combined with BCNU and radiotherapy combined with BCNU and hydroxyurea were analyzed, Levin et al. [10] found a better outcome among the glioblastoma cases when hydroxyurea was also used, but significant effects were not found for other malignant gliomas. There has also been one report [11] in which different effects were obtained in glioblastomas and other anaplastic gliomas when a comparison was made between radiotherapy combined with BCNU, on the one hand, and radiotherapy combined with BCNU, procarbazine, CCNU, and vincristine on the other.

Although the present investigation is fundamentally a historical study, we have

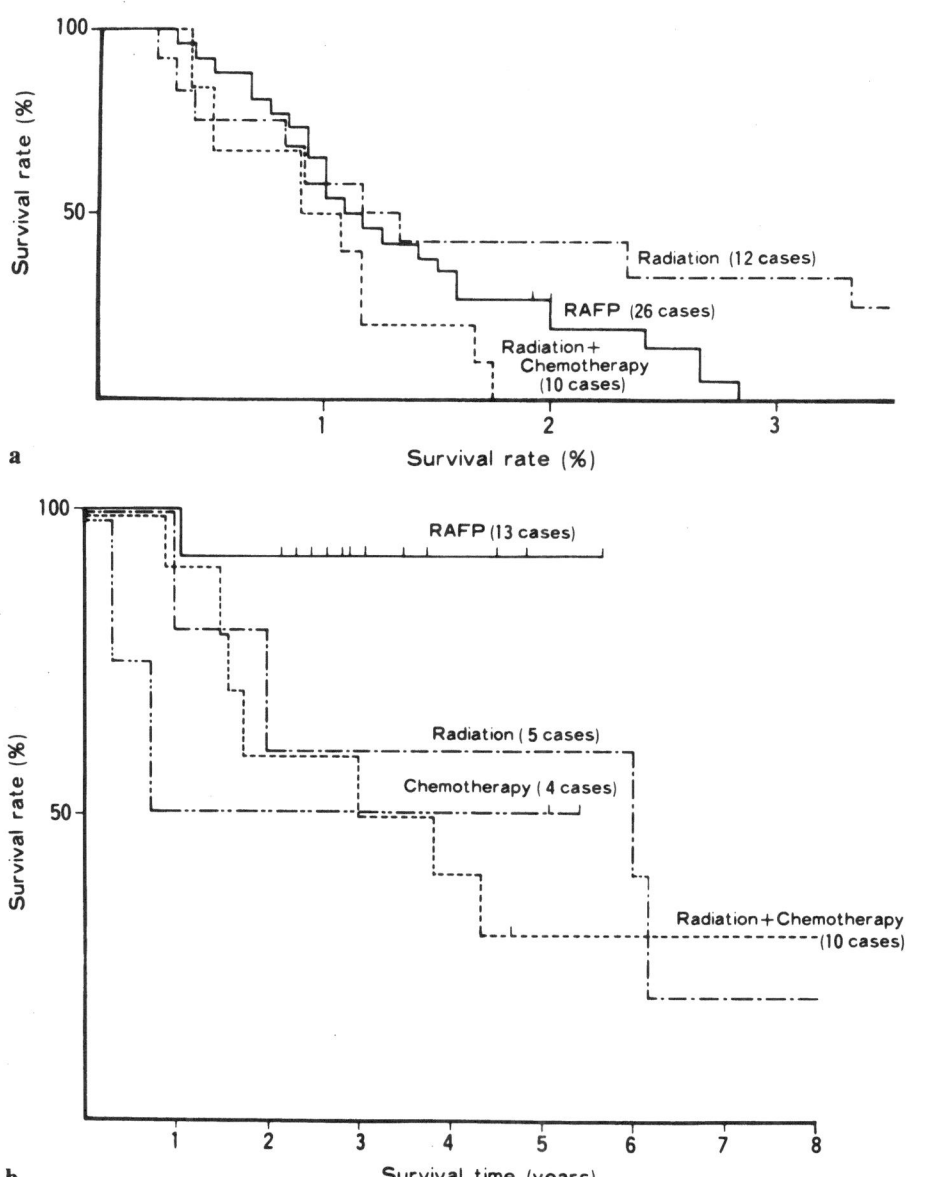

Fig. 9.10a, b. Relationship between survival rate and the method of adjuvant therapy (in totally extirpated cases). **a** Glioblastoma; **b** anaplastic astrocytoma

made a distinction between anaplastic astrocytoma and glioblastoma among the malignant gliomas for our analysis. Among the glioblastoma cases, significant differences in the survival rates were not obtained among the RAFP, radiochemotherapy, and radiotherapy only groups; however, among the anaplastic astrocytoma a cases undergoing total extirpation, the prognosis was better following

RAFP therapy than following radiochemotherapy or only radiotherapy, and the therapeutic effectiveness differed among these groups for the grade III and IV cases.

Although RAFP therapy is ineffective against the most malignant gliomas, such as glioblastoma, it was found to be effective against anaplastic astrocytoma. In comparison with anaplastic astrocytoma, the cell cycle time of glioblastoma is short, and it has a higher growth fraction [7, 8]. In the light of such facts, our results might be interpreted as follows. Although the cytotoxic effects of RAFP therapy cannot work against the rapid cell growth of glioblastoma, they may work on the relatively low-growth fraction of anaplastic astrocytoma. Moreover, in the effects of anticancer agents on solid tumors, various other factors must also be considered in addition to the dynamics of cell kinetics. Such factors include the susceptibility of tumor cells to the anticancer agents, the heterogeneity of the tumor tissues, the rate of delivery of the drug, the involvement of hypoxic cells, and the development of drug tolerance.

In any event, most previous statistical studies on adjuvant therapies have involved a small number of cases, a fact which has necessitated handling grade III and IV cases together. In the present study, we have found significant differences in the effects of adjuvant therapy in glioblastoma and anaplastic astrocytoma, suggesting that future studies should distinguish between grade III and IV cases when attempting to evaluate the effectiveness of various chemotherapies.

Finally, it is worth noting that in both the anaplastic astrocytoma and glioblastoma cases undergoing total resection of the tumor, there was significant prolongation of the survival period. This findings supports the view that removal of the tumor mass remains the single most important therapeutic step in the treatment of such gliomas.

Conclusions

A statistical study was made of the factors which influence the prognosis following radiochemotherapy based upon the results of 84 glioblastoma and 82 anaplastic astrocytoma cases.

Factors which indicate a favorable prognosis in both tumors were the age at onset (between 40 and 59 years in glioblastoma and between 20 and 39 in anaplastic astrocytoma), clinical symptoms consisting of convulsions only, a good performance status, and total resection of the tumor.

Favorable outcomes were obtained among anaplastic astrocytoma cases in which the duration of the disease was in excess of 12 months, but among the glioblastoma cases no relation between prognosis and the duration of the disease was found.

RAFP therapy was not significantly better than radiotherapy alone in the glioblastoma cases, but it was clearly superior among the anaplastic astrocytoma patients that had undergone total surgical resection of the tumor tissue.

References

1. Afra D, Kocsis B, Dobay J, Eckhardt S (1983) Combined radiotherapy and chemotherapy with dibromodulcitol and CCNU in the postoperative treatment of malignant

gliomas. J Neurosurg 59: 106–110

2. Bouchard J, Peirce CB (1960) Radiation therapy in the management of neoplasms of the central nervous system, with a special note in regard to children; twenty years' experience, 1939–1958. Am J Roentgenol 84: 610–627

3. Chin HW, Young AB, Maruyama Y (1981) Survival response of malignant gliomas to radiotherapy with or without BCNU or methyl-CCNU chemotherapy at the University of Kentucky Medical Center. Cancer Treat Rep 65: 45–51

4. Cox DR (1972) Regression model and life tables. JR Stat Soc (B) 34: 187–200

5. European Organization for Research on Treatment of Cancer(EORTC), Brain Tumor Group (1981) Evaluation of CCNU, VM-26 plus CCNU, and procarbazine in supratentorial brain gliomas. J Neurosurg 55: 27–31

6. Green SB, Byar DP, Walker MD, Pistenmaa DA, Alexander E, Batzdorf U, Brooks WH, Hunt WE, Mealey J, Odom GL, Paoletti P, Ransohoff J, Robertson JT, Selker PG, Shapiro WR, Smith KR, Wilson CB, Strike TA (1983) Comparisons of carmustine, procarbazine, and high-dose methylprednisolone as addition to surgery and radiotherapy for the treatment of malignant gliomas. Cancer Treat Rep 67: 121–132

7. Hoshino T, Wilson CB (1975) Review of basic concepts of cell kinetics as applied to brain tumors. J Neurosurg 42: 123–131

8. Hoshino T, Wilson CB, Rosenblum ML, Barker M (1975) Chemotherapeutic implications of growth fraction and cell cycle time in glioblastomas. J Neurosurg 43: 127–135

9. Kaplan EL, Meier P (1958) Nonparametric estimation for incomplete observations. J Am Stat Assoc 53: 457–481

10. Levin VA, Wilson CB, Davis R, Wara WM, Pisher TL, Irwin L (1979) A phase III comparison of BCNU, hydroxyurea, and radiation therapy to BCNU and radiation therapy for the treatment of primary malignant gliomas. J Neurosurg 51: 526–532

11. Levin VA, Wara WM, Davis RL, Vestnys P, Resser KJ, Vatsko K, Nutik S, Gutin PH, Wilson CB (1985) Phase III comparison of BCNU and the combination of procarbazine, CCNU, and vincristine administered after radiotherapy with hydroxyurea for malignant gliomas. J Neurosurg 63: 218–233

12. Nelson DF, Shoenfeld D, Weinstein AS, Nelson JS, Wasserman T, Goodman RL, Carabell S (1983) A randomized comparison of misonidazole sensitized radiotherapy plus BCNU and radiotherapy plus BCNU for treatment of malignant glioma after surgery; preliminary results of and RTOG study. Int J Rad Oncol Biol Phys 9: 1143–1151

13. Poisson M, Pouillart P, Bataini JP, Mashaly R, Pertuiset BF, Metzger J (1979) Malignant gliomas treated after surgery by combination chemotherapy and delayed radiation; I. Analysis of results. Acta Neurochirurgica 51: 15–25

14. Roth JG, Elvidge AR (1960) Glioblastoma multiforme: A clinical survey. J Neurosurg 17: 736–750

15. Scott GM, Gilbert FB (1980) Epilepsy and other factors in the prognosis of gliomas. Acta Neurol Scandinav 61: 227–239

16. Seiler RW, Greiner RH, Zimmerman A, Markwalder H (1978) Radiotherapy combined with procarbazine, bleomycin, and CCNU in the treatment of high-grade supratentorial astrocytomas. J Neurosurg 48: 861–865

17. Stage WS, Stein JJ (1974) Treatment of malignant astrocytomas. Am J Roentgenol 120: 7–18

18. Walker MD, Alexander E, Hunt WE, MacCarty CS, Mahaley MS Jr, Mealer J Jr, Norrell HA, Qwens G, Ransohoff J, Wilson CB, Gehan EA, Strike TA (1978) Evaluation of BCNU and/or radiotherapy in the treatment of anaplastic gliomas. J Neurosurg 49: 333–343

19. Weir B, MSc, FRCS(C) (1973) The relative significance of factors affecting postoperative survival in astrocytomas, grade 3 and 4. J Neurosurg 38: 448–452

Chapter 10

Clinical Analysis of Glioma: Low-Grade Astrocytoma

M. KITAHARA

Introduction

There have been many recent studies on the prognosis of malignant glioma cases following various therapies [9, 23, 24, 33], but there have been only a few sporadic reports on the therapeutic results in low-grade astrocytoma (LGA). In previous studies, the prognosis for LGA of the cerebellum has been relatively good [6, 7, 10, 16, 18, 47], but most reports have indicated a relatively poor 5-year survival rate of 40%–60% in supratentorial cases [16, 21, 22, 25, 34, 39, 46]. Moreover, there have been few investigations on the therapeutic method in such cases and definitive conclusions concerning the effectiveness of radiotherapy or chemotherapy following surgery have not yet been possible.

In this chapter, we report the therapeutic results in the LGA cases experienced by us and discuss the results of radiation, ACNU, FT-207 and PSK (RAFP) therapy with brief reference to the literature.

Materials and Methods

During the 20-year period between 1965 and 1984, we experienced 91 cases of LGA (grades I and II) in our clinic. In all cases, histological confirmation was made either at surgery or at autopsy, and the cases were classified according to the WHO histological grading system.

The site of the tumor was supratentorial in 60 cases (65.9%) and infratentorial in 31 (34.1%; Table 10.1). Both types were more frequently found among relatively young patients (Fig. 10.1). Study was made of the therapeutic results in these 91 cases according to the supratentorial, cerebellar, or brainstem lesion. Those patients who died within 1 month of surgery or who could not be followed up postoperatively were excluded from the study. The therapeutic results were expressed as a survival curve, following the method of Kaplan and Meier [17] and tests for significance were done following the Cox-Mantel method [4].

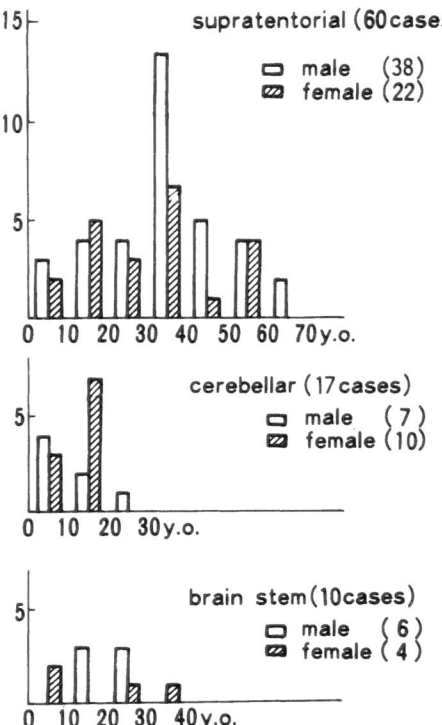

Fig. 10.1. Sex and age distribution

Table 10.1. Location of 91 cases

Location	No.
Supratentorial cases	60
Frontal lobe	27
Temporal lobe	3
Parietal lobe	3
Occipital lobe	1
Frontotemporal lobe	2
Frontoparietal lobe	1
Frontotemporoparietal lobe	5
Porietotemporal lobe	2
Temporooccipital lobe	1
Thalamus	1
Basal ganglia	2
Lateral ventricle	1
Third ventricle	1
Infratentorial cases	31
Cerebellar hemisphere	9
Cerebellar vermis	8
Pons	9
Medulla oblongata	1
C-P angle	1
Fourth ventricle	3

Results

Location of Tumor

Study was made of the 53 supratentorial, 17 cerebellar, and ten brainstem LGA cases (Fig. 10.2). In cerebellar LGA, the 10-year survival rate of 16 cases (excluding one death 2 weeks postoperatively) was 92.9%. The one patient who died 14 months after the first treatment had a solid tumor, but the prognosis for cases with mural nodules forming cysts was particularly good. All but one of the brainstem LGA cases were fatal. Eight patients died within 2 years of the first treatment and the prognosis was extremely poor in spite of radiotherapy or RAFP therapy.

In contrast, the 5- and 10-year survival rates of the supratentorial LGA cases were 61.9% and 52.1%, respectively. There was a relatively sharp fall in the survival rate over the first 3 years following initial treatment, but a slower fall between 3 and 5 years, and little change thereafter. It is thus apparent that in supratentorial LGA there are fatalities in the relatively early period following first therapy, but there is a favorable prognosis for those cases which survive for 5 years.

We next studied the relationships between the prognosis, clinical findings, and therapy in the supratentorial and cerebellar LGA cases.

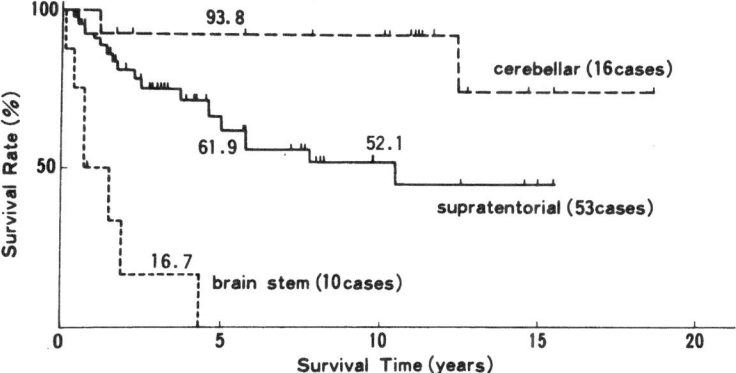

Fig. 10.2. Correlation of survival rate with location of tumor

Cerebellar LGA

Pathological findings showed 11 cystic tumors, eight of which showed the presence of mural nodules and these were histologically classified as pilocytic astrocytoma (Table 10.2). The three remaining cases were fibrillary astrocytoma. There were six solid tumor cases—five fibrillary astrocytomas and one pilocytic astrocytoma.

Of the eight cystic tumor cases with mural nodules, the mural nodules were excised in six cases, and two cases were given radiotherapy or RAFP therapy after the excision of the nodules. Three cystic tumor cases without mural nodules were excised totally. In one of these cases, there was recurrence after 7 years, but there was no recurrence in the other ten cases and the postoperative courses have been favorable.

With regard to therapy for the six solid tumor cases, total excision was done in two cases, subtotal excision in one case, total excision followed by radiotherapy in one case, and RAFP therapy only in one case. Two of these patients have subsequently died, but the outcomes have been favorable in the remaining four.

It has previously been reported that 70%–80% of cerebellar LGAs have cystic tumors and some 50%–75% of these cases have mural nodules [12, 18, 27]. It is generally thought that in cystic tumor cases with mural nodules surgical resection of the mural nodule alone will produce favorable results [5, 6, 37, 40, 45], but a poor prognosis [12, 47] has been found in solid tumor cases or cystic tumor cases with histopathological types called protoplasmic or diffuse [38].

There have been several reports on postoperative radiotherapy techniques in cerebellar LGA. Some authors maintain that radiotherapy is unnecessary [3, 20, 26, 28, 29, 43], some use radiotherapy only when subtotal resection has been done [2, 7, 8, 27], and some use it anytime when total resection including the cyst wall has not been done [8, 11, 15].

In our series, we have obtained good results by means of excision of the mural nodules in cystic tumor cases. But, among the solid tumor cases, one was fatal in the early postoperative period, suggesting that postoperative adjuvant therapy was necessary.

Table 10.2. Clinical features of 17 cases of cerebellar low-grade astrocytoma

Case no.	Age (yrs)	Sex	Location	Gross type	Histological finding	Treatment Operation	Radiotherapy (Gy)	Chemotherapy	Recurrence (interval)	Survival time (yr, mo)	Present status
1	14	F	Rt. HS	Cyst with MN	Pilocytic	Rem. MN	—	—	—	15, 5	Good
2	19	F	Lt. HS	Cyst with MN	Pilocytic	Rem. MN	45	—	—	14, 8	Good
3	22	M	Rt. HS	Cyst with MN	Pilocytic	TR	—	—	—	12, 9	Good
4	13	F	Lt. HS	Cyst with MN	Pilocytic	Rem. MN	—	—	+7 yr	12, 6	Dead
5	13	M	Lt. HS	Cyst with MN	Pilocytic	Rem. MN	—	—	—	11, 3	Good
6	13	M	Rt. HS	Cyst with MN	Pilocytic	Rem. MN	—	—	—	11, 1	Good
7	17	F	Vermis	Cyst with MN	Pilocytic	Rem. MN	—	—	+6Y5 mo	10, 0	Good
8	16	F	Vermis	Cyst with MN	Pilocytic	Rem. MN	—	—	—	7, 9	Good
9	17	F	Lt. HS	Cyst without MN	Fibrillary	TR	—	—	—	15, 8	Good
10	10	F	Vermis	Cyst without MN	Fibrillary	TR	60	—	—	11, 10	Good
11	7	M	Vermis	Cyst without MN	Fibrillary	TR	50	AFP	—	1, 11	Good
12	5	F	Vermis	Solid	Fibrillary	TR	—	—	—	10, 10	Good
13	7	M	Vermis	Solid	Fibrillary	TR	—	FT-207 + PSK	+5Y6 mo	10, 5	Good
14	6	M	Rt. HS	Solid	Fibrillary	TR	60	—	—	5, 6	Good
15	4	F	Vermis	Solid	Fibrillary	—	60	AFP	+1Y5 mo	1, 8	Fair
16	6	M	Rt. HS	Solid	Pilocytic	SR	60	—	—	1, 2	Dead
17	3	F	Vermis	Solid	Fibrillary	SR	—	—	—	2 weeks	Dead

HS cerebellar hemisphere, *MN* mural nodule, *Rem. MN* removal of mural nodule, *TR* total removal, *SR* subtotal removal, *AFP* ACNU + FT-207 + PSK

Supratentorial LGA .

Clinical findings and prognosis. In the present series, the prognosis was good in patients under the age of 19 with no neurological deficit except convulsion and whose condition had been observed for a relatively long period from onset without the emergence of neurological deficits (Fig. 10.3–10.5). These findings are in agreement with those reported by others [21, 27, 30, 39, 41, 46].

It has been reported that the prognosis of cystic tumor cases is good and that, similar to the case of cerebellar lesions, the prognosis of those with mural nodules is particularly good [13, 30, 35, 36]. In our series, we have experienced only six cases of cystic tumor, but the outcome in all cases has been good (Table 10.3).

Recurrence of tumor. At follow-up, recurrence was found to have occurred in 15 of the 53 cases (28.3%; Fig. 10.6). The timing of the recurrence was between 8 months and 14 years from the first treatment, but about half (seven cases) had recurrence

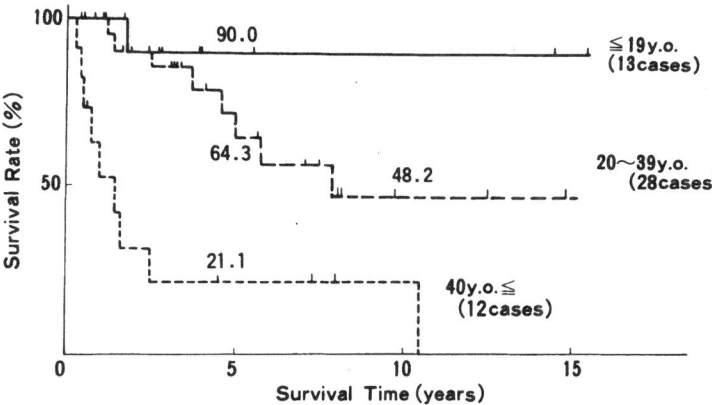

Fig. 10.3. Correlation of survival rate with age at diagnosis

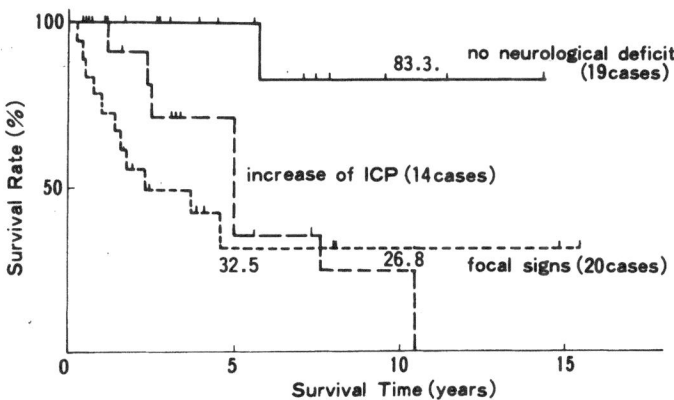

Fig. 10.4. Correlation of survival rate with neurological signs before treatment

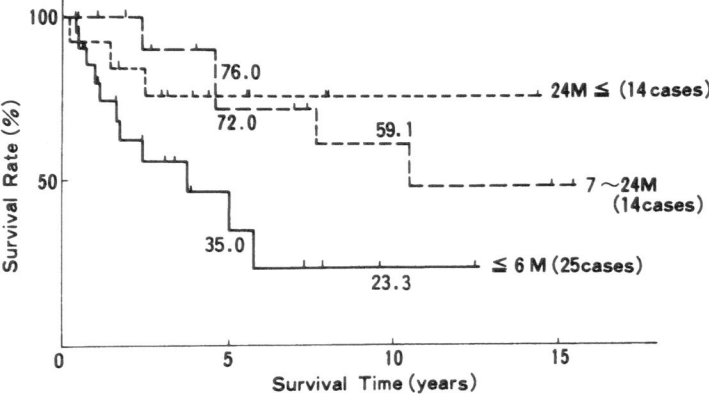

Fig. 10.5. Correlation of survival rate with duration of symptoms before treatment

Table 10.3. Summary of cystic tumors

Case no.	Age (yrs)	Sex	Location	Treatment			Recurrence (interval)	Survival time (yr, mo)	Present status
				Opera-tion	Radio-therapy (Gy)	Chemo-therapy			
1	32	F	Lt. T	SR	60	CQ	—	9, 7	Good
2	18	M	Rt. BG	SR	60	—	+(5Y6M)	5, 7	Good
3	12	F	Rt. FTP	TR	60	AFP	—	3, 10	Good
4	13	F	Rt. F	TR	50	AFP	—	2, 8	Good
5	2	M	Lt. P	TR	60	AFP	—	2, 5	Good
6	11	M	Lt. T	TR	60	AFP	—	0, 6	Good

BG basal ganglia, *F* frontal, *T* temporal, *FTP* frontotemporoparietal, *SR* subtotal removal, *TR* total removal, *AFP* ACNU + FT-207 + PSK, *CQ* carboquone

within 3 years. Among the 26 cases receiving RAFP therapy, recurrence was found in only two (7.6%) and there was a tendency for relapse not to occur in the early posttreatment period.

Histopathologically, 14 of the 15 cases of recurrence were grade II cases. The one grade I case had recurrence 5 years 6 months after subtotal resection of the lesion and radiotherapy. The histopathological findings at the time of recurrence indicated greater malignancy of the lesion in six cases, four of which were anaplastic astrocytoma and two glioblastoma.

Efficacy of postoperative radiotherapy and chemotherapy as determined by CT scan. The efficacy of postoperative radiotherapy and chemotherapy was evaluated in 18 cases using CT scans (Table 10.4; Fig. 10.7). There was complete remission in no cases, partial remission (to less than 50% of the original size of the tumor) in seven cases (38.9%), and no change (reduction to more than 50% or growth of less than 25%) in 11 cases (61.1%). Among these cases, RAFP therapy was performed in

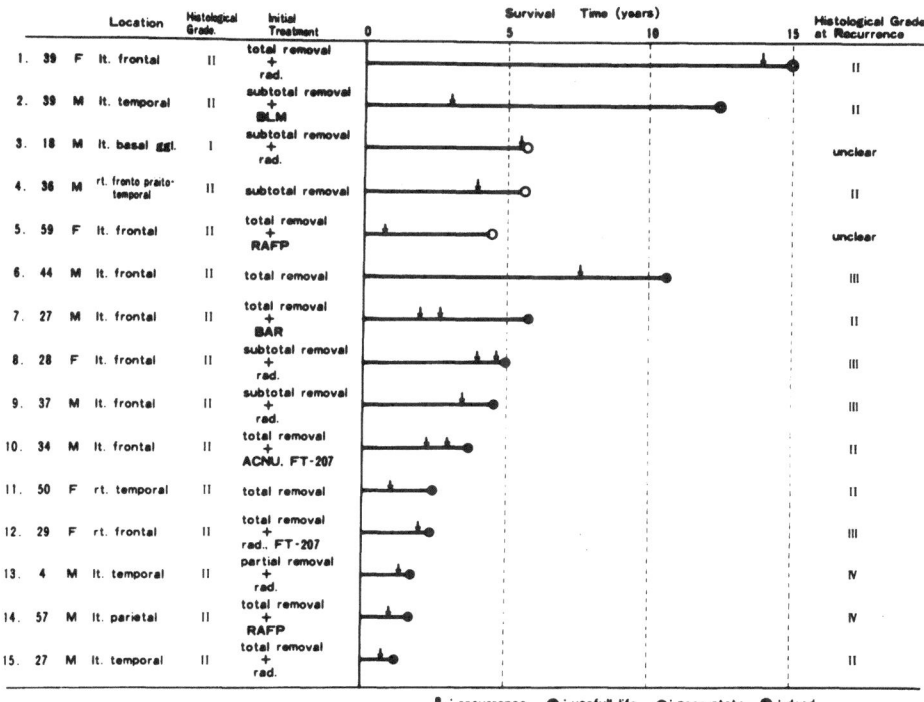

Fig. 10.6. Summary of recurrent cases

Table 10.4. Response to treatment on CT scan

	Radiation	Radiation and chemotherapy	RAFP	Total
CR	0	0	0	0
PR	1	0	6	7
NC	3	1	7	11
PG	0	0	0	0
Total	4	1	13	18

CR complete remission of mass lesion, *PR* 50% or greater decrease of mass lesion, *NC* decrease less than 50%, increase less than 25%, *PG* 25% or greater increase of mass lesion

13, resulting in partial remission in six cases (46.2%) and no change in seven (53.8%). In other words, there was a reduction in the size of the tumor in about half of the patients with RAFP therapy.

Relationship between surgery and prognosis. Comparisons were made of the prognosis in the 31 cases of total resection, 11 cases of subtotal resection, and 11 cases of partial resection, biopsy or radiotherapy, and/or chemotherapy only

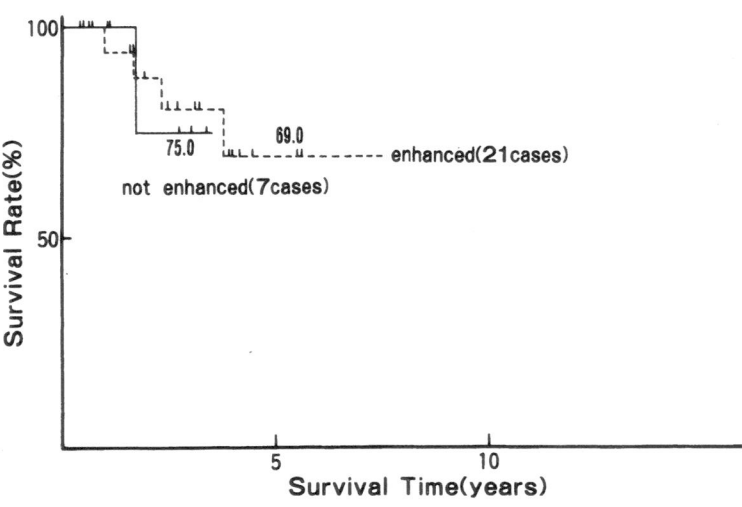

Fig. 10.7. Correlation of survival rate with CT findings

(Table 10.5). The 5- and 10-year survival rates for the total resection group were 70.6% and 64.2%, respectively, and those for the subtotal resection group were not statistically different at 71.4% and 55.8%, respectively. The prognosis for the other 11 patients was considerably worse, however, with five fatalities within 2 years. Although statistical differences between the total and subtotal cases in our series were not found, previous studies have indicated a better prognosis for total excision [7, 21]. Moreover, study of the individual cases in our series indicated that even in grade I cases, which are described as "benign" in the WHO classification, there was recurrence in one patient who did not undergo total resection. This finding strongly suggests that total resection should be performed whenever possible.

Relationship between prognosis, radiotherapy, and chemotherapy. The prognosis was also compared among four distinct therapeutic groups: those undergoing only surgical therapy (total or subtotal, six cases); those undergoing surgery and radiotherapy (seven cases); those undergoing surgery and RAFP therapy (19 cases); and those undergoing surgery and radiotherapy other than RAFP therapy (nine cases; Fig. 10.8; Table 10.5).

The 5-year survival rate was 80% in the surgery only group, 71.4% in the surgery plus radiotherapy group, and 43.1% in the group receiving surgery plus radiochemotherapy other than RAFP therapy. The 5-year survival rate in the group undergoing surgery and RAFP, however, was higher at 93.3% (Fig. 10.9). Although the differences among these groups did not reach statistical significance, it is noteworthy that one of the 19 RAFP-treated patients died within 5 years of therapy. The results of long-term follow-up of such cases would be of extreme interest.

There have been several studies reporting that postoperative radiotherapy is effective in supratentorial cases [22, 27, 42, 49], but it has also been reported that radiotherapy has no influence on the survival rate [13]. Since the location of the tumor can be identified using CT scanning, it has been reported that locally applied

Table 10.5. Treatment for 53 cases of supratentorial
low-grade astrocytoma

Treatment	No.
Total removal	3
Subtotal removal	3
Total removal and radiation	4
Subtotal removal and radiation	3
Partial removal and radiation	1
Total removal, radiation, and chemotherapy	8
Subtotal removal, radiation, and chemotherapy	1
Biopsy, radiation, and chemotherapy	2
Subtotal removal and chemotherapy	1
Biopsy and chemotherapy	1
Total removal and RAFP	16
Subtotal removal and RAFP	3
Biopsy and RAFP	7

radiation is sufficient [39] and that caution must be taken not to exceed the radiation
dose which normal brain tissue can withstand [39].

In a study of 461 cases by Laws et al. [21], it was reported that differences in the
efficacy of postoperative radiotherapy were found according to age. Specifically,
they found no improvement in the prognosis following radiotherapy in patients
under 40 years of age. In our series, there were some cases with favorable outcomes
following surgery alone, and no difference was found in the prognosis following
surgery and radiotherapy.

It should be noted, however, that a rigorous control study still needs to be done
regarding the influence of age, site of tumor, and surgical method to determine the
efficacy of radiotherapy. A detailed study is also still required, because the cytotoxic
effect and recovery from radiation damage casued by tumor cells are closely related
to the total radiation dose, radiation field, and duration of the radiation therapy.

There have been few reports on the effects of chemotherapy in supratentorial
LGA [48]. The results of our RAFP therapy indicate that such therapy is effective
in LGA, with recurrence not occurring in the early posttreatment period. The
reduction of the tumor following such therapy was 46.2% in CT scans.

Discussion

Among cases of LGA, those with cerebellar astrocytoma have favorable prognoses.
Particularly in the case of cystic tumor cases with mural nodules, good results have
been obtained by simple surgical excision of the mural nodules [5, 6, 37, 40, 45]. In
contrast, there is early recurrence in cases of supratentorial LGA and relatively
many fatalities [30, 31, 36], which makes it difficult to generalize about the prognosis
in supratentorial LGA cases as a whole (Table 10.6).

The clinical course of such patients suggests that there are two distinct groups:
one in which there is early recurrence within several years following therapy and a

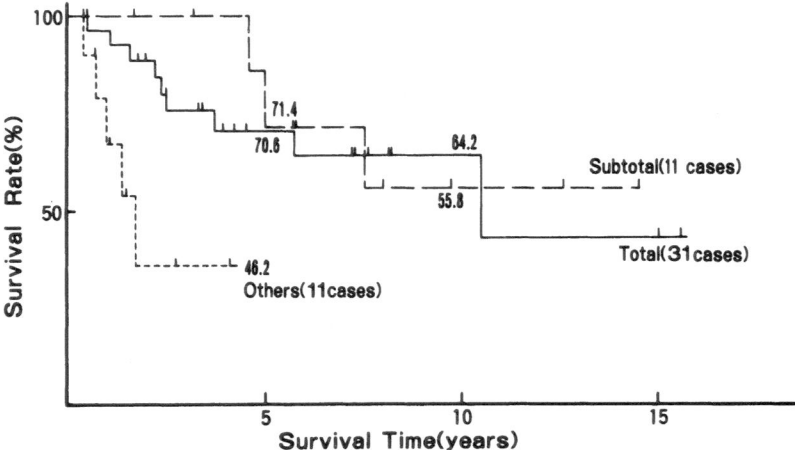

Fig. 10.8. Correlation of survival rate with surgical removal

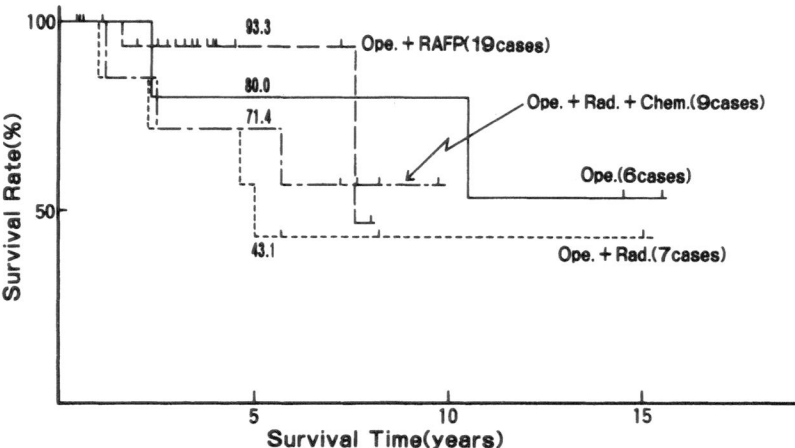

Fig. 10.9. Correlation of survival rate with radiochemotherapy

poor prognosis is indicated, and a second group in which there is no recurrence and a favorable outcome is likely. Treatment of the former group remains problematic, but RAFP therapy has been found to prevent early recurrence and is thought to be effective as the first therapy.

Even when identical histopathological findings are obtained in supratentorial and cerebellar LGA cases, their individual clinical courses may differ greatly and it has previously been pointed out that the lesion may become more malignant at the time of recurrence [1, 19, 21, 36, 44]. It is, therefore, impossible to determine the nature of the tumor solely from the histopathological findings. Nagashima et al. have determined the labeling index of tumor cells in anaplastic astrocytoma using BudR monoclonal antibodies and found that the proliferative capacity of tumor

Table 10.6. Series of supratentorial astrocytoma

Authors	No. of patients	Treatment	Survival rate (%)				
			3-year	5-year	10-year	15-year	20-year
Grant [14]	279	Surg. alone	—	27	19	11	6
Gol [13]	194	Surg. ± Rad.	—	15	9	—	—
Stage [40]	45	Surg. ± Rad.	39	25	—	—	—
Marsa[a] [27]	15	Surg. + Rad.	72	72	57	—	—
Leibel [22]	14	Total removal	100	100	100	89	88
and	37	Incomp. resect.	27	19	11	4	0
Sheline [42]	71	Incomp. resect. + Rad.	59	46	35	25	23
Laws [21]	461	Surg. ± Rad.	55	35	21	17	17
	57	Total removal	75	61	44	35	—
	404	Subtotal removal	50	33	18	13	—
	252	Surg. ± Rad. (≤40 Gy)	52	34	25	18	—
	74	Surg. + Rad. (≥40 Gy)	64	49	20	20	—
Brain Tumor Registry in Japan [34]	1056		55.8	47.1	Mean survival time was 13.3 years		
Mercuri[a] [31]	41	Surg. ± Rad.					

Surg. surgical removal, *Rad.* radiation therapy, *Incomp. resect.* incomplete resection
[a] Cases in children

tissues with identical histopathological findings can differ [32]. We believe that it is important to investigate methods for determining more objectively the labeling index, growth fraction, etc. in LGA. With the emergence of PET and MRI techniques, we believe that it should be possible to determine the specific metabolic nature of individual brain tumors and thereby distinguish between similar lesions in ways which current histopathological techniques do not allow.

Summary

We made a study of the efficacy of RAFP therapy in a series of low-grade astrocytomas experienced in our clinic. We believe that RAFP therapy is appropriate for the first treatment of such tumors, particularly in supratentorial cases in which recurrence in the early period following therapy is infrequent and the 5-year survival rate is 93.3%.

References

1. Bernell WR, Kepes JJ, Seitz EP (1972) Late malignant recurrence of childhood cerebellar astrocytoma. Report of two cases. J Neurosurg 37: 470–474
2. Biemond A (1974) Cerebellar tumors. In: Viken PJ, Bryun GW (eds) Handbook of clinical neurology, vol. 17, North-Holland Amsterdam, pp 707–718
3. Budka H (1975) Partially resected and irradiated cerebellar astrocytoma of childhood: malignant evolution after 28 years. Acta Neurochirurgica 32: 139–146
4. Cox DR (1972) Regression model and life tables. JR Stat Soc (B) 34: 187–220
5. Cushing H (1931) Experiences with the cerebellar astrocytomas. A clinical review of seventy-six cases. Surg Gynec Obstet 52: 129–204
6. Elvidge AR (1968) Long-term survival in the astrocytoma series. J Neurosurg 28: 399–404
7. Fazekas JT (1977) Treatment of grades I and II brain astrocytomas. The role of radiotherapy. Int J Radiat Oncol Biol Phys 2: 661–666
8. Geissinger JD, Bucy PC (1971) Astrocytomas of the cerebellum in children, Long-term study. Arch Neurol 24: 125–135
9. Gerosa MA, Dougherty DV, Wailson CB, Rosenbulum ML (1983) Improved treatment of a brain-tumor model: II. Sequential therapy with BCNU and 5-fluorouracil. J Neurosurg 58: 363–373
10. Gjerris F, Harmsen A, Klinken L, Reske-Nielsen E (1978) Incidence and long term survival of children with intracranial tumors treated in Denmark 1935-1959. Br J Cancer 38: 442–451
11. Gjerris F, Klinken L (1978) Long-term prognosis in children with benign cerebellar astrocytoma. J Neurosurg 49: 179–184
12. Gol A, Mckissocle W (1959) The cerebellar astrocytomas: a report on 90 verified cases. J Neurosurg 16: 287–296
13. Gol A (1961) The relatively benign astrocytomas of the cerebrum. A clinical study of 194 verified cases. J Neurosurg 18: 501–506
14. Grant FC (1956) A study of the results of surgical treatment in 2326 consecutive patients with brain tumors. J Neurosurg 13: 479–488
15. Griffin TW, Beaufait D, Blasko JC (1979) Cystic cerebellar astrocytomas in childhood. Cancer 44: 276–280
16. Jimenez J (1983) Brain tumors in children. Results of treatment in 138 patients. Neoplasma 30: 93–96

17. Kaplan EL, Meier P (1958) Nonparametric estimation for incomplete observations. J Am Stat Assoc 53: 457–481
18. Kitaoka K, Tashiro K, Abe H, Tsuru M (1980) A clinical survey of cerebellar astrocytoma—comparison between childhood and adult cases. Neurol Surg 8: 55–64 (in Japanese)
19. Kleinman GM, Schoene WC, Walshe TM III, Richardson EP Jr (1978) Malignant transformation in benign cerebellar astrocytoma, case report. J Neurosurg 49: 111–118
20. Kooth WT, Miller MH (1971) Intracranial tumors of infants and children. Thieme, Stuttgart
21. Laws ER, Taylor WF, Clifton MB, Okazaki H (1984) Neurosurgical management of low-grade astrocytoma of the cerebral hemispheres. J Neurosurg 61: 665–673
22. Leibel SA, Sheline GE, Wara WM, Boldrey EB, Nielsen SL (1975) The role of radiation therapy in the treatment of astrocytomas. Cancer 35: 1551–1557
23. Levin VA, Hoffman WF, Pischer TL, Seager ML, Boldrey EB, Wilson CB (1978) BCNU-5-fluorouracil combination therapy for recurrent malignant brain tumors. Cancer Treat Rep 62: 2071–2076
24. Levin VA, Wara WM, Davis RL, Vestnys P, Resser KJ, Yatsko K, Nutik S, Gutin PH, Wilson CB (1985) Phase III comparison of BCNU and the combination of procarbazine, CCNU, and vincristine administered after radiotherapy with hydroxyurea for malignant gliomas. J Neurosurg 63: 218–223
25. Lewy LF, Elvidge AR (1956) Astrocytoma of the brain and spinal cord. A review of 176 cases, 1940–1949. J Neurosurg 13: 413–443
26. Liebner EJ, Pretto JI, Hochhauser M, Kassraba W (1964) Tumors of the posterior fossa in childhood and adolescence. Their diagnostic and radiotherapeutic patterns. Radiology 82: 193–201
27. Marsa GW, Probert JC, Rubinstein LJ, Bagshaw MA (1973) Radiation therapy in the treatment of childhood astrocytic gliomas. Cancer 32: 646–655
28. Matson DD (1968) Surgery of posterior fossa tumors in childhood. Clin Neurosurg 15: 247–262
29. Matson DD (1969) Neurosurgery of infancy and childhood, 2nd edn. Thomas, Springfield, pp 410–479
30. Mercuri S, Russo A, Palma L (1981) Hemispheric supratentorial astrocytomas in children. Long-term results in 29 cases. J Neurosurg 55: 170–173
31. Müller W, Áfra D, Schröder R (1977) Supratentorial recurrence of gliomas. Morphological studies in relation to time intervals with astrocytomas. Acta Neurochirurgica 37: 75–91
32. Nagashima T, De Armond SJ, Murovic J, Hoshino T. (1985) Immunocytochemical demonstration of S-phase cells by anti-deoxyuridine monoclonal antibody in human brain tumor tissues. Acta Neuropathol 67: 155–159
33. The cooperative clinical trial group for malignant gliomas (1985) Evaluation of ACNU alone and combined with Tegaful as addition to radiotherapy for the treatment of malignant gliomas. Brain and Nerve 37: 999–1006 (in Japanese)
34. The committee of the brain tumor registry in Japan (1984) Brain tumor registry in Japan, vol. 5, Japanese Ministry of Health and Welfare, Tokyo
35. Palma L, Guidetti B (1985) Cystic pilocytic astrocytomas of the cerebral hemispheres. J Neurosurg 62: 811–815
36. Palma L, Russo A, Mercuri S (1983) Cystic cerebral astrocytomas in infancy and childhood: long-term results. Child's Brain 10: 79–91
37. Rubinstein LJ (1972) Tumors of the central nervous system. Atlas of tumor pathology, 2nd series, Fasc 6. AFIP, Washington
38. Russel DS, Rubinstein LJ (1977) Pathology of tumors of the nervous system, 4th edn. Arnold, London, pp 183–191
39. Scanlon PW, Taylor WF (1979) Radiotherapy of intracranial astrocytomas: analysis of 417 cases treated from 1960 through 1969, Neurosurg 5: 301–308
40. Scatliff JH, Kummer AI, Frankel SA (1962) Cystic enlargement and obstruction of the

fourth ventricle following posterior fossa surgery. Am J Roentgenol 88: 536–542
41. Sheline GE (1975) Radiation therapy of tumors of the central nervous system in childhood. Cancer 35: 957–964
42. Sheline GE (1977) Radiation therapy of brain tumors. Cancer 39: 873–881
43. Schenk VWD (1966) Congenital cavities of the posterior fossa. Acta Neuropathol 6: 117–126
44. Schmitt HP (1983) Rapid anaplastic transformation of gliomas in childhood. Neuropedatrics 14: 137–143
45. Silverberg GD (1971) Simple cysts of the cerebellum. J Neurosurg 35: 320–327
46. Stage WS, Stein JJ (1974) Treatment of malignant astrocytomas. AJR 120: 7–18
47. Tsuchida T, Fukuda M, Tanaka R (1982) Long-term results of cerebellar astrocytoma with special reference to operative procedure and radiotherapy. Neurol Med Chir (Tokyo) 22: 117–124 (in Japanese)
48. Ushio Y, Hayakawa T, Mogami H (1980) Effect of chemotherapy for benign gliomas. Neurol Med Chir (Tokyo) 20, suppl: 195–196 (in Japanese)
49. Yamashita J (1980) Radiation therapy for benign gliomas. Neurol Med Chir (Tokyo) 20, suppl: 196 (in Japanese)

Chapter 11

Clinical Analysis of Glioma: Oligodendroglioma

M. KITAHARA

Introduction

The majority of oligodendrogliomas are found in the cerebral hemispheres, primarily in the frontal lobes, and are known to be relatively benign tumors. Because of the characteristic growth patterns of oligodendrogliomas, including diffuse infiltration of the cerebral cortex and contralateral invasion through the corpus callosum, however, surgical treatment is often difficult [2]. In addition, a wide range of 5-year survival rates have been reported, varying from 40% to 100%, and early postoperative death is not infrequent [4, 6, 7, 9, 11, 13, 14, 18–20].

Many authors have previously argued that postoperative radiation therapy is necessary in oligodendroglioma, but, particularly in cases of tumors which have been confirmed histologically to be benign, decisions concerning its use are not easily made. Recently, there have been several reports indicating that postoperative radiation therapy is effective, but other reports have noted that the prognosis does not differ regardless of whether or not postoperative radiation therapy is employed. In the present chapter, we report the therapeutic results in cases of oligodendroglioma using surgical removal and radiation, ACNU, FT-207, and PSK (RAFP) therapy.

Materials and Methods

Between 1965 and 1984, we experienced a total of 41 cases of oligodendroglioma at our clinic. In all cases, the diagnosis was confirmed by histopathological study of the tissue removed at surgery. The patients included 21 males and 20 females, and ages ranged from 10 to 73 years of age with a peak in the 30s and 40s (Fig. 11.1). The site of the tumor was the frontal lobe in 27 patients (65.9%), four of whom had bilateral frontal lesions (Table 11.1).

Therapy for the 41 cases was as follows: surgical resection only in 13 cases, surgery with postoperative radiation therapy in 13 cases, surgery with postoperative radiation, FT-207 and PSK in four cases, and surgery with postoperative RAFP therapy in 11 cases (Table 11.2). Among the 28 cases receiving radiation therapy, 11 had doses of 5000–6000 rads applied locally over the site of the tumor, and the remaining 17 had 3000 rads applied locally and 3000 rads applied to the whole brain.

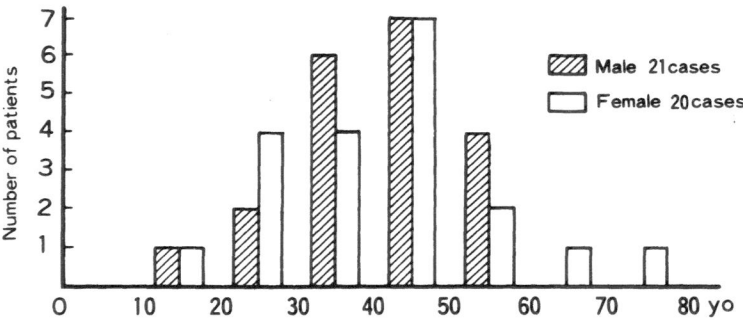

Fig. 11.1. Age and sex distribution of 41 cases

The World Health Organization (WHO) classification was followed for histopathological diagnosis. There were 32 oligodendrogliomas (grade II), four anaplastic oligodendrogliomas (grade III), and four mixed oligodendrogliomas (three grade II and one grade III). Excluding two patients who died within 1 month of surgery, analysis of the therapeutic results was done in 39 cases. The survival curve was calculated using the Kaplan and Meier method [10] and the significance tests were done following the Cox-Mantel method [5].

Results

Overall Survival Curve for the 39 Cases

The 5- and 10-year survival rates for the 39 cases were 73.1% and 32.2%, respectively, with most deaths occurring between 5 and 10 years from first therapy (Fig. 11.2). Five patients survived for more than 10 years from first therapy, but two of these patients experienced recurrence of the oligodendroglioma and died subsequent to further therapy. One additional case had recurrence after 10 years and has been successfully treated by RAFP. In previous studies of the results of therapy in oligodendroglioma, 5-year survival rates have ranged from 30% to 80%, with most reports indicating 5-year survival rates greater than 60%, but a recent study by Mørk et al. [11] reported a 5-year survival rate of only 34.2% among 175 cases.

Histopathological Findings

Five of the 39 patients showed malignant tumors in histopathological examination. Three of these five have already died and the duration of survival was 8 months after the initial treatment in one case and more than 6 years in two cases. The two remaining cases with malignant tumors have survived for 37 and 86 months without recurrence. The therapy in the malignant cases was postoperative radiation therapy in four cases and postoperative RAFP therapy in one case; therapy is thought to have been successful in all but the one early fatality.

Table 11.1. Location of 41 cases

	Left	Right	Bilateral	Total
Frontal lobe	15	8	4	27
Frontoparietal lobe	1	2		3
Temporal lobe	1			1
Temporooccipital lobe		1		1
Parietotemporal lobe	1			1
Parietooccipital lobe		2		2
Occipital lobe		1		1
Lateral ventricle	3	1		4
Corpus callosum				1

Table 11.2. Treatment of 41 cases

Treatment	No.
Total removal	5 (1)
Subtotal removal	8 (1)
Total removal and radiation	8
Subtotal removal and radiation	4
Biopsy and radiation	1
Total removal, radiation, and FT-207 · PSK	2
Subtotal removal, radiation, and FT-207 · PSK	1
Biopsy, radiation, and FT-207 · PSK	1
Total removal and RAFP	9
Subtotal removal and RAFP	1
Biopsy and RAFP	1

Figures in parentheses indicate operative death

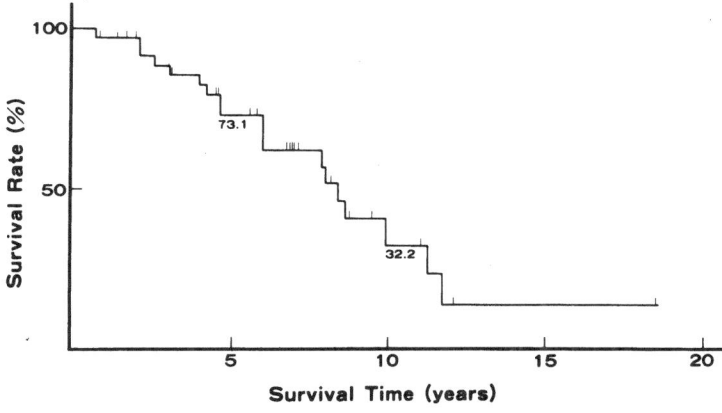

Fig. 11.2. Survival rate of 39 cases of oligodendroglioma

Table 11.3. Clinical features of recurrent cases

Case no.	Age (yrs)	Sex	Location	Histological grade	Initial Treatment			Interval (yr, mo)	Change of histological finding	Survival time (yr, mo)	Prognosis
					Surgery	Radiation (rad)	Chemotherapy				
1	26	F	Blt. frontal	II	Subtotal removal	—	—	0, 6	—	2, 7	Dead
2	43	M	Rt. frontal	II	Subtotal removal	—	—	1, 10	—	4, 2	Dead
3	47	M	Rt. frontal	II	Subtotal removal	—	—	3, 2	—	4, 8	Dead
4	34	M	Lt. frontal	II	Total removal	—	—	4, 9	—	11, 2	Good
5	53	M	Rt. frontal	II	Subtotal removal	Local brain, 6000	—	7, 6	+ (glioblastoma)	7, 11	Dead
6	44	M	Rt. fronto-parietal	III	Subtotal removal	Local brain, 6000	—	5, 0	—	6, 0	Dead
7	33	M	Lt. frontal	II	Total removal	Local brain, 6000	—	9, 2	—	11, 4	Dead
8	39	M	Blt. frontal	II	Total removal	Local brain, 6000	—	11, 1	—	11, 8	Dead
9	31	M	Rt. frontal	II	Total removal	Whole brain, 3000 Local brain, 3000	ACNU FT-207 PSK	4, 5	+ (grade III)	4, 8	Dead

Blt. bilateral, *Rt.* right, *Lt.* left

Method of Excision

A comparison of the results was made between the 23 cases in which total resection of the tumor was possible and the 13 cases in which subtotal resection was performed (Fig. 11.3). The 5- and 10-year survival rates of the former group were 84.7% and 59.6%, respectively, whereas in the latter group the 5-year survival rate was 58.3% and none of the patients survived for 10 years. The differences in these survival rates were statistically significant ($P < 0.05$). It has been known for many years that the prognosis following total resection is good [8, 15], and our results also indicate that as complete a resection as possible should be undertaken.

Radiation Therapy and Chemotherapy

Among the 23 patients undergoing total resection, there were four who received no further therapy, seven who received postoperative radiation therapy, two who received FT-207 and PSK chemotherapy, and nine who received RAFP therapy (Fig. 11.4a). One of the patients who received only surgical removal has died, but the outcome of the other three such patients has been favorable and not statistically different from the outcome of patients who also underwent radiation therapy.

There has been only one recurrence and death among the nine patients receiving RAFP therapy, but the follow-up period is as yet too short to draw firm conclusions about the effectiveness of RAFP therapy. Further study of the outcome of these patients is required.

Among the 13 patients undergoing subtotal resection of the tumor, seven had only surgical removal, four received postoperative radiation therapy, one received radiation therapy, FT-207 and PSK, and one received RAFP. All of the patients receiving only subtotal resection died between 2 years and 8 years 5 months after the initial treatment. Five died within 5 years. In contrast, the patients undergoing radiotherapy have not had early recurrence of the tumor and the one patient given RAFP therapy is currently well (Fig. 11.4b).

All the three patients who underwent only biopsy and radiation therapy or RAFP

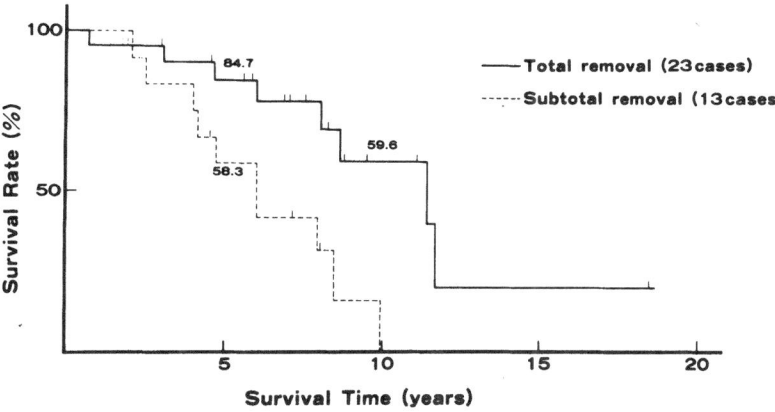

Fig. 11.3. Comparison of survival rate between total removal and subtotal removal

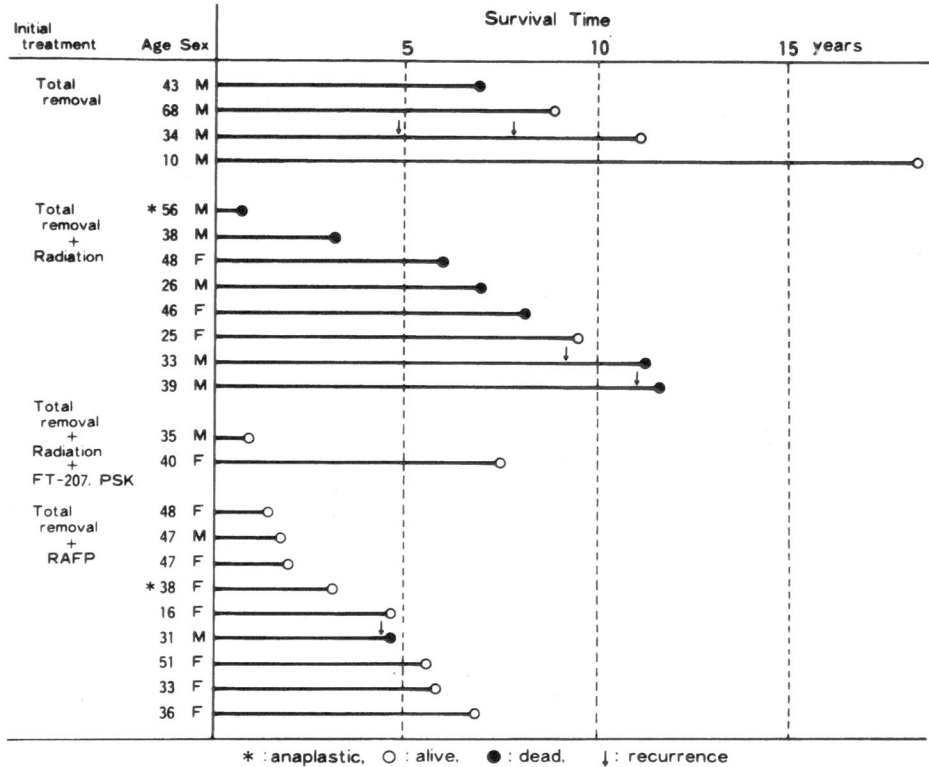

Fig. 11.4a–c. a Summary of clinical course of 23 cases with total removal. **b** Summary of clinical course of 13 cases with subtotal removal. **c** Summary of clinical course of biopsy cases

therapy have had favorable outcomes (Fig. 11.4c), suggesting that radiation therapy is effective alone or in combination with chemotherapy in cases of oligodendroglioma.

Method of Radiation Therapy

Comparison was made of the outcome in the 11 patients undergoing 5000–6000 rads of locally applied radiation therapy with that in the 17 cases receiving 3000 rads of whole-brain and 3000 rads of local irradiation (Fig. 11.5). Since the follow-up period for the latter group has been relatively short, comparisons between the groups cannot be made. Nevertheless, it was found that the 5-year survival rate among the former group was 81.8%, but recurrence after several years was relatively frequent and the 10-year survival rate was only 34.1%. In contrast, among the cases undergoing both local and whole-brain irradiation, there has been only one death thus far.

As mentioned earlier, oligodendroglioma often spreads diffusely within the cortex, so that the border of the tumor is not clear and there is a strong possibility of tumor tissue existing outside the identified field receiving radiation therapy. As

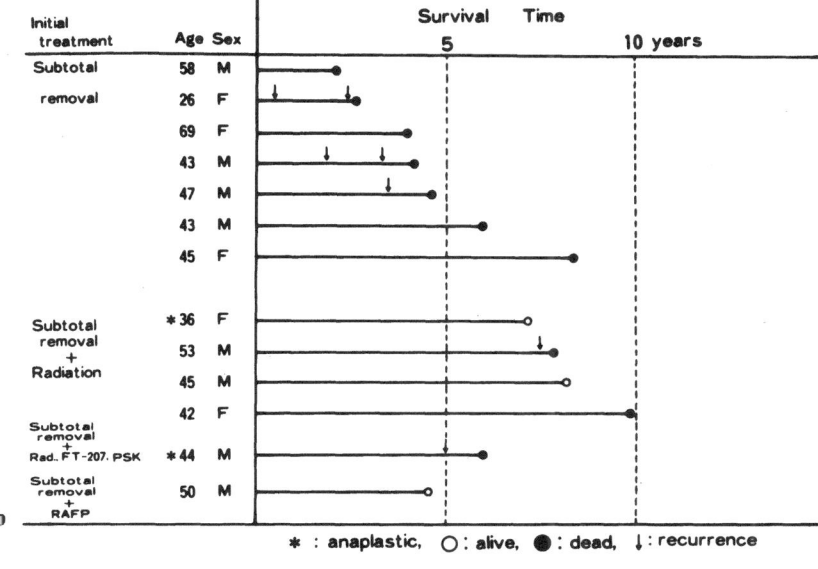

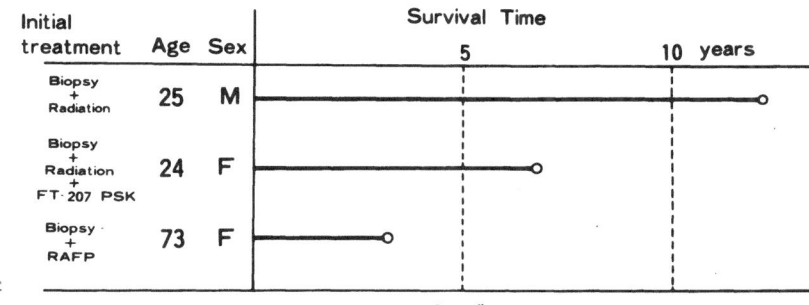

Fig. 11.4b, c.

a consequence, it is considered essential to administer whole-brain irradiation in such cases. In the present series, however, significant differences between the two groups were not found. Further study of the effectiveness of different methods of irradiation is still needed.

Recurrence

Recurrence was identified in a total of nine cases following the initial therapy (Table 11.3). The interval from initial treatment until recurrence ranged from 6 months to 11 years 1 month, with more than 5 years elapsing in four cases. Recurrence was found in four of the cases undergoing surgical resection only and in five cases undergoing postoperative radiation therapy, including one undergoing RAFP therapy. There was a tendency for the interval until recurrence to be shorter among the patients who had surgery only. In four of the five patients receiving radiation therapy and having recurrence, only local irradiation was used.

The histopathological findings at recurrence included two cases with ma-

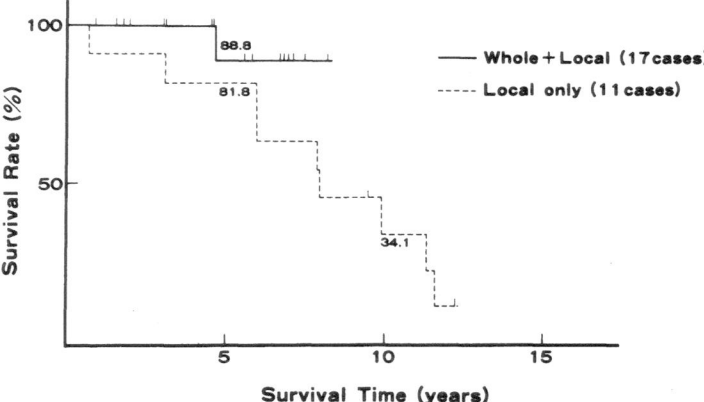

Fig. 11.5. Correlation of survival rate with whole-brain irradiation

lignant transformation relative to the original tumor, one had an anaplastic oligodendroglioma and one had a glioblastoma. Malignant transformation at recurrence has previously been reported by Áfra et al. [1], Müller et al. [12], and Barnard (3). The frequency of malignant transformation was particularly high in the reports by Müller et al. and Áfra et al. and it is necessary to bear this in mind.

Discussion

Several previous studies on the effectiveness of postoperative irradiation in oligodendroglioma have been reported (Table 11.4), but unanimity of opinion has not been reached. Sheline et al. [16] found radiation therapy to be significantly better than surgery alone with 5- and 10-year survival rates of, respectively, 85% and 55% following 2000–6000 rads of irradiation, in comparison with rates of 31% and 21% when only surgical removal was done. Roberts and German [15] reported an increase in the mean survival time of 5.2–6.2 years following surgery when radiation therapy using 6000 rads was employed. Shenkin [17] maintains that oligodendrogliomas are sensitive to radiation therapy and that a prolonged period until recurrence can be obtained by means of postoperative radiation therapy. Chin et al. [4] reported a 5-year survival rate of 100% following postoperative radiation therapy 5300–9000 rads. As treatment for oligodendroglioma, they recommend radical surgical resection followed by radiation therapy to treat the remaining microscopic lesions.

In contrast, Weir and Elvidge [19] found no positive effects from postoperative radiotherapy and are dubious about its effectiveness in such cases. From an analysis of the results in oligodendroglioma in children, Dohrmann et al. [6] reported that radiation therapy had no effects on either the survival rate or survival time. Moreover, in a recent study by Reedy et al. [14], no difference in the 5-year survival rate was found between those treated surgically only and a group of 27 cases given 2200–6500 rads postoperatively.

In our experience, we have found radiation therapy to be effective in oligo-

Table 11.4. Series of intracranial oligodendroglioma

Authors	No. of patients	Treatment	Survival rate (%)	
			5-year	10-year
Sheline et al. [16]	16	Surg. alone	31	25
	16	Surg. + Rad.	85	55
Wier and Elvidge [19]	63		41	—
Dohrmann et al. [6][a]	3	Surg. alone	67	—
	7	Surg. + Rad.	71	—
Chin et al. [4]	9	Surg. alone	81.8	—
	7	Surg. + Rad.	100	—
Reedy et al. [14]	21	Surg. alone	70	—
	27	Surg. + Rad.	68	—
Mørk et al. [11]	175		34.2	11.0
Brain Tumor Registry in Japan [13]	326		53.7	—

Surg. surgical removal, *Rad.* radiation therapy
[a] Cases in children

dendroglioma cases, but in order to draw firm conclusions concerning the effects of such therapy, it is necessary to take into consideration the influences of the total radiation dose, the fractionation of the dose, and the radiation field. A control study of these factors remains to be done.

There have not been any previous reports on the effectiveness of chemotherapy in oligodendroglioma. We have given combined radiation therapy and chemotherapy to a total of 14 cases—11 receiving RAFP therapy and three receiving radiation therapy, FT-207, and PSK therapy. Although the follow-up period for some of these cases is still short, thus far there have been only two cases of recurrence, one of which was an anaplastic oligodendroglioma. Recurrence has occurred in only one of the eleven patients treated using RAFP therapy and the results of further follow-up studies are eagerly awaited.

With regard to the recurrence of oligodendroglioma, Roberts and German [15] reported that 24 of their 38 patients undergoing only surgical resection had recurrence and the mean interval until recurrence was only 1.5 years. In contrast, Áfra et al. [1] and Müller et al. [12] studied the recurrence among 52 patients and found that it occurred after 5 or 10 years in some cases. In our series as well, recurrence was found after 7 years 6 months, 9 years 2 months, and 11 years 1 month from first therapy, thus indicating the importance of long-term follow-up studies.

Conclusion

A study of the therapeutic results in 39 cases of oligodendroglioma was made. The 5- and 10-year survival rates were 73.1% and 32.2%, respectively. Several cases showed recurrence after more than 5 years from the initial treatment and such cases indicate the importance of long-term follow-up studies.

Recurrence was infrequent in the early period following postoperative radiation therapy and such therapy is thought to be effective in the majority of oligodendroglioma cases. Statistically significant differences between groups of patients given RAFP therapy and radiation therapy alone have not been seen, but recurrence has been found in only one patient who underwent RAFP therapy.

References

1. Áfra D, Müller W, Benoist GY, Schröder R (1978) Supratentorial recurrences of gliomas. Results of reoperations on astrocytomas and oligodendrogliomas. Acta Neurochirurgica 43: 217–227
2. Bailey P, Bucy PC (1929) Oligodendrogliomas of the brain. J Pathology 32: 735–751
3. Barnard RO (1968) The development of malignancy in oligodendrogliomas. J Path Bact 96: 113–123
4. Chin HW, Hazel JJ, Kim TH, Webster JH (1980) Oligodendrogliomas. I.A clinical study of cerebral oligodendrogliomas. Cancer 45: 1458–1466
5. Cox DR (1972) Regression model and life tables. JR Stat Soc (B) 34: 187–220
6. Dohrmann GJ, Farwell JR, Flannery JT (1978) Oligodendrogliomas in children. Surg Neurol 10: 21–25
7. Earnest F, Kernohan JW, Craig WM (1950) Oligodendrogliomas. Arch Neurol Psychiatry 63: 964–976
8. Horrax G, Wu WQ (1951) Postoperative survival of patients with intracranial oligodendroglioma with special reference to radical tumor removal. A study of 26 patients. J Neurosurg 8: 473–479
9. Jimenez J, Alert J, Beldarrain L, Montalov J, Roca C (1983) Brain tumors in children. Results of treatment in 138 patients. Neoplasma 30: 93–96
10. Kaplan EL, Meier P (1958) Nonparametric estimation for incomplete observations. J Am Stat Assoc 53: 457–481
11. Mørk SJ, Lindegaard K, Halvorsen TB, Lehmann EH, Solgaard T, Hatlevoll R, Harveī S, Ganz J (1985) Oligodendroglioma; incidence and biological behavior in a defined population. J Neurosurg 63: 881–889
12. Müller W, Áfra D, Schröder R (1977) Supratentorial recurrences of gliomas. Morphological studies in relation to time intervals with oligodendrogliomas. Acta Neurochirurgica 39: 15–25
13. The committee of the brain tumor registry in Japan (1984) Brain tumor registry in Japan, vol. 5. Japanese Ministry of Health and Welfare, Tokyo
14. Reedy DP, Bay JW, Hahn JF (1983) Role of radiation therapy in the treatment of cerebral oligodendroglioma: an analysis of 57 cases and a literature review. Neurosurgery 13: 499–503
15. Roberts M, German WJ (1966) A long term study of patients with oligodendrogliomas. Follow-up of 50 cases, including Dr. Harvey Cushing's series. J Neurosurg 24: 697–700
16. Sheline GE, Boldrey E, Karlsberg P, Phillips TL (1964) Therapeutic considerations in tumors affecting the central nervous system: oligodendrogliomas. Radiology 82: 84–89
17. Shenkin HA (1965) The effect of roentgen-ray therapy on oligodendrogliomas of the brain. J Neurosurg 22: 57–59
18. Shenkin HA, Grant FC, Drew JH (1947) Postoperative period of survival of patients with oligodendroglioma of the brain. Arch Neurol Psychiatry 58: 710–715
19. Weir B, Elvidge AR (1968) Oligodendrogliomas. An analysis of 63 cases. J Neurosurg 29: 500–505
20. Wislawski J (1970) Cerebral oligodendrogliomas. Clinical manifestations, surgical treatment and histological findings in seventy cases. Polish Med J 9: 164–172

Chapter 12

Clinical Analysis of Glioma: Ependymoma

M. KITAHARA

Introduction

Ependymoma is a localized tumor and is known to be a glioma that can be completely resected. However, such tumors are often deep-seated near the ventricles, histologically malignant, or show spinal dissemination; it is not unusual for appropriate therapy to be uncertain and the prognosis poor. The results of a national survey on brain tumors in Japan [28] has indicated that the prognosis in ependymoma is not good, with the 5-year survival rate for intracranial ependymoma being 44.5% and that for malignant ependymoma 26.5%.

In recent years, however, postoperative radiation therapy has been used in such cases and several reports have indicated improved therapeutic results [10, 11, 18, 20, 21, 24–26]. In contrast, there have been very few reports on the therapeutic results in cases which have been given postoperative chemotherapy [21]. For several years, we have been treating intracranial ependymoma cases with chemotherapy— principally, ACNU, 5-FU, and FT-207—in addition to surgical resection and radiation therapy. Here, we report our therapeutic results with particular emphasis on the effectiveness of combined radiation therapy and chemotherapy, such as radiation, ACNU, FT-207, and PSK (RAFP).

Materials and Methods

A total of 30 cases of intracranial ependymoma were experienced at our clinic over the 20-year period from 1965 to 1984. All cases were histologically confirmed from tissue obtained either at surgery or autopsy. Of the patients, 14 were male and 16 female. Eight were between the ages of 0 and 4, two between 5 and 9, five between 10 and 14, three between 15 and 19, six between 20 and 29, one between 30 and 39, three between 40 and 49, and four between 50 and 59 years (Fig. 12.1). Among the juvenile cases (0–14 years), there were five with tumors of the lateral ventricles, four with intracerebral tumors, and four with tumors of the fourth ventricle. Among the adult cases (15 years and over), there were four tumors of the lateral ventricles, four intracerebral tumors, one of the third ventricle, and eight of the fourth ventricle (Table 12.1).

The histological findings, following the World Health Organization (WHO)

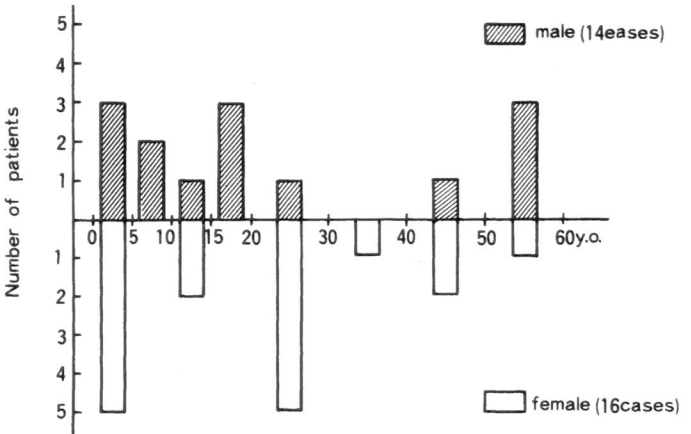

Fig. 12.1. Age and sex distribution

Table 12.1. Location of tumor

	Children (0–14 years)	Adults (≥ 15 years)	Total
Lateral ventricle	5	4	9
Cerebral hemisphere	4	4	8
Third ventricle	0	1	1
Fourth ventricle	4	8	12

classification, were as follows: 11 grade I cases, seven grade II cases, ten grade III cases, and two grade IV cases. The relationship between the histological grade, age, and site was as follows: Among the adult cases, about half (eight cases) were grade III or grade IV, and six of these were supratentorial (Table 12.2).

Among the 30 patients, three died within 1 month postoperatively, two of postoperative meningitis and one suddenly of unknown causes. The therapeutic results were studied in the remaining 24 cases.

The initial therapy in 16 cases was surgical resection (total in 11 cases, subtotal in five cases) followed by radiation therapy. In six cases, surgical resection (total in five, subtotal in one) was followed by both radiation therapy and chemotherapy. In one case, radiation therapy was given following a shunt operation and in one case radiation therapy and chemotherapy were performed following biopsy. In other words, 22 of the 24 patients underwent total or subtotal resection followed by radiation therapy and/or chemotherapy. Two received RAFP therapy.

The total radiation dose was 4000–6000 rads in all cases; 16 received radiation therapy at sites confined to the lesion itself and eight received whole-brain irradiation followed by local irradiation. The distribution of these therapeutic methods did not differ significantly among adult and juvenile cases nor according to the malignancy of the tumor (Table 12.3).

The survival curve was calculated according to the method of Kaplan and Meier [10] and tests of significance were done following the Cox-Mantel method [6].

Table 12.2. Correlation of histological diagnosis (WHO) with location and age

	Histological grade							
	Children				Adults			
	I	II	III	IV	I	II	III	IV
Supratentorial	2	4	2	1	2	1	5	1
Infratentorial	3	0	1	0	4	2	2	0
Total	5	4	3	1	6	3	7	1

Table 12.3. Treatment of 24 cases of intracranial ependymoma

	Histological grade				Total
	Children		Adults		
	I + II	III + IV	I + II	III + VI	
Removal and radiation	4	4	4	4	16
Removal, radiation, and chemotherapy	2	1	1	2	6
VPs and radiation	0	0	1	0	1
Biopsy, radiation, and chemotherapy	0	0	1	0	1

Results

Overall Survival Rate

The 5- and 10-year survival rates among the 24 patients were 44.6% and 39.7%, respectively (Fig. 12.2). Of the patients, 15 have died, 11 of them within 3 years of the initial treatment. Five patients have survived for more than 10 years from initial treatment, and four of these have not had recurrence of the tumor.

Histological Findings

The 5- and 10-year survival rates for the 14 grade I and II cases were 58.3% and 48.6%, respectively, whereas the 5-year survival rate for the ten grade III and IV patients was 26.6% (Fig. 12.3). This survival rate was significantly lower than that for the grade I and II case ($P < 0.05$).

It has previously been reported that the 5-year survival rate in cases of intracranial ependymoma is between 17% and 58% [2–5, 11, 14, 15, 22, 23, 27] (Table 12.4). For those with malignant lesions, however, the 5-year survival rate is still poorer at 10%–30% [5, 9, 14, 16–18, 27] (Table 12.5). Coulon and Till [5] reported that none of their patients under the age of 19 who had malignant lesions treated by postoperative radiation therapy survived for more than 3 years. Chin et al. [5] have stated that the prognosis is poor in cases with malignant tumors even when radiation

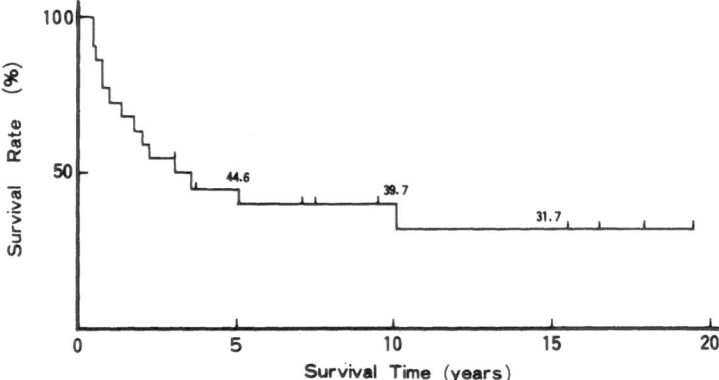

Fig. 12.2. Survival rate of 24 cases of intracranial ependymoma

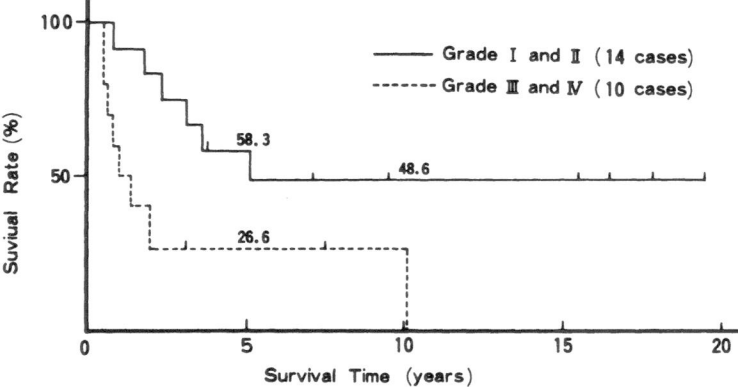

Fig. 12.3. Correlation of survival rate with histological findings

therapy is used. They maintain that large doses of irradiation or other adjunct therapy is required. As in the case of other malignant gliomas, the therapeutic technique for anaplastic ependymoma requires further study.

The 5-year survival rate among cases with histologically benign lesions has generally been reported to be above 50% (ranging from 25% to 80%), but early recurrence and death are not infrequent [5, 6, 9, 14, 16, 18, 27].

Age and Location of Tumor

Comparison was made between the results of the 11 juvenile cases and 13 adult cases (Figs. 12.4, 12.5). The 5- and 10-year survival rates were 40.0% and 30.0% among the juvenile cases, and 47.6% and 47.6% among the adult cases. These results suggest better survival among the adult patients, but the differences between the groups were not statistically significant. With regard to the site of the lesion, it is noteworthy that all three of the infratentorial tumors among the juvenile cases were fatal.

Table 12.4. Survival of patients with intracranial ependymoma

Series		Number of patients	Treatment	Survival rate (%)		
				3-year	5-year	10-year
Cushing	1932	25	Surg. alone		20	
Ringertz and Reymond	1949	54	Surg. alone		47	
Richmond	1959	50	Surg. + Rad.		50	
Bouchard and Peirce	1960	12[a]	Surg. + Rad. (≧ 50 Gy)		58	50
Kricheff et al.	1964	59	Surg. + Rad. (≧ 36 Gy)		41	
Phillips et al.	1964	22	Surg. + Rad.		56	43
		15	Surg. + Rad. (≧ 45 Gy)		87	62
Mørk and Loken	1977	12[a]	Surg. alone		17	
		16[a]	Surg. + Rad.		40	
Kim and Fayos	1977	11	Surg. + Rad.	68	45	
Glanzmann et al.	1980	15	Surg. + Rad.	60	40	
		5	Surg. + Rad. (≧ 45 Gy)	90	82	
Chin et al.	1982	7	Surg. + Rad.	71.4	71.4	
Salazar et al.	1983	17	Surg. + Rad. (local)	40	38	38
		9	Surg. + Rad. (whole brain)	75		
Brain Tumor Registry in Japan	1984	254		53.1	44.5	

Surg. surgical resection, *Rad.* radiation therapy
[a] Both of benign and anaplastic cases

Table 12.5. Survival of patients with intracranial anaplastic ependymomas

Series	Number of patients	Treatment	Survival (%)	
			3-year	5-year
Kim and Fayos [12]	21	Surgery + radiation	21	16
Glanzmann et al. [9]	9	Surgery + radiation	33	20
Chin et al. [4]	9	Surgery + radiation	33.3	22.2
Salazar et al. [23] {	14	Surgery + radiation (local)	40	25
	20	Surgery + radiation (whole CNS)	67	

Previous studies on therapeutic results in relation to the location of the tumor have produced diverse findings, but in recent years several reports have indicated slightly better outcomes among cases with infratentorial tumors (Table 12.6). There have also been, however, sporadic reports indicating that the operative mortality among infratentorial cases is high (Table 12.7). Reports concerning the relationship between age and therapeutic results have also been varied (Table 12.8) and we

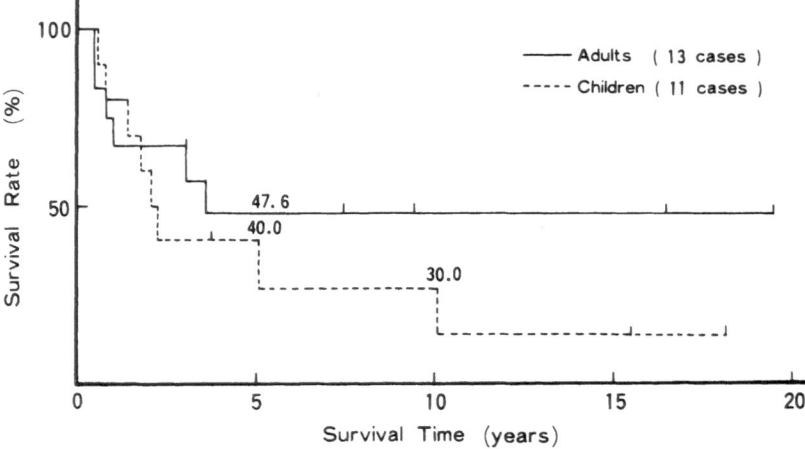

Fig. 12.4. Comparison of survival rate between adults and children

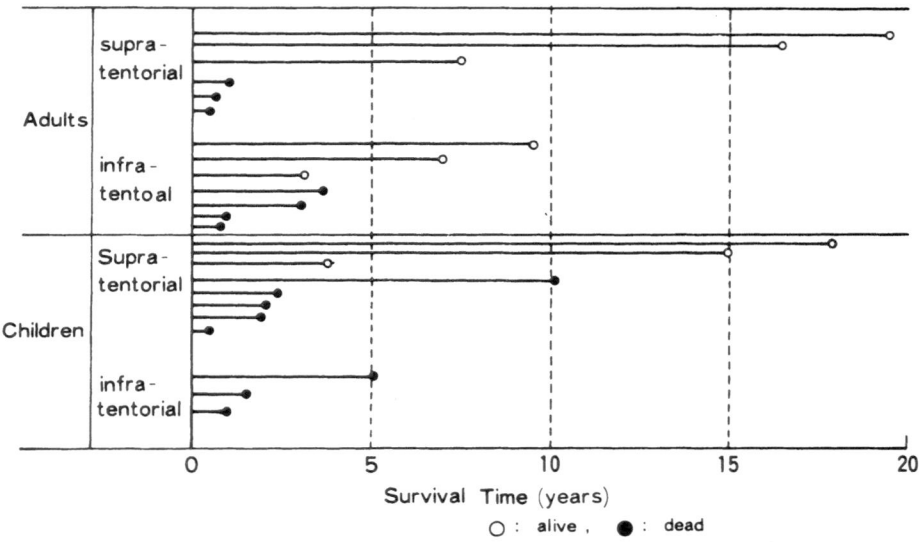

Fig. 12.5. Correlation of survival time with location

believe it is necessary to study the influence of such factors as age, location, and malignancy of the tumors.

Therapeutic Methods

Comparisons were made between two groups of patients—the sixteen patients who underwent surgical resection of the tumor followed by radiation therapy and the six undergoing surgical resection, radiation therapy, and chemotherapy (Fig. 12.6). The chemotherapy in the latter group included ACNU, FT-207, and PSK (i.e.,

Table 12.6. Considerations of survival rate correlated with location of ependymoma

Series	Treatment	5-year survival (%)		
		Supratentorial	Infratentorial	Total
Kricheff et al. [13]	Surgery + radiation	33	45	41
Dohrmann et al. [7]	Surgery alone	29	17	25
	Surgery + radiation	21	10	15
Mørk and Loken [16]	Surgery alone	0	25	17
	Surgery + radiation	33	46	40
Kim and Fayos [12]	Surgery + radiation	46	33	37
Glanzmann et al. [9]	Surgery + radiation	46	72	—
Chin et al. [4]	Surgery + radiation	34	40	37

Table 12.7. Operative mortality in different series of intracranial ependymoma

Series	Total		Supratentorial		Infratentorial	
	Percent	No.	Percent	No.	Percent	No.
Ringertz and Reymond [21]	40	(19/48)	22	(4/18)	50	(15/30)
Kricheff et al. [13]	20	(13/65)	—		—	
Barone and Elvidge [2]	32	(15/47)	—		—	
Mørk and Loken [16]	22	(8/36)	17	(2/12)	25	(6/24)
Glanzmann et al. [9]	12.5	(3/24)	—		—	

Table 12.8. Considerations of survival rate correlated with age of patients

Series	5-year survival (%)			
	Adults		Children	
	Supratentorial.	Infratentorial.	Supratentorial.	Infratentorial.
Dohrmann et al. [7]	31	33	27	10
Coulon and Till [5]	—	—	9.9	22.2
Chin et al. [4]	17[a]		50[a]	
Salazar et al. [23]	18[a]		45[a]	
Read [20]	40	67	15	28

[a] Combined supratentorial and infratentorial cases

RAFP therapy) in two cases, FT-207 only in two cases, 5-FU only in one case, and BAR (BudR + antimetabolite + radiation) therapy in one case. In one of the two patients given FT-207, an intrathecal injection of 5 mCi ^{198}Au was also given.

The 5-year survival rate in the group receiving only surgery and radiation therapy was 35.7% and the 10-year survival rate was 28.5%. In contrast, in the group also receiving radiochemotherapy, there were no deaths within 2 years of first therapy and the 5-year survival rate (66.7%) was significantly higher ($P < 0.05$) than that of

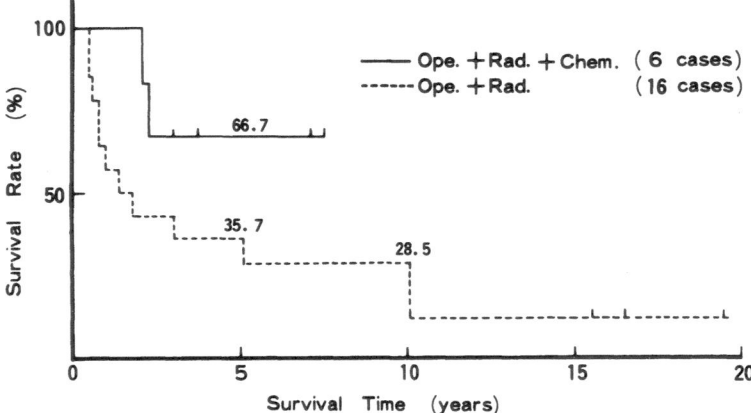

Fig. 12.6. Comparison of survival rate between postoperative radiotherapy and radio-chemotherapy

the group not receiving radiochemotherapy.

The two patients receiving RAFP therapy were grade II and III and both have survived for 3–4 years without recurrence of the tumor. No differences in the results were found between the patients given local irradiation versus those given local and whole-brain irradiation.

Long Survival Cases

All five of the patients surviving for more than 10 years from first therapy were relatively young patients (3–29 years of age) with tumors located supratentorially (lateral ventricle, frontal lobe, or frontoparietal region; Table 12.9). Histopathologically, one was grade I, three were grade II, and one was grade III.

In all fives cases, surgical resection was followed by radiation therapy, but chemotherapy was not used. Recurrence has not been found in four of the five patients; in one case, recurrence of a malignant meningioma followed after 9 years at the site of the therapy. The new lesion in this patient was again treated by surgical removal and radiation therapy, but the patient subsequently died [13].

Recurrence

Recurrence has been found in 9 of the 24 cases (Table 12.10). These include three grade I lesions, one grade II, four grade III, and one grade IV. All three cases of grade I were located in the fourth ventricle. In six cases, the initial therapy was surgical resection and radiation therapy, and in two cases chemotherapy was also used. In one case, radiation therapy was used following a shunt operation. The period from first therapy until recurrence was as follows: less than 1 year in three cases, 1–2 years in three cases, and 2–3 years in three cases. Recurrence was relatively early even among grade I and II cases and, with the exception of one case, death followed between 2 months and 4 years after recurrence (averaging 11.8

Table 12.9. Clinical features of long-survival cases

Case	Age (years)	Sex	Location	Histological grade	Operation	Radiation (^{60}Co, rad)	Recurrence	Survival (years)	Present status
1	29	F	Rt. frontal lobe	II	Total removal	4500	(−)	19.5	Good
2	3	M	Rt. lateral ventricle	II	Total removal	5500	(−)	17.8	Good
3	23	F	Rt. frontoparietal lobe	I	Subtotal removal	5000	(−)	16.5	Good
4	12	M	Lt. lateral ventricle	II	Total removal	5000	(−)	15.5	Good
5	3	F	Rt. frontal lobe	III	Total removal	3650	Malignant meningioma	10	Died

Table 12.10. Clinical features of recurrent cases

Case	Age (years)	Sex	Location	Histological grade	Initial treatment	Interval (months)	Extracranial metastasis	Survival time (months)	Present status
1	23	F	Fourth ventricle	I	Total removal + 5500 rad	30	(−)	37	Died
2	14	F	Fourth ventricle	I	Total removal + 4100 rad	14	Spinal dissemination	61	Died
3	17	M	Fourth ventricle	I	VIPS + 7000 rad	25	(−)	43	Died
4	2	M	Rt. lateral ventricle	II	Subtotal removal + 4500 rad	18	(−)	22	Died
5	49	M	Rt. temporal lobe	III	Total removal + 6000 rad	9	(−)	12	Died
6	13	F	Fourth ventricle	III	Total removal + 5000 rad	12	(−)	17	Died
7	26	M	Lt. frontal lobe	III	Total removal + 6000 rad + FT-207	36	(−)	84	Poor
8	2	F	Ft. lateral ventricle	III	Subtotal removal + 5000 rad + 5-FU	16	(−)	25	Died
9	3	F	Rt. fronto-parietal lobe	IV	Total removal + 5000 rad	4	Intraperitoneal dissemination	6	Died

months). The recurrence was a focal lesion in seven cases, but in one case it was due to spinal dissemination of tumor cells and in another case it involved both a focal lesion and an intra-abdominal metastasis, thought to have occurred via the shunt tube. The histological nature of the recurrence was not malignant in any case.

Discussion

Various reports on the effectiveness of radiation therapy in cases of intracranial ependymoma have been made, but in recent years a large number have indicated improved survival rates obtained by means of postoperative radiation therapy [10, 11, 18, 20, 24, 25]. There have also been reports that radiation therapy is effective in benign tumors [18, 19, 21, 24, 25] and that the prognosis is favorable when a dose of more than 4500 rads is used [11, 20]. Moreover, there have also been reports that the prognosis is better when whole-brain, rather than local irradiation only is employed [e.g., 25].

In our series of patients, radiation therapy was used in all cases, so that comparisons with surgery alone are not possible. In addition, significant differences in the prognosis have not yet been found between our patients undergoing local irradiation only and those undergoing local and whole-brain irradiation.

The spinal dissemination of tumor cells is an important factor influencing the prognosis [24, 25] (Table 12.11). It is known that such dissemination occurs in approximately 3% of intracranial ependymoma cases and is particularly numerous among those with subtentorial lesions. Most such tumors are found to be malignant, but there have also been reports of benign tumors among such cases [10, 14, 19]. Even when neurological symptoms are not present, cytological study of the CSF sometimes reveals tumor cells and Coulon and Till [6] reported five such cases out of 43 without neurological symptoms. Salazar et al. [25] reported that 32 of 108 autopsy cases (30%) had foci due to spinal dissemination. Since the prognosis in such cases is particularly poor, there have also been reports of preventive irradiation of the spinal cord. According to Salazar et al. [25], the 3-year survival rate of anaplastic ependymoma cases given whole-brain radiation followed by spinal irradiation was 70%, whereas it was only 35% among those given only whole-brain irradiation. Read [21] also reported good results in juvenile cases given spinal irradiation.

In contrast, Kricheff et al. [15] reported no positive effects among patients given preventive spinal irradiation. They maintain that further study of the use of spinal irradiation as a preventive measure is still needed. In our series, we had one patient with spinal dissemination, despite the fact that the original lesion was grade I. For this reason, we believe it is essential to study the postoperative course of ependymoma cases with this possibility in mind.

There have been a few previous studies on the effects of chemotherapy on intracranial ependymoma [5, 21]. Read [21] used chemotherapy in a total of 15 cases but concluded that its effectiveness was uncertain. Among our patients, a distinct trend toward better outcomes was seen when chemotherapy was used: The 5-year survival rate following postoperative radiation therapy was 35.7%, whereas that following postoperative radiation therapy and chemotherapy was 66.7%. These results strongly indicate the need for further study of the effectiveness of chemotherapy.

Table 12.11. Spinal seeding

Authors	Infratentorial			Supratentorial		
	Benign	Malignant	Total	Benign	Malignant	Total
Bloom et al. (1975)	1/13	4/7	5/20			0/11
Kim and Fayos (1977)	1/8	5/13	6/21	0/3	1/8	1/11
Oi and Raimondi (1980)	1/13	3/7	4/20	0/6	2/7	2/13
Svien et al. (1975)	0/21	0/12	0/33	0/9	0/12	0/21

Both in our series and in the cases reported in the literature, it is apparent that recurrence, even among cases with histologically benign lesions, is not rare and that the vast majority occur within 3 years after the initial treatment. There have also been reports of malignant transformation at the time of recurrence [1]. These findings indicate that the choice of therapy used in the initial treatment of the tumor is an important factor in the ultimate prognosis. In light of the fact that recurrence in the early period following postoperative radiation therapy and chemotherapy was not observed, we believe that the use of both radiation therapy and chemotherapy in the initial treatment will play an important role in achieving improvements in the outcome of cases of intracranial ependymoma.

Conclusion

We studied therapeutic results in 24 of 30 cases of intracranial ependymoma we experienced in which the effects of therapy could be evaluated. In 22 of the 24 cases, postoperative radiation therapy with or without chemotherapy was used and it was found that the prognosis was better when chemotherapy was employed. In light of the fact that recurrence in a relatively early period following initial treatment was not frequently found, we consider that postoperative radiation therapy together with chemotherapy is effective in such cases.

References

1. Áfra D, Müller W, Slowik F, Wilcke O, Budka H, Turoczy L (1983) Supratentorial lobal ependymomas: Reports on the grading and survival periods in 80 cases, including 46 recurrences. Acta Neurochirurgica 69: 243–251
2. Barone BA, Elvidge AR (1970) Ependymomas: a clinical survey. J Neurosurg 33: 428–438
3. Bloom HJG (1982) Intracranial tumors: response and resistance to therapeutic endeavors, 1970–1980. Int J Radiat Oncol Biol Phys 8: 1083–1113
4. Bouchard J, Peirce CB (1960) Radiation therapy in the management of neoplasms of the central nervous system, with a special note in regard to children: twenty years experience, 1939–1958. Am J Roentgenol 84: 610–628
5. Chin HW, Maruyama Y, Markesbery W, Young AB (1982) Intracranial ependymoma. Cancer 49: 2276–2280
6. Coulon RA, Till K (1977) intracranial ependymomas in children: a review of 43 cases.

Child's Brain 3: 154–168

7. Cox DR (1972) Regression model and life tables. J R Stat Soc (B) 34: 187–220
8. Cushing H (1932) Intracramial tumors. Notes upon a series of two thusand verified cases with surgical mortality, percentages pertaining thereto. Charles C Thomas, Springfield, IL, p 56
9. Dohrman GJ, Farwell JR, Flannery JT (1976) Ependymomas and ependymoblastomas in children. J Neurosurg 45: 273–283
10. Fokes EC Jr, Earle KM (1969) Ependymomas: clinical and pathological aspects. J Neurosurg 30: 585–594
11. Glanzmann CH, Horst W, Schiess K, Friede R (1980) Considerations in the radiation treatment of intracranial ependymoma; prognosis in 24 own cases and results in published series after different techniques of radiation treatment. Strahlentherapie 156: 97–101
12. Kaplan EL, Meier P (1958) Nonparametric estimation from incomplete observations. J Am Stat Assoc 53: 457–481
13. Katakura R, Ohara H, Sakurai Y (1978) Malignant meningioma following irradiation therapy for ependymoma, a case report. Neurol Surg 6: 935–939 (in Japanese)
14. Kim YH, Fayos J (1977) Intracranial ependymomas. Radiology 124: 805–808
15. Kricheff II, Becker M, Schneck SA, Taveras JM (1964) Intracranial ependymomas: a study of survival in 65 cases treated by surgery and irradiation. Am J Roentogenol 91: 167–175
16. Mabon RF, Svien HJ, Kernohan JW, Craig W Mck (1949) Proceedings of the staff meetings of the Mayo Clinic. 24: 65–71
17. MeiLiu H, Boggs J, Kidd J (1976) Ependymomas of childhood. child's Brain 2: 92–110
18. Mørk SJ, Loken AC (1977) Ependymoma: a follow-up study of 101 cases. Cancer 40: 907–915
19. Oi S, Raimondi AJ (1980) Brain tumors in infants and children—Factors affecting prognosis: I Ependymoma. Neurol Surg 8: 1049–1055 (in Japanese)
20. Phillips TL, Sheline GE, Boldrey E (1964) Therapeutic consideration in tumors affecting the central nervous system: ependymomas. Radiology 83: 98–105
21. Read G (1984) The treatment of ependymoma of the brain or spinal canal by radiotherapy: A report of 79 cases. Clin Radiol 35: 163–166
22. Richmond JJ (1953) Radiotherapy of intracranial tumors in children. J Fac Radiologists 4: 180–189
23. Ringertz N, Reymond A (1949) Ependymomas and choroid plexus papillomas. J Neuropathol Exp Neurol 8: 355–380
24. Salazar OM, Rublin P, Bassano D, Marcial V (1975) Improved survival of patients with intracranial ependymomas by irradiation: dose selection and field extension. Cancer 35: 1563–1573
25. Salazar OM, Castro-Vita H, Van Houtte P, Rubin P, Aygun C (1983) Improved survival in cases of intracranial ependymoma after radiation therapy. Later report and recommendations. J Neurosurg 59: 652–659
26. Sheline CE (1975) Radiation therapy of tumors on the central nervous system in childhood. Cancer 35: 957–964
27. Svien HJ, Mabon RF, Kernohan JW, Craig W Mck (1953) Ependymoma of the brain: pathologic aspects. Neurology 3: 1–15
28. The committee of the brain tumor registry in Japan (1984) Brain tumor registry in Japan, vol. 5. Japanese Ministry of Health and Welfare, Tokyo

Chapter 13

Clinical Analysis of Glioma: Medulloblastoma

Y. Takahashi

Introduction

Although progress in the treatment of medulloblastoma has been made in recent years [1-6, 9, 10, 12, 14, 15, 21, 23], it is still one of the types of brain tumor with a poor prognosis. Since 1979, we have used radiation therapy combined with chemotherapy using ACNU, FT-207, and PSK (RAFP) to treat medulloblastomas. In this way, we have obtained a 5-year survival rate of 82.5% [20, 22] (Fig. 13.1). Here, we discuss the prognosis and factors influencing the prognosis among the cases experienced at our clinic thus far.

Materials and Methods

Between 1948 and February 1985, a total of 67 cases of medulloblastoma were treated in the Divisions of Neurosurgery of Tohoku University and Sendai National Hospital. Of the patients, 41 were male (61.2%) and 26 female (38.8%). The age at onset ranged between 3 months and 41 years, with a mean age of 10.2 years. In the case of those patients in whom treatment was evaluated and a follow-up study was made, factors influencing the prognosis were examined. The therapies of the 40 cases were surgery alone (eight cases), surgery and radiation therapy (17 cases), and RAFP therapy (15 cases; Table 13.1). The items of investigation were as follows.

Prognosis and Tumor Size

The tumor-metastasis (TM) classification of medulloblastomas of Chang et al. [7] was used and the correlation between the size of the tumor and prognosis was studied for each therapy group (Table 13.2). Of the 40 cases, the size of tumor could be determined in 31 cases at the time of diagnosis on the basis of computed tomography) (CT) scans, cerebral angiography, ventricular imaging, and operative findings. These included 17 patients undergoing surgery and radiation therapy (eight T3a stage, six T3b stage, and three T4 stage cases). Study was made of the survival rate for each T stage in both groups. Spinal fluid examination before the beginning of the therapy was done in only a few cases, and so MO stage comparisons were not made.

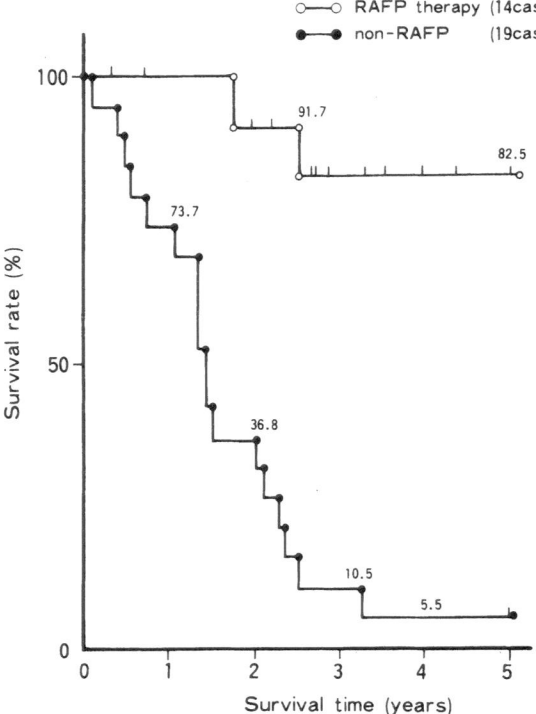

○──○ RAFP therapy (14cases)
●──● non-RAFP   (19cases)

Fig. 13.1. Survival rate of medulloblastoma treated by RAFP therapy

Prognosis and Chemotherapy

There have been some reports indicating that therapeutic results in cases of medulloblastoma are improved if chemotherapy is used in addition to radiation therapy [2]. A comparison was therefore made of the survival rates in a group of 15 patients receiving both radiation therapy and chemotherapy and those in a group of 16 patients not receiving chemotherapy.

Site of Recurrence and Irradiation Dose in RAFP Therapy

We studied ten cases of recurrence of the 14 that could be followed after the completion of the RAFP therapy. The number of cases was examined in which first recurrence of the tumor was located in the posterior fossa, supratentorium, and spinal cord. We investigated the relationship between recurrence and the total irradiation applied to the posterior fossa in the initial treatment. We also studied the correlation between supratentorial recurrence and the total irradiation applied to the supratentorium upon initial treatment in cases receiving more than 50 Gy to the posterior fossa and more than 20 Gy to the spinal cord.

Time-Dose Fractionation with Recurrence, Survival Time, and Event-Free Survival

Even when the total radiation dose among patients is the same, the radiobiological effects often differ due to differences in the duration of the radiation therapy, the

Table 13.1. Method of treatment for medulloblastomas

	No. of cases
Operation only	
Total removal	4
Subtotal removal	1
Partial removal, biopsy	2
Shunt drainage	1
Total	8
Radiation and operation	
Total removal	5
Subtotal removal	8
Partial removal, biopsy	4
Total	17
Radiation, chemotherapy, and/or operation	
Total removal	2
Subtotal removal	1
Shunt ~ Drainage	9
Operation (—)	3
Total	17
Total	40

Table 13.2. Chang staging system for posterior fossa medulloblastoma. After Chang et al. [7]

Stage	Definition
Tumor stage	
T-1	Tumor less than 3 cm in diameter, limited to midline position in vermis, roof of fourth ventricle, and, less frequently to cerebellar hemispheres
T-2	Tumor more than 3 cm in diameter, further invading one adjacent structure or partially filling fourth ventricle
T-3	
T-3a	Tumor invading two adjacent structures or completely filling fourth ventricle with extension into aqueduct of Sylvius, foramen of Magendie, or foramen of Luschka, producing internal hydrocephalus
T-3b	Tumor arising from floor of fourth ventricle or brain stem and filling fourth ventricle
T-4	Tumor further spreading through aqueduct of Sylvius to involve third ventricle or midbrain or tumor extending to upper cervical cord
Metastasis stage	
M-0	No evidence of gross subarachnoid or hematogeneous metastasis
M-1	Microscopic tumor cells found in cerebrospinal fluid
M-2	Gross nodule seedings demonstrated in cerebellar, cerebral subarachnoid space, or third or lateral ventricles
M-3	Gross nodule seedings in spinal subarachnoid space
M-4	Extraneuroaxial metastasis

fraction number of the total dose, the dose per fraction, and discontinuity in the radiation therapy. For this reason, the so-called time-dose fractionation (TDF) value for expressing the actual level of the effects of the irradiation has been devised. According to Orton and Ellis [18], the TDF values of the whole therapeutic course can be expressed as:

$$TDF = TDF_1 \times (T/(T + R))^{total} + TDF_2$$

where TDF_1 and TDF_2 are the TDF values of the first and second halves of the therapeutic course, respectively, T is the number of days in the first half of the course, and R is the interval. In actual practice, therapy is designed to approach a TDF value of 100.

For the evaluation of therapeutic effectiveness, there is, in addition to the survival time, the event-free survival time (EFS), which expresses the period from remission until recurrence. In the present study, in order to investigate further the correlation between the prognosis and the TDF, we examined the correlation between the survival time and the TDF, and between the EFS and the survival time. The survival time was defined as the period from the completion of the initial RAFP therapy and the EFS was defined as the period from then until recurrence on CT scan.

In order to examine the relationship between the TDF value and recurrence, study was made of the incidence of recurrence in relation to the TDF value of the supratentorium, the posterior fossa, and the spinal cord. Study was also made of the influence which the TDF value had on the survival rate and the EFS period.

Results

Prognosis and Size of Tumor at Time of Diagnosis

Among the ten patients who underwent both surgery and radiation therapy, nine died within 3 years (Fig. 13.2). Regardless of the T stage, none of the patients survived for more than 4 years. In contrast, among the patients undergoing RAFP therapy, 12 are still alive and, excepting the two T2 stage cases, the 3-year survival rate for the T3a, T3b, and T4 stage cases was 100%. Moreover, the 5-year survival rate for the T3a and T4 stage cases was 100%. A clear tendency was found for the prognosis to be better in the RAFP group for T3a, T3b, and T4 stage lesions, but such results were not statistically significant when the individual T stages were compared across the therapeutic groups.

Prognosis and Chemotherapy

The survival rates in the group receiving both radiation therapy and chemotherapy were as follows: 100% 1-year survival, 92.3% 2-year survival, 83.9% 3-year survival, and 83.9% 4-year survival (Fig. 13.3). In contrast, in the group receiving radiation therapy alone these survival rates were 73.3%, 26.7%, 6.7%, and 0%, respectively. Clearly, the group with chemotherapy tended to have longer survival rates, but again the results were not statistically significant.

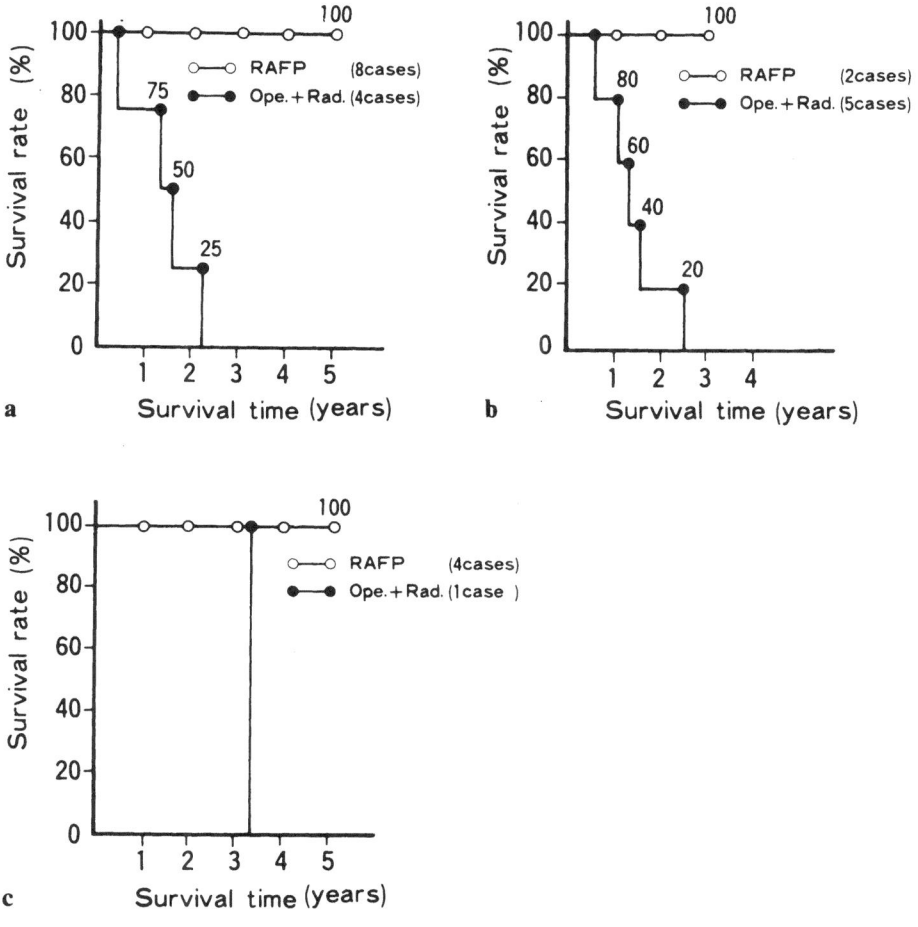

Fig. 13.2a–c. Comparison of survival rate between RAFP therapy group and operations plus radiotherapy (*Ope + Rad*) group by each T stage. **a** T3a stage; **b** T3b stage; **c** T4 stage

Total Radiation Dose and Site of Recurrence with RAFP

First recurrence. Among the 14 patients who completed RAFP therapy, recurrence was found in ten (Table 13.3). Four cases had recurrence in the posterior fossa near the original lesion, five had recurrence in the supratentorium, and one had recurrence simultaneously in the posterior fossa and spinal cord. Equal numbers of recurrence in the posterior fossa and the supratentorium were thus found, with the frequency of metastasis to the supratentorium being particularly noteworthy [18–20]. There were also two cases of recurrence in the frontal lobe at the frontal base, but in these cases it is thought that the base of the frontal lobe was considered beyond the limits of the radiation field because of the danger of irradiation to the eyes. We have more recently performed radiation therapy with this problem in mind, and have had no subsequent recurrences in the frontal base [18–20].

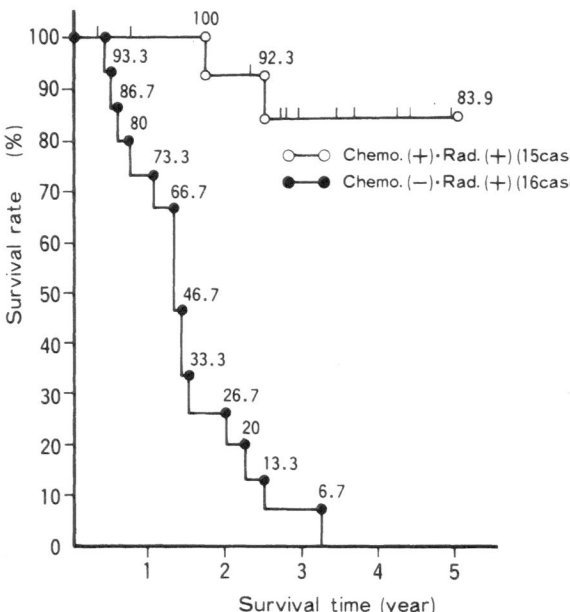

Fig. 13.3. Comparison of survival rate with or without chemotherapy

Recurrence in posterior fossa and total dose to posterior fossa in initial RAFP therapy. In RAFP therapy, attempts were made to give total doses of 60 Gy, 30 Gy, and 30 Gy to the posterior fossa, supratentorium, and spinal cord, respectively, but in practice it was often found necessary to terminate the radiation therapy due to myelosuppression. Instead of a constant dose to the posterior fossa, therefore, total doses ranging between 35 and 68 Gy were applied. It was thus possible to study the correlation of the total dose with the recurrence.

Recurrence in the posterior fossa was found in five cases, the total dose to the posterior fossa in the initial RAFP therapy being 50 Gy in two cases, 51.8 Gy in one case, 55 Gy in one case, and 60 Gy in one case (a mean total dose of 56.8 Gy). Among the four cases in which recurrence was not found, the total dose to the posterior fossa was 60 Gy in three cases and 50 Gy in one case (a mean total dose of 57.5 Gy). The difference in the total doses was not statistically significant.

Recurrence in superatentorium and total dose to supratentorium in initial RAFP therapy. Similar to the posterior fossa, it was found that the total dose to the supratentorium ranged between 25 and 50 Gy. Among the five cases with recurrence in the supratentorium, three had received a total of 30 Gy. In contrast, the four cases without recurrence had been given 40 Gy. There was thus a tendency for the cases without recurrence to have had higher doses to the supratentorium.

TDF and RAFP Patients and Recurrence, Survival Time, and EFS

TDF and recurrence. Among the four cases without recurrence, the total dose to the posterior fossa was greater than 50 Gy and the TDF of the posterior fossa was

Table 13.3. Site of first recurrence and total doses of initial RAFP therapy in recurrent cases

Case no.[a]	Age (years)	Sex	Site of recurrence	Total dose to posterior fossa (Gy)	Total dose to supratentorium (Gy)	Total dose to spinal cord (Gy)
1 (Y. M.)	1	F	Aqueductus Sylvi, pineal region	51.8	30.6	24
2 (F. M.)	7	F	Vermis	50	30	30
3 (T. Y.)	8	F	Fourth ventricle, lumbar cord	55	25	13
4 (M. K.)	21	F	Lt. cerebellar hemisphere	60	30	45
5 (T. T.)	9	F	Fourth ventricle	50	25	20.4
6 (M. S.)	16	M	Ant. horn of rt. lat. ventricle	52	30	30
7 (K. K.)	9	F	Lt. frontal lobe	60	30	18
8 (S. H.)	2	M	Wall of rt. lat. ventricle	50	30	20
9 (M. O.)	13	M	Lt. frontal lobe	60	30	40
10 (K. A.)	7	M	Wall of bil. lat. ventricles	35	35	(−)

Lt. left, *Ant.* anterior, *rt.* right, *lat.* lateral, *bil.* bilateral

[a] Cases 1–5, posterior fossa recurrent cases; cases 6, 7 supratentorial recurrent cases

greater than 90 in three of the four cases (a mean TDF value of 88.6 in the four cases; Table 13.4). In contrast, the mean TDF value in the ten cases with recurrence was 71.6, a value well below that in the former group. With regard to irradiation of the supratentorium, all four of the cases without recurrence showed total irradiation doses in excess of 30 Gy and the mean TDF was 57.8. The mean TDF among the ten cases with recurrence was 40.1, well below the value in the cases without recurrence. But a constant trend was not found with regard to irradiation of the spinal cord: There were cases without recurrence in whih no spinal cord irradiation was done and cases in which a low TDF value was obtained. On the other hand, there were also cases with recurrence in which high TDF values were obtained.

TDF and EFS. In the two fatalities due to recurrence, the TDF values for the posterior fossa, supratentorium, and spinal cord were low. The TDF values for the posterior fossa were in the 50s and those for the supratentorium were in the 20s. Among the five cases surviving for 3 or more years, TDF values were obtained in four. The values for the posterior fossa in these four were 91.5, 77.0, 63.6, and 87.4 (a mean of 79.9) and the TDF values for the supratentorium were 46.6, 34.4, 45.2, and 40.4 (a mean of 41.7). Both of these mean TDF values were higher than those in the fatal cases.

Study of the relationship between TDF and EFS values showed high TDF values (around 90) and total posterior fossa irradiation above 50 Gy in the four cases with EFS in excess of 2 years. Three of these four cases had total irradiation doses to the supratentorium in excess of 30 Gy and high TDF values in excess of 40. Although nine of the ten cases with EFS of less than 2 years had a total dose to the posterior fossa in excess of 50 Gy, the mean TDF value was low at 73.0. Nevertheless, the TDF value for supratentorial irradiation was higher than that of the former group (46.0). A clear correlation between EFS and TDF values for spinal cord irradiation was not found.

Discussion

There have recently been many reports on the treatment of medulloblastoma in which surgical excision of the tumor, followed by radiation therapy and immuno-chemotherapy for the remaining tumor tissue has been advocated [5, 7–11, 16]. Controversy continues, however, concerning when and what degree of surgical excision should be performed in medulloblastoma [5, 7, 8, 13, 17, 24, 25]. Although a minority view, the opinion has been expressed that good therapeutic results can be obtained if only partial resection of the tumor is done, followed by radiation therapy and chemotherapy [16]. Favorable results have also been reported in cases where, first, ventricular drainage is performed, followed by radiation therapy and immuno-chemotherapy, rather than direct surgery on the tumor [24].

We also have studied the influence of the surgical method on the outcome of medulloblastoma, but we have found no significant effects on the period of post-operative survival. Even in relatively advanced stages (T_3–T_4), there are cases in which good reduction or disappearance of the tumor can be obtained with radiation therapy and immunochemotherapy (i.e., RAFP therapy), and long-term survival thereby found. It can be concluded, therefore, that when excising an untreated

Table 13.4. TDF, recurrence, survival time and EFS in RAFP therapy cases

Case no.	Recurrence	Survival time (yr, mo)	EFS (yr, mo)	Total dose to posterior fossa[a] (Gy)	Total dose to supratentorium[a] (Gy)	Total dose to spinal cord[a] (Gy)
1	(−)	0, 9	0, 9	60 (94.5)	40 (63.1)	30 (43.5)
2	(−)	0, 4	0, 4	50 (76.7)	50 (76.7)	30 (47.0)
3	(−)	3, 6	3, 6	68 (91.5)	30 (46.6)	30 (29.3)
4	(−)	2, 11	2, 11	60 (91.8)	30 (44.9)	0
5	(+)	3, 11	1, 6	52 (77.0)	30 (45.2)	30 (44.5)
6	(+)	2, 11	1, 5	60 (94.2)	30 (47.0)	18 (26.4)
7	(+)	2, 8	0, 10	52.2 (78.9)	30.6 (46.0)	24 (38.5)
8	(+)	4, 11	0, 10	50 (63.6)	30 (34.4)	20 (22.5)
9	(+)	2, 3	1, 6	60 (84.5)	30 (44.2)	40 (45.6)
10	(+)	2, 8	0, 8	35 (46.3)	35 (46.3)	0
11	(+)	6, 3	3, 9	50 (?)	25 (?)	13 (?)
12	(+)	4, 4	3, 6	60 (87.4)	30 (40.4)	45 (52.5)
13[b]	(+)	1, 9	1, 5	50 (55.9)	25 (27.1)	20.4 (20.4)
14[b]	(+)	2, 6	0, 12	50 (58.6)	30 (29.9)	30 (31.0)

[a] TDF given in *parentheses*

[b] Fatal

tumor which has shown continued active proliferation, great care must be paid to the possibility of disseminating tumor tissue during surgery and, furthermore, to avoiding the use of unnecessary shunts which can provide pathways for metastasis.

In our experience, we have found that when RAFP therapy is used in hydrocephalus cases, there is a decrease in the intracranial pressure together with a reduction in tumor size, and it is therefore unnecessary to do the shunt operation. We consequently use RAFP therapy for the initial treatment in all cases except those in which there is severe intracranial hypertension due to extreme hydrocephalus or the tumor is very large and the patient is thought unlikely to withstand the radiation therapy. However, for cases in which part of the tumor remains following therapy, we perform surgical excision. Using that technique, we have obtained favorable results, with a 5-year survival rate of 82.5%. Thus, while favorable results due to RAFP therapy can be obtained, possible improvement in radiotherapeutic techniques and the development of new chemotherapeutic agents must be kept in mind.

In the treatment of medulloblastoma, radiation therapy is most important. For this reason, we have studied the relationship between the outcome and recurrence and TDF values, the latter being a means of expressing the effects of irradiation while taking differences in the method of irradiation and the total dose into consideration. We conclude that in order to obtain the maximal EFS in medulloblastoma cases treated with radiation therapy, the following target values should be aimed for: (a) The total dose of irradiation to the posterior fossa should exceed 55 Gy and a TDF of more than 90 should be obtained. (b) The total dose to the supratentorium should be between 30 and 40 Gy and a TDF value of more than 45 should be obtained. (c) The total dose to the spinal cord should be between 30 and 35 Gy and the TDF value should exceed 45. (d) The entire central nervous system should be irradiated simultaneously or irradiation of the posterior fossa, supratentorium, and spinal cord should be done with few or no graps in the therapeutic course.

Conclusion

Favorable outcomes and a 5-year survival rate of 82.5% were obtained using RAFP therapy in 15 cases of medulloblastoma. Study of the factors which influence the outcome in cases of medulloblastoma showed the following: (a) There is little chance that the surgical method or the choice of whether or not to operate will have any influence on the outcome of such cases. (b) It is essential to perform the radiation therapy on the entire central nervous system. The radiation dose aimed for should be more than 55 Gy to the posterior fossa and a TDF above 90, 30–40 Gy to the supratentorium and a TDF above 45, and 30–35 Gy to the spinal cord and a TDF above 45. (c) Improved therapeutic results can be expected when radiation therapy is used in combination with immunochemotherapy.

References

1. Aoki Y (1986) Radiotherapy of medulloblastoma combined with OK-432 (Picibanil ®)—Utilization of its alleviating action on the radiation-induced myelosuppression. J Jpn Soc Cancer Ther 21: 1376–1385 (in Japanese)

2. Berry MP, Jenkin RDT, Keen CW, Nair BD, Simpson WJ (1981) Radiation treatment of medulloblastoma, 21-year review. J Neurosurg 55: 43–51
3. Bloom HJG (1979) Recent concepts in the conservative treatment of intracranial tumors in children. Acta Neurochirur 50: 103–116
4. Bloom HJG (1982) Medulloblastoma in children; increasing survival rates and further prospects. Int J Radiat Oncol Biol Phys 8: 2023–2027
5. Bongarts EB, Bamberg M, Nau HE, Schmitt G, Bayindir C (1979) Optimal therapy in medulloblastoma. Acta Neurochirur 50: 117–125
6. Caputy AJ, McCullough DC, Manz HJ, Patterson K, Hammock MK (1987) A review of the factors influencing the prognosis of medulloblastoma. J Neurosurg 66: 80–87
7. Chang CH, Housepian EM, Herberg C (1969) An operative staging system and a megavoltage radiotherapeutic technique for cerebellar medulloblastomas. Radiology 93: 1351–1359
8. Choux M, Lena G (1982) Medulloblastoma. Neurochirur [suppl] 28: 117–212
9. Edwards MS, Levin VA, Wilson CB (1980) Chemotherapy of pediatric posterior fossa tumors. Child's Brain 7: 252–260
10. Farwell JR, Dohrmann GJ, Flannery JT (1984) Medulloblastoma in childhood: an epidemiological study. J Neurosurg 61: 657–664
11. Gerosa MA, Stefano E, Olivi A, Carteri A (1981) Multidisciplinary treatment of medulloblastoma: A 5-year experience with the SIOP trial. Child's Brain 8: 107–118
12. Harisiadis L, Chang CH (1977) Medulloblastoma in children: A correlation between staging and results of treatment. Int J Radiat Oncol Biol Phys 2: 833–841
13. Jereb B, Reid A, Ahuja RK (1982) Patterns of failure in patients with medulloblastoma. Cancer 50: 2941–2947
14. Kopelson G, Linggood RM, Kieinman GM (1982) Medulloblastoma in adults: improved survival with supervoltage radiation therapy. Cancer 49: 1334–1337
15. Kopelson G, Linggood RM, Kieinman GM (1983) Medulloblastoma; the indetification of prognostic subgroups and implications for multimodality management. Cancer 51: 312–319
16. Mazza C, Pasqualin A, Da Pian R (1981) Treatment of medulloblastoma in children. Long-term results following surgery, radiation and chemotherapy. Acta Neurochirur 57: 163–175
17. Mealey J, Hall PV (1977) Medulloblastoma in children. Survival and treatment. J Neurosurg 46: 56–63
18. Orton CG, Ellis F (1973) A simplification in the use of the NSD concept in practical radiotherapy. Br J Radiol 46: 529–537
19. Paterson E, Farr RF (1953) Cerebellar medulloblastoma: Treatment by irradiation of whole central nervous system. Acta Radiol 39: 323–336
20. Quinlan RA, Franke WW (1983) Molecular interactions in intermediate-sized filaments revealed by chemical cross-linking. Heteropolymers of vimentin and glial filament protein in cultured human glial cell. Eur J Biochem 132: 477–484
21. Raimondi AJ, Tomita T (1979) Medulloblastoma in childhood: Comparative results of partial and total resection. Child's Brain 5: 310–328
22. Silverman CL, Simpson JR (1982) Cerebellar medulloblastoma: The importance of posterior fossa dose to survival and patterns of failure. Int J Radiat Oncol Biol Phys 8: 1869–1876
23. The committee of Tohoku brain tumor registry (1985) Tohoku brain tumor registry, vol. 1
24. Tokars RP, Sutton HG, Greim ML (1979) Cerebellar medulloblastoma. Results of a new method of radiation treatment. Cancer 43: 129–139
25. Tomita T, Mclone DG (1986) Medulloblastoma in childhood; results of radical resection and low-dose neuraxis radiation therapy. J Neurosurg 64: 238–242

Chapter 14

Side Effects of RAFP Therapy

M. KITAHARA

Introduction

There have been many reports in recent years on the effectiveness of combined radiation therapy and chemotherapy in brain tumors, especially malignant gliomas [2, 3, 6] and combined radiochemotherapy has become popular. However, although combined therapy accelerates the damage to tumor cells, it also produces deficits in normal tissues and can give rise to acute toxicity due to myelosuppression or gastrointestinal complications. In the present chapter, we report a study of the side effects due to radiation therapy combined with ACNU, FT-207, and PSK (RAFP) therapy.

Materials and Methods

Study was made of 153 cases receiving RAFP therapy and 31 cases receiving combined radiation therapy and FT-207. Among the RAFP patients, 88 were male and 65 were female; 28 were between the ages of 0 and 19 years of age, 42 between 20 and 39, 54 between 40 and 59, and 29 were 60 or older. Among the patients receiving radiation therapy and FT-207, 21 were male and ten were female; eight were between 0 and 19 years of age, five between 20 and 39, 12 between 40 and 59, and six were 60 or older (Table 14.1).

The incidence and severity of the side effects were investigated.

Results

Incidence of Side Effects

The features of the side effects in the 153 patients receiving RAFP therapy were as follows: 105 cases (68.6%) had leukocytopenia of less than 4000/mm^3 and 99 (64.7%) had thrombocytopenia of less than $12.5 \times 10^4/mm^3$ (Table 14.2). There were also 23 cases (15%) with anemia of less than $350 \times 10^4/mm^3$ and seven (4.5%) with severe anemia (less than $300 \times 10^4/mm^3$). Among these patients, because of severe myelosuppression, radiation therapy was temporarily or permanently discontinued in ten cases (6.5%).

Table 14.1. Sex and age distribution of 184 patients

Age (years)	RAFP			Radiation + FT-207		
	Male	Female	Total	Male	Female	Total
0–19	15	13	28	5	3	8
20–39	21	21	42	4	1	5
40–59	31	23	54	10	2	11
≥60	21	8	29	2	4	6
Total	88	65	153	21	10	31

Among side effects of the gastrointestinal system, loss of appetite was frequently found. Instillations and antiemetics were required in 25 cases (16.3%) with loss of appetite, nausea, and/or vomiting. Diarrhea was present in three cases. Nausea and vomiting within several hours of ACNU injection were seen in 14 cases (9.2%). Examinations of the liver function revealed disorders in 34 patients (22.2%). Complications of the skin or the mucous membranes, such as rash and oral aphtha, were seen in four patients (2.6%). In total, 127 patients (83.0%) had side effects of some kind and only 26 patients (17.0%) were unaffected.

In contrast, among the patients treated with FT-207, ten (32.3%) had leukocytopenia, ten (32.3%) thrombocytopenia, and one anemia. In comparison with the groups treated with RAFP, the incidence of myelosuppression was low. Conversely, symptoms of nausea and vomiting were more frequent in the FT-207-treated patients (six cases, 19.4%), as was true for abnormalities of the mucous membranes (three cases or 9.6%). It is, therefore, thought that FT-207 has relatively greater effects on the gastrointestinal tract and mucous membranes. In this group, however, none showed liver dysfunction and no side effects of any kind were evident in a total of seven patients (22.6%).

Severe side effects were observed in several patients treated with RAFP. In one patient, severe leukocytopenia of less than $1000/mm^3$ was seen, but recovery followed transfusion with fresh blood. A hemorrhagic tendency was apparent in three patients with thrombocytopenia, one of whom showed intratumor bleeding. Moreover, three patients treated with RAFP died due to interstitial pneumonitis. It is uncertain whether this was directly related to the RAFP therapy, but it has previously been reported that nitrosourea administration has such effects [17] and caution is needed in this regard.

Among the side effects due to radiation therapy, radiation necrosis is known to have delayed effects, and this was confirmed in one RAFP case in which an autopsy was performed 2 years after RAFP therapy.

Age and Incidence of Side Effects

Study of the incidence of side effects was also made by dividing the 153 cases with RAFP therapy into four age-groups: 0–19, 20–39, 40–59, 60 years and above (Table 14.3). The incidence in these groups was similar—89.3%, 78.6%, 83.3%, and 82.8%, respectively. Moreover, the incidence was similar when the myelosuppression and gastrointestinal complications were studied separately.

Table 14.2. Side effects of 184 cases

	No. of patients	Leukocytopenia					Thrombocytopenia				Anemia			Liver dysfunc-tion	Nausea, vomiting	Diarrhea	Skin eruption, ersion of mucous membrane	No dis-order
		3900 – 3000	2900 – 2000	1900 – 1000	900/mm³	Total	12.4 – 10.0	9.9 – 5.0	4.9 × 10⁴/mm³	Total	349 – 300	299 × 10⁴/mm³	Total					
RAFP ACNU 1 mg/kg	14	1	4	2	0	7	6	1	0	7	3	1	4	2	2	1	0	2
2	67	10	27	11	0	48	20	21	7	48	8	4	12	20	12	1	4	9
3	28	8	6	5	1	20	11	5	4	20	1	2	3	4	4	1	0	6
4	44	17	9	4	0	30	23	1	0	24	2	0	2	8	7	0	0	9
Total	153	36	46	22	1	105	60	28	11	99	16	7	23	34	25	3	4	26
Radiation + FT-207	31	9	1	0	0	10	7	3	0	10	1	0	1	0	6	0	3	7

Table 14.3. Correlation of side effect caused by RAFP therapy with age

Age (years)	Leukocytopenia			Thrombocytopenia			Liver dysfunction	Nausea, vomiting	No disorder
	Total	3900 – 2000 (/mm³)	2000 > (/mm³)	Total	12.4 – 7.5 (× 10⁴/mm³)	7.5 > (× 10⁴/mm³)			
0–19	22 (78.6%)	14	8	17 (60.7%)	16	1	3 (10.7%)	6 (21.4%)	3 (10.7%)
20–39	32 (76.2%)	27	5	27 (64.3%)	24	3	9 (21.4%)	8 (19.0%)	9 (21.4%)
40–59	37 (68.5%)	30	7	37 (68.5%)	29	8	17 (31.5%)	9 (16.7%)	9 (16.7%)
≥60	14 (48.3%)	11	3	18 (62.1%)	13	5	5 (17.2%)	2 (6.9%)	5 (17.2%)
Total	105 (68.6%)	82	23	99 (64.7%)	82	17	34 (22.2%)	25 (16.3%)	26 (17.0%)

Study was also made of the leukocytopenia and thrombocytopenia which occurred with relatively high incidence in the RAFP patients.

Leukocytopenia

Among the 105 patients with leukocytopenia, 37 (34.9%) had levels of 3000–3900/mm^3 and 46 (43.4%) had levels of 2000–2900/mm^3, but there were 22 cases (21.0%) with severe leukocytopenia of less than 2000/mm^3, one of which had less than 1000/mm^3 (Table 14.2). In all cases, recovery followed within 2–3 weeks.

The onset of leukocytopenia was approximately 6 weeks after the beginning of RAFP therapy in most cases and ACNU is thought to have been the direct cause. There were, however, several cases in which such symptoms appeared after only 2 weeks, or after 2 or more months (Table 14.4).

The relationship between the dose of ACNU and the incidence of leukocytopenia was as follows. Doses of 1, 2, 3, and 4 mg/kg produced leukocytopenia in, respectively, 50% (7 of 14), 71.6% (48 of 67), 71.4% (20 of 28), and 68.2% (30 of 44) of the patients.

In comparison with the other groups, those given 2 mg/kg ACNU had a tendency for early onset of leukocytopenia following the beginning of treatmet and symptoms persisted for a relatively long period. As a concequence, ACNU could not be administered more than 2 mg/kg. Conversely, in the cases that showed relatively less early leukocytopenia and rapid recovery, four doses of 1 mg/kg of ACNU had been administered (Table 14.4; Fig. 14.1).

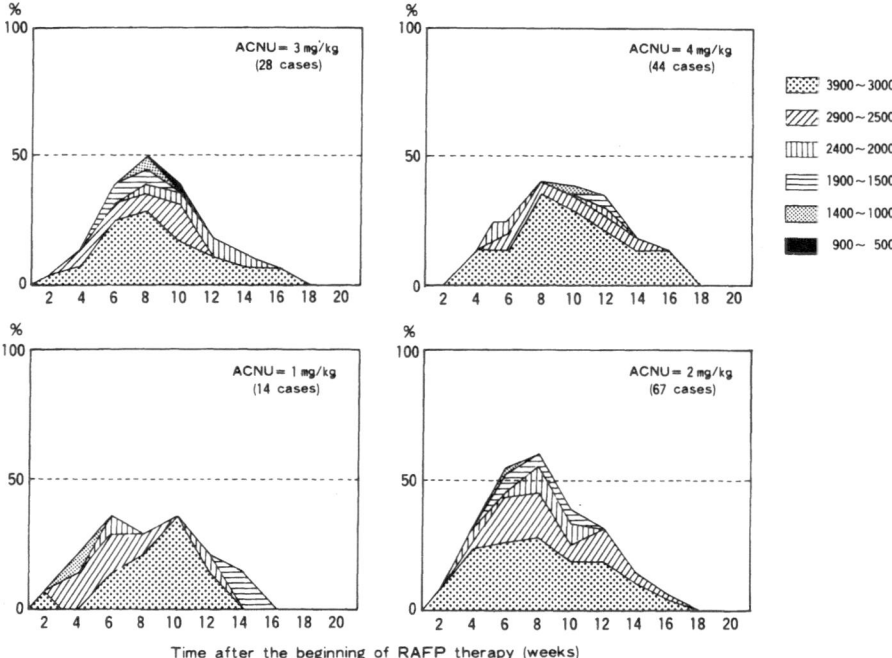

Fig. 14.1. Correlation of leukocytopenia with dose of ACNU

Table 14.4. Beginning of leukocytopenia

	No. of patients	Time (weeks)[a]								
		0–1	2–3	4–5	6–7	8–9	10–11	12–13	14–15	16–17
RAFP										
ACNU 1 mg/kg	7	0	1	2	2	0	2	0	0	0
2	48	0	4	17	16	8	1	1	1	0
3	20	0	1	3	7	6	3	0	0	0
4	30	0	0	6	5	10	2	6	1	0
Total	105	0	6	28	30	24	8	7	2	0
Radiation + FT-207	10	0	0	1	2	4	1	1	1	0

[a] Time after the beginning of treatment

Thrombocytopenia

Among the 99 cases with thrombocytopenia, 60.6% (60 cases) had thrombocyte levels of $12.4 - 10.0 \times 10^4/mm^3$, 22.2% (22 cases) had levels of $7.5 - 9.9 \times 10^4/mm^3$, 6.1% (six cases) had levels of $5.0 - 7.4 \times 10^4/mm^3$, and 11.1% (11 cases) had levels of $2.5 - 4.9 \times 10^4/mm^3$ (Table 14.2). In nearly all cases, definite improvements were seen within 1–2 weeks, but, as mentioned above, a hemorrhagic tendency was seen in three cases.

The onset of thrombocytopenia was 4–6 weeks after the beginning of RAFP therapy in most cases—somewhat earlier than the appearance of leukocytopenia (Table 14.5). This finding is consistent with a previous study reporting that thrombocytopenia due to ACNU precedes leukocytopenia by 1–2 weeks [10, 11].

The relationship between the incidence of thrombocytopenia and the ACNU dosage was as follows. Symptoms arose in 50%, 71.6%, 71.4%, and 54.5% of the cases who were given, respectively, 1, 2, 3, and 4 mg/kg. If only those cases with levels less than $7.5 \times 10^4/mm^3$ are considered, the incidence was 0%, 25%, 17.9%, and 0% for the four groups.

Similar to the onset of leukocytopenia, that of thrombocytopenia was relatively early in the group given 2 mg/kg ACNU and recovery was somewhat delayed. In the group given 4mg/kg, the onset of thrombocytopenia was late and symptoms were mild (Table 14.5; Fig. 14.2).

Discussion

In recent years, treatment of malignant glioma has predominantly combined radio-chemotherapy, and several reports of improved therapeutic results are to be found in the literature [2, 3, 5, 6, 15]. It is, however, well known that serious side effects, particularly myelosuppression, can occur due to radiochemotherapy.

In previous studies on the side effects due to such therapy in brain tumor cases, high incidences of myelosuppression have been reported—leukocytopenia in 35%–

Table 14.5. Beginning of thrombocytopenia

	No. of patients	Time (weeks)[a]								
		0–1	2–3	4–5	6–7	8–9	10–11	12–13	14–15	16–17
RAFP										
ACNU 1 mg/kg	7	0	0	3	2	0	1	1	0	0
2	48	0	7	17	18	5	1	0	0	0
3	20	0	1	9	2	6	1	0	1	0
4	24	0	1	3	8	6	2	2	0	2
Total	99	0	9	32	30	17	5	3	1	2
Radiation + FT-207	10	0	0	2	1	1	5	0	1	0

[a] Time after the beginning of treatment

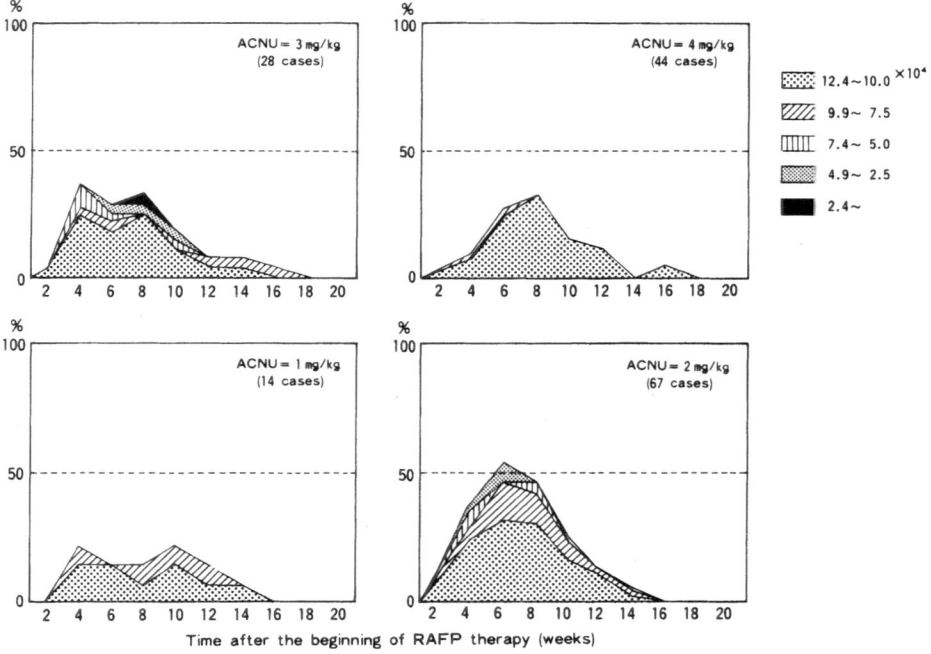

Fig. 14.2. Correlation of thrombocytopenia with dose of ACNU

88% and thrombocytopenia in 16%–84% of all cases (Table 14.6) [7, 13, 14, 16]. Since the effectiveness of radiation therapy is strongly influenced by the dose of radiation per fraction and the interval between fractions, temporary interruption of the therapy can greatly reduce the effect of radiation therapy [4, 8, 12]. As a consequence, it is of importance to be able to regulate the chemotherapy to such a level that severe myelosuppression does not occur.

Table 14.6. Side effects of radiochemotherapy for malignant gliomas

Authors	Treatment	No. of patients	Leukocytopenia	Thorombocytopenia	Nausea, vomiting (%)	Liver dysfunction (%)	Skin eruption (%)	Neuropathy (%)
Wier et al. [15]	Rad. + CCNU	13	6/13	7/13	—	—	—	—
Walker et al. [14]	BCNU	51	79%	84%	—	—	—	—
	Rad. + BCNU	72	88%	64%	—	—	—	—
Levin et al. [7]	Rad. + hydroxyurea BCNU	76	63%	50%	40	—	—	0
	Rad. + hydroxyurea Vincristin	72	80%	56%	47	—	—	38
Ushio et al. [13]	Rad. alone	48	10%	2%	4	0	0	—
	Rad. + ACNU	38	39%	26%	24	5	0	—
	Rad. + ACNU FT-207	37	35%	16%	11	0	8	—

In order to reduce the side effects and thereby undertake therapy without interrupting the therapeutic schedule, radiochemotherapy is carried out using various methods [1, 11]. In radiation therapy of the whole brain and spinal cord for medulloblastoma, Aoki [1] reduced the incidence of leukocytopenia by the combined use of OK-432 and was able to maintain the intended radiation therapy schedule. Aoki reported good therapeutic results using this technique. Attempts at bone marrow transplantation have also been made using high doses of anticancer drugs [9], but this technique is not yet established or widely employed.

Although the incidence is low, other serious side effects include interstitial pneumonitis. In our series, there were possibly three such cases. Bleomycin is known to have such side effects and the possibility of nitrosourea having similar effects has been reported [10, 17], thus suggesting that care with regard to interstitial pneumonitis should be taken when using ACNU.

In the treatment of malignant glioma, combined radiochemotherapy is essential, but the patient's condition must be monitored to prevent the onset of various side effects, particularly myelosuppression. It is thought that the chemotherapeutic agents are in fact the primary factor in the onset of myelosuppression, but in our series there were large individual differences in the onset of myelosuppression and its severity. For this reason, it is difficult to recommend an optimal dose and therapy must be undertaken in conjunction with repeated serological examinations to determine the patient's bone marrow condition.

Conclusion

A study was made of the side effects occurring in 153 patients undergoing RAFP therapy. A high incidence of myelosuppression was found, with 68.6% showing leukocytopenia and 64.7% showing thrombocytopenia. Among these patients, myelosuppression was so severe that therapy was interrupted in ten cases (6.5%). Other side effects included gastrointestinal disorders and liver dysfunction; 26 patients (17.0%), however, had no side effects due to RAFP therapy.

References

1. Aoki Y (1984) Radiotherapy combined with OK-432 for medulloblastoma and alleviating action of OK-432 on the myelosuppression in mice induced by whole body body irradiation. Proceedings of Japan Cancer Association, The 43rd Annual Meeting, October 3 (Fukuoka), p 457 (in Japanese)
2. Edwards MS, Levin VA, Wilson CB (1980) Brain tumor chemotherapy: an evaluation of agents in current use for phase II and III trials. Cancer Treat Rep 64: 1179–1205
3. Fewer D, Wilson CB, Boldrey EB, Enot KJ, Powell MR (1972) The chemotherapy of brain tumors. Clinical experience with carmustine (BCNU) and vincristine. JAMA 30: 549–552
4. Kiga M (1965) Radiological approach in fractionated irradiation. Nippon Acta Radiol 24: 1283–1285
5. Levin VA, Edwards MS, Wright DC, Seager ML, Schimberg TP, Townsend JJ, Wilson CB (1980) Modified procarbazine, CCNU, and vincristine (PCV 3) combination chemotherapy in the treatment of malignant brain tumors. Cancer Treat Rep 64: 237–241

6. Levin VA, Hoffman WF, Pischer TL, Seager ML, Boldrey EB, Wilson CB (1978) BCNU-5-fluorouracil combination therapy for recurrent malignant brain tumors. Cancer Treat Rep 62: 2071–2076

7. Levin VA, Wara WM, Davis RL, Vestnys P, Resser KJ, Yatsko K, Nutik S, Gutin PH, Wilson CB (1985) Phase III comparison of BCNU and the combination of procarbazine, CCNU, and vincristine administered after radiotherapy with hydroxyurea for malignant gliomas. J Neurosurg 63: 218–223

8. Maciejewski B, Preuss-Bayer G, Trott KR (1982) The influence of the number of the fractions and of overall treatment time on local control and late complication rate in squamous cell carcinoma of the larynx. Int J Radiat Oncol Biol Phys 8: 1471–1489

9. Phillips GL, Wolf SN, Fay JW (1986) Intensive 1,3-Bis (2-chloroethyl)-1-nitrosourea (BCNU) monochemotherapy and autologous marrow transplantation for malignant glioma. J Clin Oncel 4: 639–644

10. Saito T, Yokoyama M, Himori T, Ujiie S, Sugawara N, Sugiyama Z, Kitada K (1977) Phase I and phase II study of 1-(4-amino-2-methyl-5-pyrimidinyl)methyl-3(2-chloroethyl)-3-nitrosourea hydrochloride (ACNU) administered by intermittent dose schedule. Jpn J Cancer Chemother 4: 991–1004 (in Japanese)

11. Saito Y, Hori T, Takami M, Muraoka K, Hokama Y, Numata H (1983) The study on postoperative local chemotherapy of malignant brain tumors using ACNU and PSK. Jpn J Cancer Chemother 10: 1963–1971 (in Japanese)

12. Thames HD Jr, Peters LJ, Withers HR, Fletcher GH (1983) Accelerated fractionation vs hyperfractionation: Rationales for several treatments per day. Int J Radiat Oncol Biol Phys 9: 127–138

13. Ushio Y, Abe H, Suzuki J, Tanaka R, Kitamura K, Miwa T, Matsutani M, Takeuchi K, Takakura K, Nomura K, Yamamoto S, Kageyama N, Handa H, Mogami H, Matsumoto S, Nishimura A, Uozumi T, Hori T, Mori T, Mori K, Matsukado Y (1985) Evaluation of ACNU alone and combined with Tegaful as additions to radiotherapy for the treatment of malignant gliomas—A cooperative clinical trial. Brain and Nerve 37: 999–1006 (in Japanese)

14. Walker MD, Alexander E, Hunt WE, MacCarty CS, Mahaley MS Jr, Mealey J Jr, Norrell HA, Owens G, Ransohoff J, Wilson CB, Gehan EA, Strike JA (1978) Evaluation of BCNU and/or radiotherapy in the treatment of anaplastic gliomas. A cooperative clinical trial. J Neurosurg 49: 333–343

15. Walker MD, Green SB, Byar DP, Alexander, E Jr, Batzorf U, Brooks WH, Hunt WE, MacCarty CS, Mahaley MS Jr, Mealey J Jr, Owens G, Ransohoff J II, Robertson JT, Shapiro WR, Smith KR Jr, Wilson CB, Strike TA (1980) Randomized comparisons of radiotherapy and nitrosoureas for the treatment of malignant glioma after surgery. N Engl J Med 303: 1323–1329

16. Weir B, Band P, Urtasun R, Blain G, Mclean D, Wilson F, Mielke B, Grace M (1976) Radiotherapy and CCNU in the treatment of high-grade supratentorial astrocytomas. J Neurosurg 45: 129–134

17. Weiss RB, Muggia FM (1980) Cytotoxic drug-induced pulmonary disease; Update 1980. Am J Med 68: 259–266

Chapter 15

Clinical Study Using MRI in Patients Treated with RAFP Therapy

S. FUJIWARA

Introduction

Subsequent to the well-known paper of Damadian on the magnetic resonance imaging (MRI) of brain tumors [1], many studies have dealt with the relaxation times (RTs) used in the MRI technique. Damadian argued that the RT in malignant tumor tissue was prolonged and many others have since reported that RTs are longer the greater the malignancy of the tumor. Currently, however, the dominant view is that there is no relation between RT and the histological type of the tumor. Moreover, it is now maintained that without contrast media such as Gadolinium diethylenetriamine-pentaacetic-acid (Gd-DTPA) it is impossible to distinguish between the tumor itself and perifocal edema in MRI scans.

In studies concerned with brain imaging techniques, it has been shown that the spatial extent of benign glioma often cannot be determined in X-ray computed tomography (CT) scans except for calcification, but the extent is easily determined by MRI, despite the fact that some edemous normal brain tissue may be included. Furthermore, there are many cases in which determination of a tumor of the brainstem, posterior fossa, or base of the skull is difficult using X-ray CT scans because of bone artifacts, but in which MRI is satisfactory for detecting the tumor.

Although there has been one report of ^{31}P-spectroscopy concerning the relationship between brain tumors and radiochemotherapy [6], there have been only scattered references to ^{1}H-MRI studies on a similar condition (radiation necrosis).

From an MRI study of the relationship between histological malignancy and RTs in 201 cases of brain tumor (295 images), we have found that the RTs in meningioma and neurinoma cases were shorter than those in glioma cases, but that those in metastatic tumors were similar to those in benign glioma. We therefore concluded that study should be made of the RTs of extracerebral tumors (including metastatic tumors), and compared with gliomas.

Since the present study is concerned with gliomas, we first examined the relationship between RTs and the degree of histological malignancy and then investigated the nature of the changes in RT, X-ray CT scans, and clinical symptoms before and after RAFP therapy.

Clinical Materials and Methods

The clinical cases are those detailed in Table 15.1. There were 12 cases in the benign glioma group (cases 1–12) and 15 in the malignant glioma group (cases 13–27). Six were female and 21 were male, with a mean age of 42.1 years (range 13–70 years). MRI studies before and after the RAFP therapy in the benign group were done in seven cases in the benign group (cases 1–7) and in ten cases in the malignant group (cases 13–22) (Table 15.2).

The MRI equipment was a resistive-type magnet, 0.15-T BNT-1000J model from Bruker (West Germany). The pulse sequencing was based on the Carr-Purcell-Meiboom-Gill (CPMG) method, which is a variation on the spin-echo method (Fig. 15.1) Repetition times (Tr) of 1.0 and 3.0 s were used for measurements in each slice. From the signal intensities, the T1 and T2 relaxation times were measured (a) for the ROI (A) images from the X-ray CT images and the enhanced area of the enhanced X-ray CT images in the same slice, and (b) for the ROI (B) images from the entire abnormally high signal-intensity area in the T2-weighted image, including the

Table 15.1. Cases with gliomas examined by MRI

Case no.	Age (years)	Sex	Site	Pathological diagnosis
Benign group				
1	62	M	Left ventricle	Astrocytoma G1
2	45	M	Right frontal	Astrocytoma G2
3	37	M	Right frongal	Astrocytoma G2
4	49	M	Left parietal	Astrocytoma G2
5	37	F	Right parietal	Astrocytoma G2
6	18	M	Left thalamus	Astrocytoma G2
7	30	M	Left temporoparietal	Astrocytoma G2
8	34	M	Right frontotemporal	Astrocytoma G2
9	13	M	Left occipital	Astrocytoma G2
10	38	M	Right frontal	Astrocytoma G2
11	33	M	Left parietooccipital	Astrocytoma G2
12	35	M	Left frontal	Oligodendroglioma G2
Malignant group				
13	60	M	Right frontoparietal	Astrocytoma G3
14	39	F	Right frontoparietal	Astrocytoma G3
15	41	M	Left parietoocipital	Astrocytoma G3
16	52	M	Right parietooccipital	Astrocytoma G3
17	63	M	Left frontoparietal	Astrocytoma G3
18	44	F	Right frontoparietal	Astrocytoma G3
19	70	M	Bilateral frontal	Glioblastoma
20	45	M	Right parietooccipital	Glioblastoma
21	23	M	Left parietal	Glioblastoma
22	47	F	Left thalamus	Glioblastoma
23	38	M	Left temporal	Astrocytoma G3
24	43	M	Bilateral frontal	Astrocytoma G3
25	70	M	Right frontotemporal	Glioblastoma
26	23	F	Right frontotemporal	Glioblastoma
27	48	F	Left frontoparietal	Oligodendroglioma G4

Table 15.2. Correlation between clinical course, X-ray CT, prognosis at 6 months after treatment and rate of change in relaxation times evaluated by ROI (A)

Case no.	Symptoms[a]	X-ray CT	Prognosis	Rate of change (%)	
				T_1	T_2
1	I	U	G	22.3	9.6
2	U	U	F	9.5	1.4
3	I	I	F	10.7	16.9
4	U	I	F	24.3	32.7
5	U	U	F	10.1	11.5
6	I	U	F	9.3	10.5
7	I	U	F	4.6	2.5
13	I	I	P	18.5	16.4
14	A	I	F	35.7	61.9
15	A	I	D	16.4	6.3
16	A	A	D	2.6	28.5
17	A	U	F	3.8	5.6
18	A	U	P	136.8	106.2
19	A	U	P	57.9	5.9
20	A	U	G	67.7	29.0
21	I	I	G	18.2	3.6
22	I	I	F	0.3	1.6

I improved, *U* unchanged, *A* aggravated, *G* good, *F* fair, *P* poor, *D* dead
[a] Compared with before initiation of therapy

tumor (Fig. 15.2). The MRI study following RAFP therapy was done within 2 weeks of the completion of therapy.

Results and Discussion

Sequential MRIs

In Figs. 15.3 and 15.4, the upper row of images shows the enhanced CT scans, the middle row the T2-weighted images, and the bottom row the T1-weighted images. The images in the left-hand column were obtained prior to RAFP therapy, those in the middle column during 3000 rad of whole-brain irradiation, and those in the right-hand column after the completion of the RAFP therapy.

In the benign glioma group (Fig. 15.3) prior to RAFP therapy, only the low-density area was depicted in the enhanced X-ray CT scans, whereas in the T2 images there was a distinct high singal-intensity area, i.e., a T2-prolonged area. In the T1 images, there was a faint high signal-intensity area. It should be noted that in the MRI, particularly in the T2 image, it is not always the case that all abnormal images are an indication of the tumor itself; peritumoral edema can also often be included. Nevertheless, even in cases where the presence or extent of a lesion in X-ray CT scans is uncertain, it is distinctly depicted in MRI scans.

Following therapy, a slight reduction in the size of the lesion can be seen in X-ray CT scans, but in both the T1 and T2 MRI images, there is a distinct reduction in the

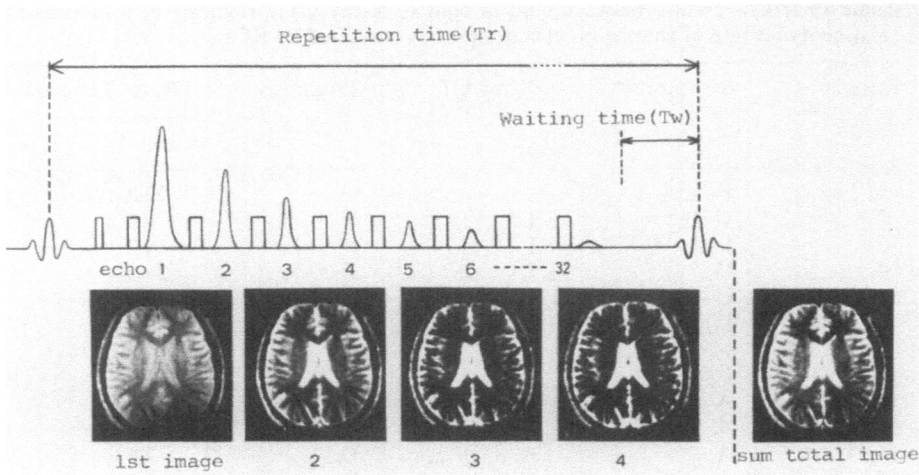

Fig. 15.1. Pulse sequence of Carr-Purcell-Meiboom-Gill (CPMG) method

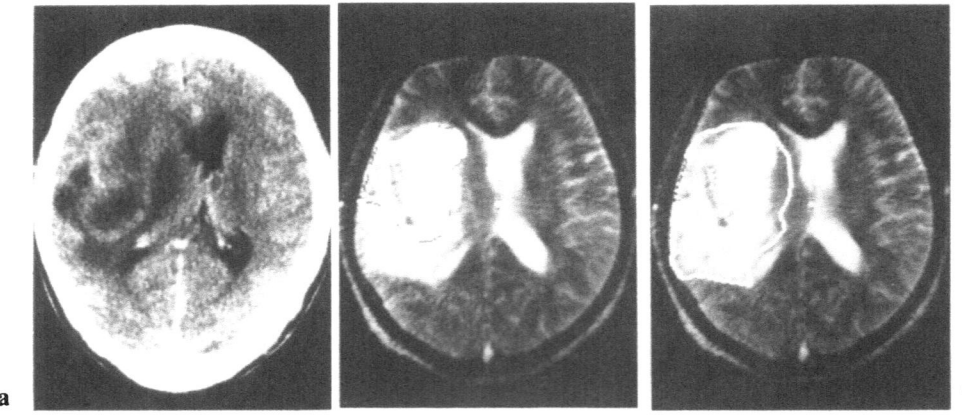

Fig. 15.2a–c. a Enhanced X-CT of case 17. **b** ROI (A) in T_2-weighted MRI image. **c** ROI (B) in T_2-weighted MRI image of the same patient

size of the lesion and a tendency toward normalization of the Tr of the signal intensity. These findings indicate that following RAFP therapy in cases of benign glioma, MRI scans are more useful than X-ray CT scans in evaluating the effectiveness of the therapy.

In contrast, in the malignant glioma cases (Fig. 15.4), the lesion was depicted and a ring-enhanced area with a perifocal low-density region was seen in enhanced X-ray CT scans prior to therapy. The T2 image, however, showed a high signal-intensity area over the entire region and the tumor could not be distinguished from the surrounding tissue.

In the T1 images, only the regions depicted as ring-enhanced areas in the X-ray

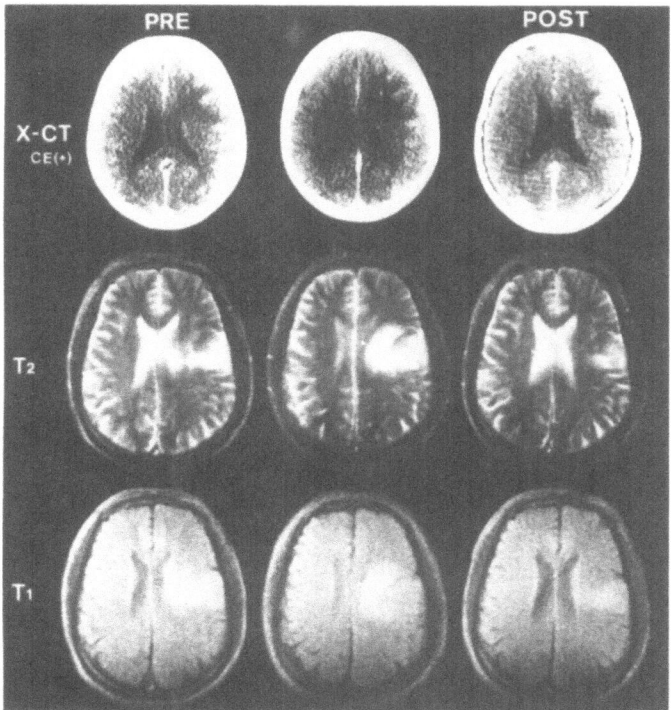

Fig. 15.3. X-ray CT-, T_1-, and T_2-weighted MRI images of a benign glioma case. *Left* pretreatment, *middle* during treatment, *right* posttreatment

CT scans were shown as low signal-intensity areas, and other portions were seen as mildly high signal-intensity areas. Following therapy in the malignant glioma case, there were some clinical improvements due to RAFP therapy, and X-ray CT scans showed a reduction in the tumor itself and a further clarity in the perifocal low-density area. In contrast, however, there was an expansion in the size of the high signal-intensity area in the MRI scans. These effects are thought to be due to brain edema caused by the therapy, but they may also reflect an enlargement in the region of the necrotic tissue. Whatever the case may be, these findings indicate that in malignant glioma cases, it is difficult to distinguish between the tumor itself and peritumoral edema using MRI scans if contrast media such as Gd-DTPA are not used. Since tumor tissues often contain various components, such as cysts, necrotic tissue, and hematomas, evaluation of MRI scans before and after therapy is difficult and indicates the current limits of the ^{1}H-MRI technique.

Study of Tr of Tumors in ROI(A)

Tr prior to RAFP therapy. The mean Tr in the benign glioma group was 717 ms for T1 and 194 ms for T2, whereas these values in the malignant glioma group were 841 ms and 250 ms, respectively (Fig. 15.5). Although the variability of the Tr values

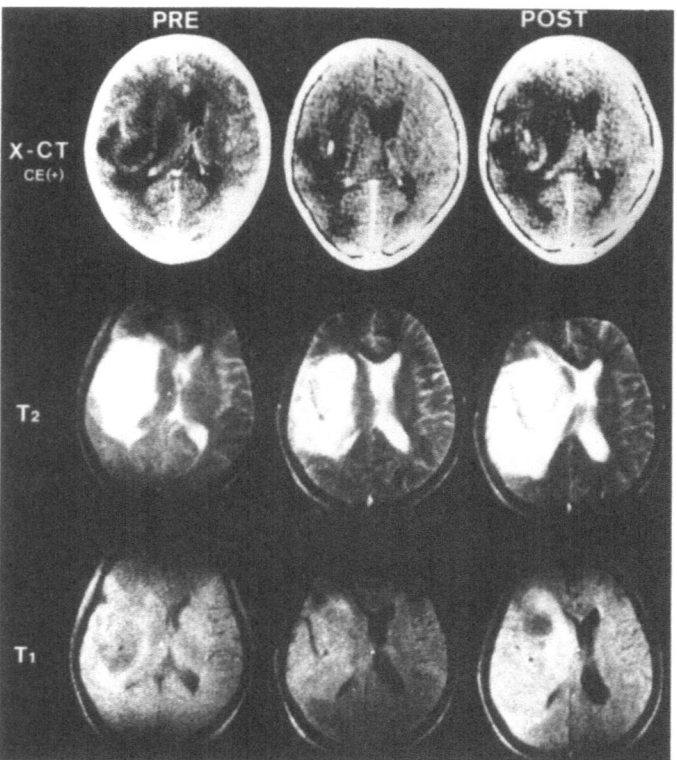

Fig. 15.4. X-ray CT-, T_1-, and T_2-weighted MRI images of a malignant glioma case. *Left* pretreatment, *middle* during treatment, *right* posttreatment

among these patients was large, there was a tendency for the Tr in malignant tumors to be greater than in benign tumors. There were, however, many cases in both groups with similar Tr values and, statistically, the differences were not significant.

It should be noted, however, that the wide distribution of Tr values, particularly in the malignant glioma group, may reflect the presence of various components within the tumor tissue, such as necrosis and cyst formation. The wide distribution of Tr values is characteristic of malignant glioma tissue; conversely, the narrower distribution of Tr values in the benign glioma cases may reflect the uniformity of the tissue.

Tr values before and after RAFP therapy. In the benign glioma cases, the mean changes in T1 and T2 values before and after RAFP therapy were 23.8% and 22.8%, respectively, whereas they were 35.8% and 26.5% in the malignant cases (Figs. 15.6, 15.7). There may have been varied responses in the malignant glioma cases, including an expansion in the region of the cysts and necrosis or glioma formation and, consequently, increased edema. Although the majority of these cases showed prolonged Tr values following therapy, some also showed reductions. Such findings are of particular interest because they indicate different susceptibility or responsivity to therapy in cases with identical histopathological lesions.

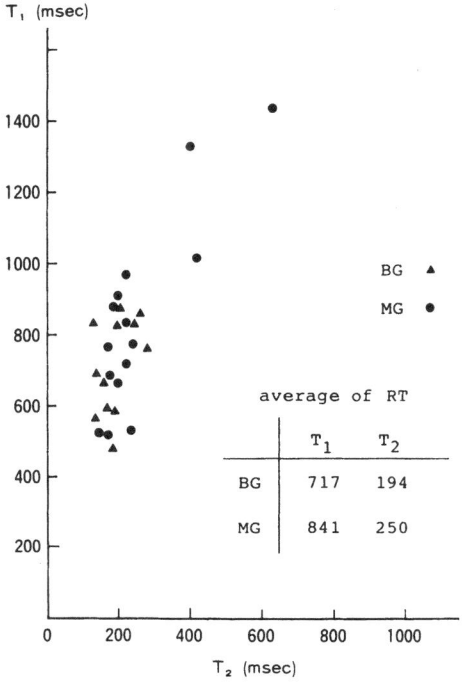

Fig. 15.5. Relaxation times in benign and malignant glioma groups evaluated at ROI. (A) prior to therapy

	average of RT	
	T_1	T_2
BG	717	194
MG	841	250

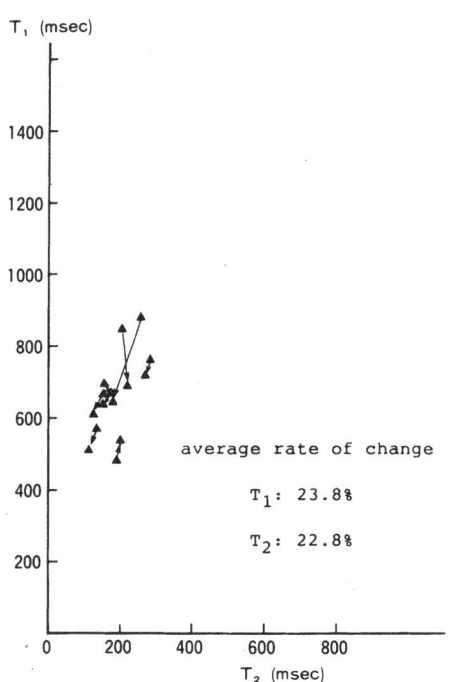

Fig. 15.6. Sequential changes of relaxation times evaluated at ROI (A) in benign glioma group between pre- and posttreatment

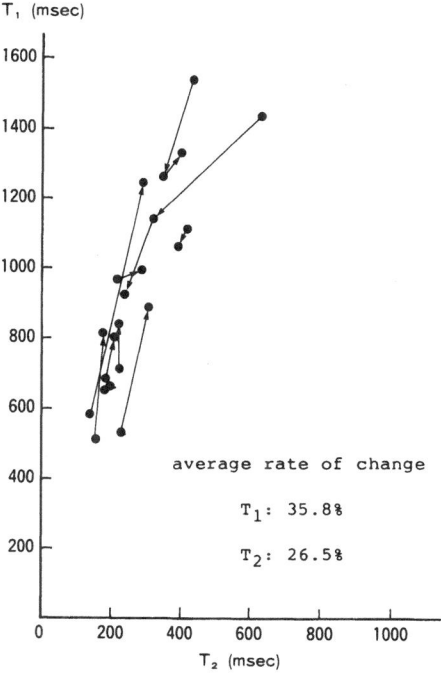

Fig. 15.7. Sequential changes of relaxation times evaluated at ROI (A) in malignant glioma group between pre- and post-treatment

Tr Values in ROI(B) Images Before and After RAFP Therapy

The mean changes in T1 and T2 values were 14.6% and 12.0%, respectively, in the benign glioma group and 24.0% and 46.6% in the malignant glioma group (Figs. 15.8, 15.9). Since this measuring technique includes perifocal edema, the evaluation of such results is problematical, but it is thought that the influence of brain edema is important in producing large changes in T2 values following RAFP therapy, as seen in the malignant group.

Prognosis from Tr Values Before and After RAFP Therapy

Study was next made of the changes in Tr values in ROI(A) in the benign and malignant glioma cases in relation to clinical symptoms, X-ray CT findings, and the outcome 6 months following therapy (Table 15.2). No notable correlations among these variables were found, however. The fact that there were some malignant cases in which large changes in Tr values were seen and others in which only small changes were seen suggests that the correlations among the parameters in such cases should be examined with independent groups. Further study certainly is required, since the number of cases in the present investigation was too small.

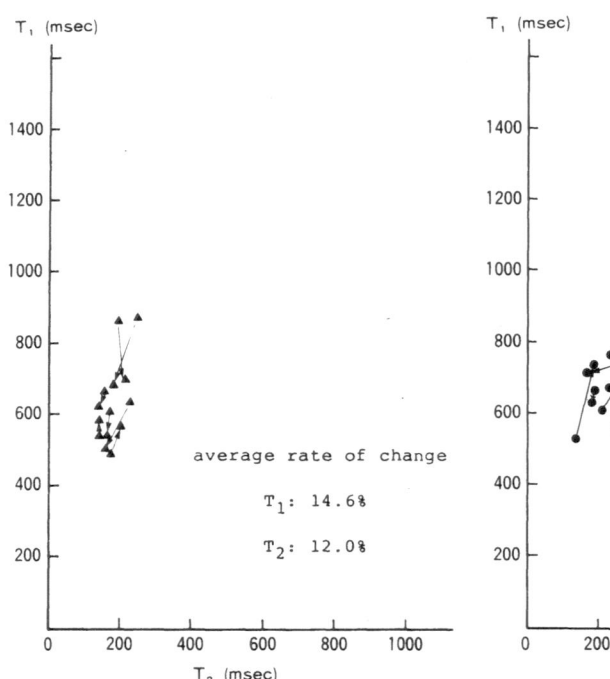

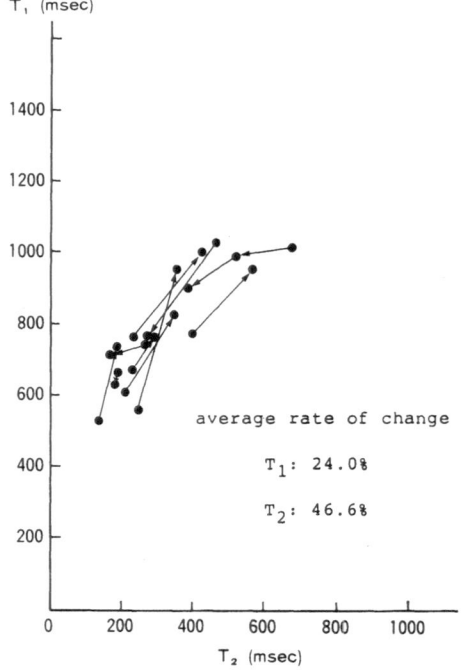

Fig. 15.8. Sequential changes of relaxation times evaluated at ROI (B) in benign glioma group between pre- and posttreatment

Fig. 15.9. Sequential changes of relaxation times evaluated at ROI (B) in malignant glioma group between pre- and post-treatment

Conclusion

Although there have been many reports on MRI scans in brain tumors, there have been only scattered conference reports [e.g., 5] on changes in such images before and after radiochemotherapy. Such reports have been concerned with only one or two cases and there has been only one report on sequential changes, that of Naruse et al. [6] using experimental tumors in laboratory animals. Since the work of Damadian [1] it has been known that the water content of malignant tumors is higher than that of benign tumors and normal tissue [2–4, 7]. Indeed, Damadian was the first to draw a connection between malignancy and water content in MRI scans. Related findings by others have led us to the present study, using the ^{1}H-MRI technique, of the changes before and after RAFP therapy in tumor Tr values, which are now known to be influenced by the water content of brain tissue.

The results of our own study on the relationship between malignancy and Tr values before and after RAFP therapy indicated that although there is a tendency for malignant gliomas to have somewhat prolonged Tr values, there is no strong correlation. It can be said, however, that the malignant glioma group characteristically had a wider spread of Tr values.

Particularly in the benign glioma group, the changes in images before and after RAFP therapy were more easily seen in the MRI scans than in the X-ray CT scans, indicating the appropriateness of the former technique for the evaluation of RAFP therapy. On the other hand, however, even among the successfully treated malignant glioma cases, there was an increase in the region of T2 prolongation in MRI scans. Such findings suggest that the influences of radiation or increases in necrosis and cyst formation are diverse and complex, and therefore that current MRI techniques will be of limited value in evaluating therapeutic results among malignant glioma cases.

The changes in Tr values brought about by RAFP therapy were found to be large in most of the malignant glioma cases and small or zero in most of the benign glioma cases. A clear relationship between such findings and clinical symptoms, X-ray CT findings, or outcome was not found. Since there were some cases showing prolongation and others with reduction of Tr values following therapy, it will be necessary to increase the number of cases for separate study of these groups in future investigations.

In the near future, it may become possible to determine the sensitivity to radiochemotherapy of individual cases prior to therapy by means of magnetic resonance spectroscopy and/or MRI scanning using various isotopes (^{13}C, ^{23}Na, or ^{31}P). The use of such techniques before therapy would be of enormous value in the treatment of various forms of brain tumor.

References

1. Damadian R (1971) Tumor detection by nuclear magnetic resonance. Science 171: 1151–1153
2. Hazlewood CF, Cleveland G, Medina D (1974) Relationship between hydration and proton nuclear magnetic resonance relaxation times in tissues of tumor-bearing and non-tumor-bearing mice: Implication for cancer detection. J Natl Cancer Inst 52: 1849–1853

3. Inch WR, McCredie JA, Knispel RR, Thompson RT, Pintar MM (1974) Water content and proton spin relaxation time for neoplastic and non-neoplastic tissues from mice and humans. J Natl Cancer Inst 52: 353–356
4. Kirikuta IC, Simplaeanu V (1975) Tissue water content and nuclear magnetic resonance in norma and tumor tissues. Cancer Research 35: 1164–1167
5. Mano I, Yoshida H, Ohmachi H, Miyagawa, S, Iio M (1985) MRI for the tumor and its application to radiation therapy. J NMR Medicine 5: 97–103 (in Japanese)
6. Naruse S, Higuchi T, Horikawa Y, Tanaka C, Nakanura K, Hirakawa K (1986) RF hyperthermia and simultaneous monitoring of its effects on the phosphate metabolism of tumor using ^{31}P-NMR spectrometer. J NMR Medicine 6: 30–37 (in Japanese)
7. Saryan LA, Hollis DP, Economou JS, Eggleston JC (1974) Brief communication: Nuclear magnetic resonance studies of cancer. IV. Correlation of water content with tissue relaxation times. J Natl Canner Inst 52: 599–602

Subject Index

ACNU   37, 40, 49, 56, 65, 68, 87, 95, 97, 100, 109, 118, 138, 155
–, blood concentration of   111
– concentration-survival curve   62
–, CSF concentration of   109
– (Nimustin)   139
–, pharmokinetics of   109
Adjuvant chemotherapy   153
– therapy   155, 163
AEV   14
Age distribution   4
– – of anaplastic astocytoma   156
– – – glioblastoma   156
– and location of tumor   200
Anaplastic astrocytoma   6, 9, 149, 153
– –, age distribution of   156
– – case, duration of disease in   160
– – –, site of lesion in   157
– –, overall survival rate of   157
Anaplastic oligodendroglioma   188
Anemia   221
Angiotensin II   119
Arterial oxygen pressure, see PaO_2
Astrocytoma   126
Autoradiography   39
Autoregulation in brain tumor tissue   117
Avian erythroblastoses virus, see AEV

Bailey   21
–, classification of   3
BAR therapy   155
Basidiomycete   142
BCNU   29, 59, 100, 109, 168
Biological response modifier, see BRM
Biphasic exponential function   39
– survival curve   60
BLM   155
Blood-brain barrier   19, 109, 139

Blood concentration of ACNU   111
– types   13
Brachytherapy   27
Brain stem   154
Brainstem LGA   174
Brain tumor, statistical analysis of   3
BRM   142

C_0 39, 76
C_q 39, 76
$_1C_0$ 39, 78
$_2C_0$ 39, 78
CCNU   29, 59, 100, 109, 151, 168
$CD_{0.5}$ 70, 74
$CD_{0.5(exp)}$ 49, 70, 71
Cell cycle-specific (CCS) drug   140
– kinetics   138
– – of malignant tumors   137
Cerbellum   9, 154, 173
Cerebrospinal fluid, see CSF
Cerebellar LGA   174, 175
Chemical substance   13
Chemotherapy   37, 117, 221
Classification of Bailey   3
– – Cushing
–, ECOG   155
–, Kernohan and Sayre   3
Clinical finding and prognosis   177
– grade   12
– symptom   154, 160
Colony-forming efficiency   39, 41
Combined therapy   37
Computed tomography, see CT
Concentration-survival curve   50
Control probability curve   49
– – of spheroid   40
CQ   155
CSF   109, 139

– concentration of ACNU   109
CT   18, 149, 231
Cumulated Index Medicus   17
Current List of Medical Literature   17
Cushing   21
–, classification of   3

D_0 39, 60, 71
D_q 39, 77
Diagnostic method   11
DNA type   14
Dose-control probability of spheroid   68
Dose-survival curve   54, 59, 68
Doubling time   42
Duration of disease   154
– – – in anaplastic astrocytoma   160
– – – in glioblastoma case   160

Eastern Cooperative Oncology Group,
    see ECOG
ECOG   22
– classification   155
EFS   216
EGF   14
– recepter   14
Emission CT   137
Endogenous factor   12
Enhancement ratio   94, see also ER
Ependymoma   6, 149, 197
–, recurrent cases of   204
Epidemiology   3
Epidermal growth factor, see EGF
ER   65-67, 71
– ratio   67
erb-B oncogene   14
Ethylnitrosourea   13
Event-free survival   210
Exogenous factor   12
Expected value   49
Exponentially growing cell   37
Extensive surgery   26
Extent of extirpation   163
Extracranial metastasis   26

Fibrillary astrocytoma   6, 11, 175
Focal neurological sign   12
Fourth ventricle   9
Frontal lobe   9, 154
FT-207   138, 155
– (Futraful)   140
5-FU   37, 40, 52, 74, 82, 87, 89, 95, 97,
    101

– concentration-survival curve   74, 82
– -induced PLD   99
– masked compound of   138
– time-survival curve   84

G_0 cell   138
G_1/S border   77, 82
– boundary   92
GB A-7 cell   38, 47, 52, 57, 61, 63, 68
– – – shperoid   38
GMB   17, see also Glioblastoma
Gemistocytic astrocytoma   6
Geographical locality   8
Glioblastoma   6, 9, 17, 126, 149, 153,
    155
–, age distribution of   156
– case, duration of disease in   160
– –, site of lesion in   157
–, overall survival rate of   157
Glioma, incidence of   3
Gliosarcoma   155
Growth factor   12
– fraction   42

Head trauma   12
Hereditary factor   12
HF   77, 78
High-grade astrocytoma   7
Histological distribution   4/5
– findings   199
^{3}H-thymidine labeling   41
Hyperbaric oxygenation therapy   128
Hyperbaric therapy   27
Hyperfractionation   27
Hypoxic cell   37, 41, 46, 61, 66, 67
– – radiosensitizer   128
– – within tumor tissue   125
– fraction, see HF

Incidence of glioma   3
Induced hypertension   68, 117
Infratentorial glioma   5, 8
Interleukin   142
Interstitial pneumonitis   222
Intra-abdominal metastasis   206
Intra-arterial administration   68
Intracarotid injection   143
Intracranial hypertension   12
Isobologram   74
– analysis   94

Japan Brain Tumor Registry   7

Karnofsky performance scale   24
KEG-1 cell   117
Kernohan   21
– and Sayre classification   3

Labeling index   41, 42, 52
Large spheroid   47, 71
Laser   26
Leukocytopenia   221, 224
Low-grade astrocytoma   7, 149, 173

Macrophage   142
Magnetic resonance imaging, see MRI
Malignant ependymoma   197
– glioma   109, 153, 232
– transformation   7, 194
– tumor   231
Mannitol   143
Masked compound of 5-fluorouracil   140
MeCCNU   100
Medulloblastoma   6, 11, 149, 209
–, tumor-metastasis classification of   209
Megavoltage therapy   27
Meningioma   12, 231
Metastatic brain tumor   126
Method of excision   191
Methylcholantren   13
Metronidazole   67
Microsurgical technique   137
Migration inhibitory factor (MIF)   142
Mixed oligodendroglioma   188
Mongoloid race   13
Monolayer cell   37, 42, 56, 59, 62, 74,
   82, 87, 89, 91, 95
– – in exponential phase   57, 61
– – in plateau phase   57, 61
– culture   38
MRI   137, 231
Multicellular spheroid   38
Multitarget, single-hit model   39
Mural nodule   175
Myelosuppression   121, 143, 221

Natural killer (NK) cell   142
Negroes   14
Neurinoma   12, 231
9L cell spheroid   52
Nitrosourea   19, 28
– agent   137

Nonproliferating pool cell, see G_0 cell

Occipital lobe   9, 154
OER   47
OK-432   228
Oligodendrocytoma   149
Oligodendroglioma   6, 11, 126, 187, 188
–, recurrence cases of   193
Oncogene   12, 14
Oncogenesis of glioma   12
Optimal dose of X-rays and ACNU   65
Overall survival rate   157
– – – of glioblastoma   157
– – curve   188
Oxygen enhancement ratio, see OER
– extraction fraction   130
– pressure, see PO_2

PaO_2 125
Parietal lobe   9, 154
PDGF   14
Performance status   155, 163
Phacomatosis   12
– disorders   12
Pharmacokinetics   137
– of ACNU   109
Pilocytic astrocytoma   6, 11, 175
Plateau phase   52
Platelet-derived growth factor, see PDGF
PLD   47, 84
– recovery   49, 52, 54, 70, 71, 74
PO_2 125
Potentially lethal damage, see PLD
Procarbazine   151, 168
Prognosis for the glioblastoma   157
Proliferating cell   42
– pool cell   138
Protoplasmic astrocytoma   6
Prostaglandin I_2 142
PSK   138, 155
– (Krestin)   142
– therapy   155, see also RAFP therapy

Q cell   52, 57, 66, 67, 99
Quarterly Cumulation Index   17
Quiescent cell   42, see also Q cell

Racial factor   13
Radiation dose   39
– necrosis   26
– therapy   137, 138, 221

– – and chemotherapy   191
Radiation Therapy Oncology Group
    (RTOG)   22
Radiochemotherapy   137
Radioresistance   45
Radiosensitivity   130
Radiosensitizer   27
Radiotherapy   12, 37
RAFP therapy   138, 149, 155, 173, 187,
    203, 209, 210, 221, 232
Randomized studies   153
Rat glioma cell, see RG C-6 cell
Recklinghausen's disease   12
Recurrence case   193
– – of ependymoma   204
– – of oligodendroglioma   193
– of tumor   177
Regeneration   46
Relationship between prognosis,
    radiotherapy, and chemotherapy   180
– – surgery and prognosis   179
Relaxation time   231
Remission rate   150
Repetition time   232
Resistant fraction   87, see also RF
RF   54, 78, 89, 93
RG C-6 cell   38, 45, 50, 56, 59, 62, 70
– – – spheroid   38, 139
RNA type   14
Rous sarcoma virus   14

Sequential trypsinization   99
Sex distribution   4
Side effect   221
Simian sarcoma virus   14
Single-strand break   59
Site of lesion in anaplastic astrocytoma
    cases   157
– – – in glioblastoma cases   157
sis-oncogene   14
SLD   62, 67, 75, 84
Small spheroid   47, 70
Soft agar assay   41
Spheroid   42, 56, 60, 63, 77, 82, 87, 89,
    91, 94, 95, 141
–, control probability of   40
Spin-echo method   232
Spinal cord irradiation   216
– dissemination   197, 206
src-oncogene   15
Statistical analysis of brain tumors   3
Steroid   143
Subcutaneously transplanted rat glioma
    38, 40, 46

Subependymal giant cell astrocytoma   6
Sublethal damage, see SLD
Supratentorial glioma   5, 8
– LGA   174, 177
Surgery   17
– and chemotherapy   17
– and radiotherapy   17
Surgical excision   155
– microscope   26
Survival rate   19
– time   210
Surviving fraction   39
Synchronization   139
– of tumor cell   138

T1 and T2 relaxation times   232
TDF   143, 210, 214
Temporal lobe   9, 154
Thalamus   154
Therapeutic ratio   66
– result   17
Thrombocytopenia   221, 225
Thromboxan A_2 142
Time dose fractionation, see TDF
Time-survival curve   50, 52
Timing of combination   56
TNF   142
Tohoku Brain Tumor Registry   3
Treatment with fast neutron   27
Tumor, age and location of   200
– cord structure   41
– -metastasis (TM) classification of
    medulloblastoma   209
– necrotizing factor, see TNF
– tissue oxygen preessure (TuO_2)   125
– –, oxygen pressure within   125

Ultrasonic surgical aspirator   26

Vincristin   138, 151, 168
Vinyl chloride   13
Viral infection   7
V-sis   14

Water-soluble nitrosourea   139
White Americans   13
Wistar King Aptekman rat   117
WHO classification   4, 21
– – of glioma   3

Xenon (Xe) 137
X-irradiation 82
X-ray 56, 65, 68, 74
– and ACNU, optimal dose of 65
– dose-survival curve 45, 47, 59, 82